Blood & Circulatory Disorders Sourcebook

Basic Information about Disorders Such As Anemia, Hemorrhage, Shock, Embolism, and Thrombosis, along with Facts Concerning Rh Factor, Blood Banks, Blood Donation Programs, and Transfusions

Edited by Linda M. Ross. 600 pages. 1998. 0-7808-0203-9. $75.

Burns Sourcebook

Basic Information about Heat, Chemical, Electrical, and Sun Burns, along with Facts about Burn Treatment and Recovery, and Reports on Current Research Initiatives

Edited by Allan R. Cook. 600 pages. 1998. 0-7808-0204-7. $75.

Cancer Sourcebook

Basic Information on Cancer Types, Symptoms, Diagnostic Methods, and Treatments, Including Statistics on Cancer Occurrences Worldwide and the Risks Associated with Known Carcinogens and Activities

Edited by Frank E. Bair. 932 pages. 1990. 1-55888-888-8. $75.

"This publication's nontechnical nature and very comprehensive format make it useful for both the general public and undergraduate students."
— *Choice, Oct '90*

"This compact collection of reliable information, written in a positive, hopeful tone, is an invaluable tool for helping patients and patients' families and friends to take the first steps in coping with the many difficulties of cancer." — *Medical Reference Services Quarterly, Winter '91*

"An important resource for the general reader trying to understand the complexities of cancer."
— *American Reference Books Annual, '91*

Cancer Sourcebook for Women

Basic Information about Specific Forms of Cancer That Affect Women, Featuring Facts about Breast Cancer, Cervical Cancer, Ovarian Cancer, Cancer of the Uterus and Uterine Sarcoma, Cancer of the Vagina, and Cancer of the Vulva; Statistical and Demographic Data; Treatments, Self-Help Management Suggestions, and Current Research Initiatives

Edited by Allan R. Cook and Peter D. Dresser. 524 pages. 1996. 0-7808-0076-1. $75.

"This timely book is highly recommended for consumer health and patient education collections in all libraries." — *Library Journal, Apr '96*

"The availability under one cover of all these pertinent publications, grouped under cohesive headings, makes this certainly a most useful sourcebook."
— *Choice, Jun '96*

"Laudably, the book portrays the feelings of the cancer victim, as well as her mate . . . .both benefit from the gold mine of information nestled between the two covers of this book. It is hard to conceive of any library that would not want it as part of its collection. Recommended."
— *Academic Library Book Review, Summer '96*

". . . written in easily understandable, non-technical language. Recommended for public libraries or hospital and academic libraries that collect patient education or consumer health materials."
— *Medical Reference Services Quarterly, Spring '97*

New Cancer Sourcebook

Basic Information about Major Forms and Stages of Cancer, Featuring Facts about Primary and Secondary Tumors of the Respiratory, Nervous, Lymphatic, Circulatory, Skeletal, and Gastrointestinal Systems, and Specific Organs; Statistical and Demographic Data, Treatment Options, and Strategies for Coping

Edited by Allan R. Cook. 1,313 pages. 1996. 0-7808-0041-9. $75.

"This book is an excellent resource. The dialogue is simple, direct, and comprehensive."
— *Doody's Health Sciences Book Review, Nov '96*

"The amount of factual and useful information is extensive. The writing is very clear, geared to general readers. Recommended for all levels."
— *Choice, Jan '97*

Cardiovascular Diseases & Disorders Sourcebook

Basic Information about Cardiovascular Diseases and Disorders, Featuring Facts about the Cardiovascular System, Demographic and Statistical Data, Descriptions of Pharmacological and Surgical Interventions, Lifestyle Modifications, and a Special Section Focusing on Heart Disorders in Children

Edited by Karen Bellenir and Peter D. Dresser. 683 pages. 1995. 0-7808-0032-X. $75.

". . . comprehensive format provides an extensive overview on this subject." — *Choice, Jun '96*

"Easily understood, complete, up-to-date resource. This well executed public health tool will make valuable information available to those that need it most, patients and their families. The typeface, sturdy nonreflective paper, and library binding add a feel of quality found wanting in other publications. Highly recommended for academic and general libraries."
— *Academic Library Book Review, Summer '96*

Continues next page

Communication Disorders Sourcebook

Basic Information about Deafness and Hearing Loss, Speech and Language Disorders, Voice Disorders, Balance and Vestibular Disorders, and Disorders of Smell, Taste, and Touch

Edited by Linda M. Ross. 533 pages. 1996. 0-7808-0077-X. $75.

"This is skillfully edited and is a welcome resource for the layperson. It should be found in every public and medical library."
— *Doody's Health Sciences Book Review, May '96*

Congenital Disorders Sourcebook

Basic Information about Disorders Acquired during Gestation, Including Spina Bifida, Hydrocephalus, Cerebral Palsy, Heart Defects, Craniofacial Abnormalities, Fetal Alcohol Syndrome, and More, along with Current Treatment Options and Statistical Data

Edited by Karen Bellenir. 607 pages. 1997. 0-7808-0205-5. $75.

Consumer Issues in Health Care Sourcebook

Basic Information about Consumer Health Concerns, Including an Explanation of Physician Specialties, How to Choose a Doctor, How to Prepare for a Hospital Visit, Ways to Avoid Fraudulent "Miracle" Cures, How to Use Medications Safely, What to Look for when Choosing a Nursing Home, and End-of-Life Planning

Edited by Wendy Wilcox. 600 pages. 1998. 0-7808-0221-7. $75.

Contagious & Non-Contagious Infectious Diseases Sourcebook

Basic Information about Contagious Diseases like Measles, Polio, Hepatitis B, and Infectious Mononucleosis, and Non-Contagious Infectious Diseases like Tetanus and Toxic Shock Syndrome, and Diseases Occurring as Secondary Infections Such As Shingles and Reye Syndrome, along with Vaccination, Prevention, and Treatment Information, and a Section Describing Emerging Infectious Disease Threats

Edited by Karen Bellenir and Peter D. Dresser. 566 pages. 1996. 0-7808-0075-3. $75.

Diabetes Sourcebook

Basic Information about Insulin-Dependent and Noninsulin-Dependent Diabetes Mellitus, Gestational Diabetes, and Diabetic Complications, Symptoms, Treatment, and Research Results, Including Statistics on Prevalence, Morbidity, and Mortality, along with Source Listings for Further Help and Information

Edited by Karen Bellenir and Peter D. Dresser. 827 pages. 1994. 1-55888-751-2. $75.

"Very informative and understandable for the layperson without being simplistic. It provides a comprehensive overview for laypersons who want a general understanding of the disease or who want to focus on various aspects of the disease."
— *Bulletin of the MLA, Jan '96*

Diet & Nutrition Sourcebook

Basic Information about Nutrition, Including the Dietary Guidelines for Americans, the Food Guide Pyramid, and Their Applications in Daily Diet, Nutritional Advice for Specific Age Groups, Current Nutritional Issues and Controversies, the New Food Label and How to Use It to Promote Healthy Eating, and Recent Developments in Nutritional Research

Edited by Dan R. Harris. 662 pages. 1996. 0-7808-0084-2. $75.

"It is so refreshing to find a reliable and factual reference book. Recommended to aspiring professionals, librarians, and others seeking and giving reliable dietary advice. An excellent compilation."
— *Choice, Feb '97*

"Recommended for public and medical libraries that receive general information requests on nutrition. It is readable and will appeal to those interested in learning more about healthy dietary practices."
— *Medical Reference Services Quarterly, Fall '97*

Ear, Nose & Throat Disorders Sourcebook

Basic Information about Disorders of the Ears, Nose, Sinus Cavities, Tonsils, Adenoids, Pharynx, and Larynx, along with Statistical and Demographic Data and Reports on Current Research Initiatives

Edited by Linda M. Ross. 600 pages. 1998. 0-7808-0206-3. $75.

Endocrine & Metabolic Diseases & Disorders Sourcebook

Basic Information for the Layperson about Disorders Such As Graves' Disease, Goiter, Cushing's Syndrome, and Hormonal Imbalances, along with Reports on Current Research Initiatives

Edited by Linda M. Ross. 600 pages. 1998. 0-7808-0207-1. $75.

Continues on back end sheets

Men's Health Concerns
Concerns
SOURCEBOOK

Health Reference Series

Volume Thirty-eight

Men's Health Concerns
SOURCEBOOK

Basic Information about Health Issues that Affect Men, Featuring Facts about the Top Causes of Death in Men Including Heart Disease, Stroke, Cancers, Prostate Disorders, Chronic Obstructive Pulmonary Disease, Pneumonia and Influenza, Human Immunodeficiency Virus and Acquired Immune Deficiency Syndrome, Diabetes Mellitus, Stress, Suicide, Accidents and Homicides; and Facts about Common Concerns for Men Including Impotence, Contraception, Circumcision, Sleep Disorders, Snoring, Hair Loss, Diet, Nutrition, Exercise, Kidney and Urological Disorders, and Backaches

Edited by
Allan R. Cook

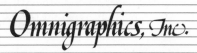
Omnigraphics, Inc.

Penobscot Building / Detroit, MI 48226

RR
RA
776.5
.M457
1998

Bibliographic Note

Edited by
Allan R. Cook

Peter D. Dresser, Managing Editor, Health Reference Series
Karen Bellenir, Series Editor, Health Reference Series

Omnigraphics, Inc.

Matthew P. Barbour, Manager, Production and Fulfillment
Laurie Lanzen Harris, Vice President, Editorial Director
Peter E. Ruffner, Vice President, Administration
James A. Sellgren, Vice President, Operations and Finance
Jane J. Steele, Marketing Consultant

Frederick G. Ruffner, Jr., Publisher

Library of Congress Cataloging-in-Publication Data

Men's health concerns sourcebook / edited by Allan R. Cook.
     p. cm. -- (Health reference series ; v. 38)
     Consists of reprints from various sources. Includes bibliographical
     references and index.
     ISBN 0-7808-0212-8 (lib. bdg. ; alk. paper)
     1. Men -- Health and hygiene -- Popular works.
     I. Cook, Allan R.   II. Series.
     [DNLM: 1. Men collected works. 2. Health collected works.
     W1HE506R v. 38 1998]
     RA776.5.M457 1998
     613' .04234 -- dc21
     DNLM/DCL
     for Library of Congress   98-33612
                                                                      CIP

∞

Printed in the United States of America

39361572

Table of Contents

Part III: Family Planning Decisions

Part IV: Circumcision

Part V: Sleep Disorders

Preface

About This Book

Many of the health concerns that affect men differ significantly from those faced by women. While issues of the reproductive organs perhaps present the most obvious differences, others also exist. For instance, two-thirds of all lung cancer victims are men, 84 percent of all AIDS cases are men, and unintentional injuries claim twice as many men as women. And, even though the rates are growing closer, men, on average still die approximately seven years younger than women. The reason for this disparity may have less to do with gender differences than with lifestyle factors, such as alcohol consumption, diet and exercise, smoking, and the fact that women consult their doctors more often than men.

The articles in this volume offer introductory and basic information on the health concerns that most often and distressingly affect men. They also suggest ways for meeting and minimizing those challenges. Other volumes in the *Health Reference Series* treat some of these concerns in more detail. To help the reader locate sources of more in-depth information, the final section of this Preface includes references to other pertinent volumes in the *Health Reference Series*.

How to Use This Book

This book is divided into parts and chapters. Parts focus on broad areas of interest and chapters on specific topics within those areas.

Part I: Introduction: Gender Focus offers statistics and comparisons of health concerns by gender. One chapter identifies and explains the transformative effect of testosterone which begins to reconstruct the fetus at six weeks.

Part II: Top Ten Causes of Death in Men introduces in order the health concerns identified by the National Institutes of Health as prevalent in terms of morbidity and mortality. It also discusses common symptoms, causes, risk factors, treatments, and avoidance and coping strategies.

Part III: Family Planning Decisions answers the most common concerns about reproduction, fertility, and impotence.

Part IV: Circumcision focuses on the difficult decision faced first by parents of male children of whether to circumcise their child or not and then by that child later in life about the value of circumcision reversal.

Part V: Sleep Disorders includes information on these serious and life-threatening conditions that affect far more people than is commonly believed.

Part VI: Diet, Nutrition, and Fitness provides information on lifestyle issues and concerns including hair loss, weight control, diet, exercise, and abuse of alcohol, tobacco, and other drugs.

Part VII: Gender, No Guarantee of Immunity explains that while some disorders like breast cancer, osteoporosis, eating disorders, and urinary tract infections, may be more prevalent in women, they still affect a significant number of men. Often by classifying these as "women's problems" men and health professionals fail to treat the disorders in a timely or effective manner until it is too late.

Part VIII: Other Common Concerns gives some introductory information on two other common health issues of concern to men: kidney and urologic disorders, the tenth most common cause of death in both men and women, and backaches, an affliction that strikes some 80 percent of men sometime in their lives.

Bibliographic Note

This volume contains individual documents and excerpts from periodic publications issued by the following government agencies: Agency for Health Care Policy and Research (AHCPR), National

Institute of Arthritis and Musculoskeletal and Skin Diseases (NIAMS), National Institutes of Health (NIH), Food and Drug Administration (FDA), U.S. Department of Health and Human Services (DHHS), the National Center for Research Resources (NCRR), the National Heart Lung and Blood Institute (NHLBI), the National Institute on Aging (NIA), the National Institute of Neurological Disorders and Stroke (NINDS), and the National Institute of Diabetes and Digestive and Kidney Diseases.

This volume also includes copyrighted materials reprinted with permission from the following sources: American Academy of Otolaryngology–Head and Neck Surgery; American Hair Loss Council; American Lung Association; American No-Scalpel Vasectomy Association; American Psychiatric Association; Avanstar Communications; Cathy Young; Columbia-Presbyterian Medical Center, Department of Urology; Emphysema Foundation; Lippincott-Raven; Mayo Foundation for Medical Education and Research; Brian J. Morris, PhD, Dsc.; National Association of Social Workers; National Osteoporosis Foundation; and Tuft's University *Diet & Nutrition Letter*.

All copyrighted material is reprinted with permission. Document numbers where applicable and specific source citations are provided on the appropriate page of each chapter. Every effort has been made to secure all necessary rights to reprint the copyrighted material. If any omissions have been made, please contact Omnigraphics to make corrections for future editions.

Acknowledgements

Many people and organizations have contributed the material in this volume. The editor gratefully acknowledges the assistance and cooperation of the American Academy of Otolaryngology–Head and Neck Surgery; American Hair Loss Council; American Lung Association; American No-Scalpel Vasectomy Association; American Psychiatric Association; Avanstar Communications; Cathy Young; Columbia-Presbyterian Medical Center, Department of Urology; Emphysema Foundation; Lippincott-Raven; Mayo Foundation for Medical Education and Research; Brian J. Morris, PhD, Dsc.; National Association of Social Workers; National Osteoporosis Foundation; Tuft's University *Diet & Nutrition Letter*.

Special thanks to Margaret Mary Missar for her patient search for the documents that make up this volume, Karen Bellenir for her technical assistance and advice, Bruce the Scanman for his pixel perambulations, and Valerie Cook for her sharp-eyed text verification.

Note from the Editor

This book is part of Omnigraphics' Health Reference Series. The series provides basic information about a broad range of medical concerns. It is not intended to serve as a tool for diagnosing illness, in prescribing treatments, or as a substitute for the physician/patient relationship. All persons concerned about medical symptoms or the possibility of disease are encouraged to seek professional care from an appropriate health care provider.

Notes on the Health Reference Series

Further information on a variety of diseases and disorders can be found in the following *Health Reference Series* volumes:

- *Diabetes Sourcebook* (Volume 3)—comprehensive disease and statistical information about diabetes mellitus, the eighth most prevalent cause of death for men.

- *AIDS Sourcebook* (Volume 4)—symptoms, treatments, and preventative measures as well as statistical and historical data on the seventh most common cause of death for men.

- *Cardiovascular Diseases and Disorders Sourcebook* (Volume 5)—in-depth information about the most common cause of death in men.

- *Respiratory Diseases and Disorders Sourcebook* (Volume 6)—extensive information on respiratory illnesses including Chronic Obstructive Pulmonary Disorders, the fifth leading cause of death in men, pneumonia and influenza, the sixth leading cause of death in men, and asthma.

- *Mental Health Disorders Sourcebook* (Volume 9)—information on other mental health concerns including information on sexual abuse and spouse abuse as well as on suicide, the ninth most common cause of death for men.

- *Cancer Sourcebook for Women* (Volume 10)—although intended primarily for women, this volume contains a section that offers advice for the partner of a woman with breast cancer.

- *Communications Disorders Sourcebook* (Volume 11)—useful information on hearing loss.

- *The New Cancer Sourcebook* (Volume 12)—extensive information on all forms of cancer, the second most common cause of death in men.

- *Genetic Disorders Sourcebook* (Volume 13)—information and resource listings for sex-linked genetic disorders.

- *Substance Abuse Sourcebook* (Volume 14)—information on drug abuse, intervention, and prevention.

- *Diet and Nutrition Sourcebook* (Volume 15)—essential information on nutrition, healthy eating habits, and weight control.

- *Gastrointestinal Diseases and Disorders Sourcebook* (Volume 16)—information on problems of the digestive system including ulcers, lactose intolerance, and cirrhosis of the liver.

- *Immune System Disorders and Sourcebook* (Volume 17)—information on gender differences in immune system functioning and more information on HIV and AIDS.

- *Allergies Sourcebook* (Volume 19)—information on occupational and environmental asthma and other respiratory problems.

- *Fitness and Exercise Sourcebook* (Volume 20)—detailed information on exercise and fitness along with data about specific activities and recent research efforts.

- *Kidney and Urinary Tract Disorders Sourcebook* (Volume 21)—discusses urinary tract disorders including liver diseases and bladder disorders.

- *Back and Neck Disorders Sourcebook* (Volume 24)—information on back and neck injuries, treatment, coping, and rehabilitation.

- *Sexually Transmitted Diseases Sourcebook* (Volume 26)—extensive information on common sexually transmitted diseases, their treatment and prevention.

- *Environmentally Induced Disorders Sourcebook* (Volume 28)—information on disorders associated with environmental and occupational exposures.

- *Pain Sourcebook* (Volume 32)—information on common forms of pain including headache and backache along with treatment and coping strategies.

Part One

Introduction: Gender Focus

Chapter 1

Testosterone:
Key to Masculinity and More

From the first glance at the newborn, the evidence is obvious—a tiny penis and a scrotum enclosing the testes. No doubt about it: a male child.

But his gender wasn't always so clear. For the first six weeks or so of gestation, this new baby boy appeared identical to a girl. He had embryonic gonadal cells that looked like they could quite normally develop into ovaries. He had tissue apparently capable of forming fallopian tubes, a uterus, and vagina.

At about seven weeks of gestational age, testes began to form from cells that otherwise might have become ovaries. The hormone testosterone, produced by the testes beginning in the eighth week, initiated a cascade of actions and reactions causing remarkable changes in embryonic cells that had been on the road to becoming female organs and tissue. Testosterone promoted development of the penis and scrotum, formation of the structures involved in sperm production, and regression of tissue that, without testosterone, would have become fallopian tubes, uterus, and vagina. The result is announced at birth, "It's a boy!"

Testosterone (one of the masculinizing hormones called androgens) continues to exert a spectrum of influences—sometimes quietly, sometimes furiously—throughout a lifetime. Little wonder that this powerful hormone has been approved by the Food and Drug Administration for the treatment of serious health problems caused by a deficiency

FDA Consumer, May 1995.

3

or absence of naturally occurring androgens and that physicians and scientists here and abroad are trying to demonstrate other beneficial uses for the hormone.

Fluctuating Hormones

At birth, baby boys normally have testosterone blood levels close to those of adolescent and young adult males. But the level soon falls and remains relatively low until puberty, when testosterone and other hormone levels rise sharply. About 99 per cent of American boys begin puberty between 9 and 14 years of age.

The earliest sign of puberty is enlargement of the testes. Other changes—the appearance of pubic and other body hair, muscle and bone growth, deepening of the voice, and often acne—tell the world, to say nothing of the boy himself, that sexual maturation is well under way.

After puberty and into adulthood, a complex interaction among the testes, the adrenal glands (which also produce testosterone), and the pituitary and hypothalamus (located at the base of the brain) regulates levels of testosterone and other androgens. In adulthood, testosterone is thought to play a role, not only in sexual function, but in common adult male traits, such as loss of scalp hair and accumulation of abdominal fat—the all-too-familiar "spare tire."

Testosterone levels decline with advancing age, but some men retain essentially youthful testosterone levels well into their seventies and eighties.

The presence of presumably normal amounts of testosterone is believed to be associated with some potentially dangerous changes in men. For example, it probably stimulates excessive growth of the prostate, which can lead to urinary disorders and prostate cancer, the second most common cancer in American men. (See "Prostate Cancer: New Tests Create Treatment Dilemmas" in the December 1994 *FDA Consumer* and reprinted in this Sourcebook.)

A number of problems, collectively called "hypogonadism," result from failure of the testes to function normally because of genetic defect, illness, or injury. Unless an obvious abnormality is present at birth, delayed puberty may be the first indication that the testes are producing insufficient amounts of testosterone. If the malfunction occurs before the twelfth week of gestation, male genitalia may not form fully or properly. When testosterone levels fall below normal after birth but before the normal onset of puberty, boys may begin puberty late or not at all, exhibit reduced growth of genitalia and body hair, retain a high-pitched voice, and show atypical bone growth and body proportions.

The consequences of hypogonadism beginning after puberty depend largely on the degree and duration of below-normal testosterone levels. Typical effects are diminished libido, potency, sperm production, and overall strength. If the condition persists for a long time, the testes atrophy, fine wrinkles appear around the eyes and mouth, and body hair becomes sparse.

Testosterone Replacement

An estimated 150,000 to 200,000 boys and men in the United States are currently receiving testosterone to treat hypogonadism, although many more cases are thought to be undiagnosed and untreated. FDA has approved both oral and injectable testosterone products for use in hormone replacement therapy for boys and men who have hypogonadism. Testosterone is not readily absorbed and used by the body when taken by mouth. Most patients receive the drug by injection for their entire lives. An external patch that delivers the hormone through the skin of the scrotum has been approved by FDA for use in men 18 and older.

Carefully monitored testosterone replacement therapy, combined with other medical and psychological support, can help in cases of delayed puberty by inducing essentially normal growth and maturation. Mature men whose testosterone output is impaired because of illness, including chronic alcoholism, or injury also benefit from testosterone replacement and other medical treatment that can improve sexual and reproductive function.

Not to Be Taken Lightly

Testosterone exerts powerful effects on human bodies, helping make them stronger and bigger. It also increases sex drive and function in men (and, according to some studies, in women—although this possibility is still uncertain). Not surprisingly, some young American men obtain testosterone illegally. And so, it seems, do athletes, including both men and women Olympic competitors who apparently use the hormone to improve performance. This use violates Olympic rules—and it's dangerous.

Androgens, such as testosterone, taken by injection or by mouth during early puberty can cause abnormal bone growth, including premature growth stoppage. At inappropriate doses, testosterone can disturb fluid and mineral balances; cause nausea and other gastrointestinal problems, including life-threatening liver disease and tumors; induce male breast enlargement; interfere with blood clotting; cause increased or decreased libido, headache, anxiety, and depression; raise cholesterol levels; and—especially if taken over a long period—suppress normal testosterone production.

Like anabolic steroids, many testosterone products, including the skin patch formulation known as Testoderm, are schedule III controlled substances because of the potential for abuse. Testosterone is nothing to fool around with.

Chapter 2

Facts and Figures: Rates and Comparisons of Injury and Disease by Gender, Race, and Age

Leading Causes of Death—Snapshots

Mortality

- In 1995 injury death rates were higher for males than for females in every age group except infancy. At ages 20–24 years, the injury death rate for males was 4.6 times the rate for females. Beginning at ages 10–14 years and for all subsequent 5- and 10-year age groups, the ratio was at least 2 to 1.

- In 1995 unintentional injury accounted for 61 percent of all injury deaths, suicide for 21 percent, and homicide for 15 percent. Unintentional injury mortality and suicide rates were highest for the elderly, and homicide rates were highest at 20–24 years of age.

- In 1994–95 at 15–34 years of age, unintentional injury death rates and suicide rates were higher for American Indians than for other racial or ethnic groups, and homicide rates were higher for the black population than for other groups. Among persons 75 years and over, injury mortality was lower for Hispanic persons than for other groups primarily as a result of their lower unintentional injury death rates due to falls and suffocation.

Selected from NIH Publication *Injury Chartbook* and NHLBI FY 1996 Fact Book, Chapter 4.

Table 2.1. Leading Causes of Death and Numbers of Deaths, According to Sex.

Male

	All causes	1,075,078	All causes	1,172,959
1	Diseases of heart	405,661	Diseases of heart	362,714
2	Malignant neoplasms	225,948	Malignant neoplasms	281,611
3	Unintentional injuries	74,180	Cerebrovascular diseases	61,563
4	Cerebrovascular diseases	69,973	Unintentional injuries	61,401
5	Chronic obstructive pulmonary diseases	38,625	Chronic obstructive pulmonary diseases	53,938
6	Pneumonia and influenza	27,574	Pneumonia and influenza	37,787
7	Suicide	20,505	Human immunodeficiency virus infection	35,950
8	Chronic liver disease and cirrhosis	19,768	Diabetes mellitus	26,124
9	Homicide and legal intervention	19,088	Suicide	25,369
10	Diabetes mellitus	14,325	Homicide and legal intervention	17,740

Female

	All causes	914,763	All causes	1,139,173
1	Diseases of heart	355,424	Diseases of heart	374,849
2	Malignant neoplasms	190,561	Malignant neoplasms	256,844
3	Cerebrovascular diseases	100,252	Cerebrovascular diseases	96,428
4	Unintentional injuries	31,538	Chronic obstructive pulmonary diseases	48,961
5	Pneumonia and influenza	27,045	Pneumonia and influenza	45,136
6	Diabetes mellitus	20,526	Diabetes mellitus	33,130
7	Atherosclerosis	17,848	Unintentional injuries	31,919
8	Chronic obstructive pulmonary diseases	17,425	Alzheimer's disease	13,607
9	Chronic liver disease and cirrhosis	10,815	Nephritis, nephrotic syndrome, and nephrosis	12,287
10	Certain conditions originating in the perinatal period	9,815	Septicemia	11,974

8

- The degree of urbanization is associated with injury mortality rates. In 1994 the age-adjusted unintentional injury death rate in non-metropolitan counties was 1.6 times the rate in metropolitan counties while homicide rates in large core metropolitan counties were 2–3 times the rates in other types of counties.

- Motor vehicle traffic injuries and firearm injuries were the two leading causes of injury death in the United States in 1995, accounting for 29 and 24 percent of all injury deaths. Poisoning was the third leading cause of injury death, accounting for 11 percent of all injury deaths.

- Among children 1–14 years of age, motor vehicle traffic injuries were the leading cause of death in 1995. Among infants, suffocation was the leading cause of injury death. The five leading causes of injury death among infants and children under 15 years of age—motor vehicle traffic injuries, fires and burns, drowning, suffocation, and firearms—accounted for 80 percent of injury deaths.

- Among teenagers 15–19 years of age and young adults 20–24 years of age, motor vehicle traffic-related injuries and firearm-related injuries were the two leading causes of death in 1995. For older adults 65–74 years, motor vehicles and firearms were the two leading causes of injury deaths accounting for one-half of injury mortality. At ages 75–84 years, motor vehicles and falls were the cause of close to one-half of all injury deaths. For those 85 years and over, falls caused one-third of injury deaths.

- Age-adjusted motor vehicle traffic injury death rates declined 15 percent from 1985 to 1993 with a more rapid decline among males than females. During the same period firearm injury death rates increased 22 percent, with larger increases occurring among males than females. During the most recent period 1993–95, the age-adjusted motor vehicle traffic injury death rate increased 2 percent while the firearm injury death rate declined 11 percent.

- Between 1985 and 1993 the firearm injury death rate among persons 15–34 years of age increased 44 percent primarily as a result of increases in the firearm homicide rate, followed by an 11-percent decline in the firearm injury death rate by 1995. On

10 Leading Causes of Death: Death Rates, U.S., 1995

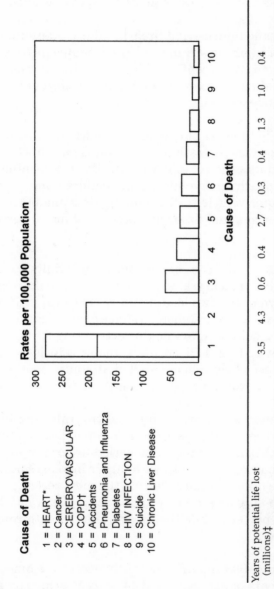

Cause of Death

1 = HEART*
2 = Cancer
3 = CEREBROVASCULAR
4 = COPD†
5 = Accidents
6 = Pneumonia and Influenza
7 = Diabetes
8 = HIV INFECTION
9 = Suicide
10 = Chronic Liver Disease

Years of potential life lost (millions)‡	3.5	4.3	0.6	0.4	2.7	0.3	0.4	1.3	1.0	0.4

* Includes 184 deaths per 100,000 population from CHD.
† COPD and allied conditions (including asthma).
‡ Based on the average remaining years of life up to age 75 years.
Note: Capitalization indicates diseases addressed in Institute programs.
Source: Vital statistics of the U.S., NCHS (provisional).

Figure 2.1.

the other hand, the motor vehicle traffic injury death rate declined 18 percent in this age group from 1985 to 1993 and was relatively stable through 1995. From 1985 to 1995 the alcohol-related traffic injury death rate declined 32 percent.

- Motor vehicle injury death rates among white males and black males 20 years of age are generally higher in the South and lower in the Northeast than in other geographic areas of the United States.

- In 1994 the firearm injury death rate among males 15–24 years in the United States was 32 percent higher than the motor vehicle traffic injury death rate. An international comparison shows that in none of 10 comparison countries did the firearm injury death rate exceed the motor vehicle traffic injury death rate for young males. The motor vehicle traffic injury death rate among young males 15–24 years of age was higher in New Zealand than in the other countries.

- In 1994–95 transportation-related incidents accounted for 41 percent of all occupational injury fatalities and assaults and violent acts accounted for 20 percent. Occupational injury death rates for fishers, timber cutters, and airplane pilots were more than 20 times the national average.

- In 1995 life expectancy at birth was 75.8 years, slightly longer than in 1994 and matching the record high attained in 1992. In 1995 white females continued to have the highest life expectancy at birth (79.6 years), followed by black females (73.9 years), white males (73.4 years), and black males (65.2 years).

- Years of potential life lost (YPLL) per 100,000 population under 75 years of age is a measure of premature mortality. In 1995 YPLL for malignant neoplasms, heart disease, and unintentional injuries accounted for 21 percent, 17 percent, and 13 percent of all YPLL and HIV infection accounted for 7 percent. The age-adjusted YPLL rate for HIV infection increased 55 percent between 1990 and 1994 and remained stable in 1995.

- Educational attainment is inversely associated with mortality. In 1995 the age-adjusted death rate for persons 25–64 years of age who had not graduated from high school was 2.4 times the

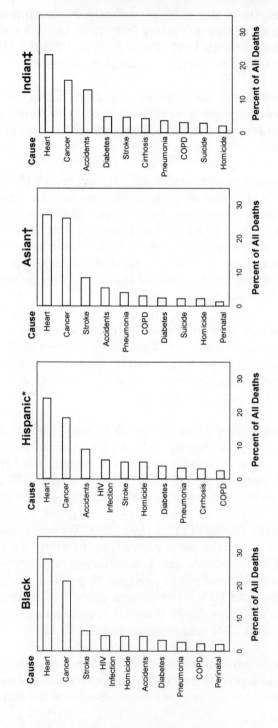

10 Leading Causes of Death Among Minority Groups, U.S., 1993

* Data for 49 reporting states and the District of Columbia.

† Includes deaths among individuals of Asian extraction and Asian-Pacific Islanders.

‡ Includes deaths among Aleuts and Eskimos.

Source: Vital statistics of the U.S., NCHS.

Figure 2.2.

rate for persons with more than a high school education and the death rate for high school graduates was double that for persons with more than a high school education.

- Between 1990 and 1995 the age-adjusted death rate for heart disease, the leading cause of death, decreased 9 percent to 138.3 deaths per 100,000 population. The average annual decline during 1990–95 (1.9 percent) was slower than during 1980–90 (2.8 percent). Compared with white Americans, heart disease mortality was 41 percent lower for Asian Americans and 49 percent higher for black Americans in 1995.

- The long term downward trend in the age-adjusted death rate for stroke, the third leading cause of death, was interrupted in 1993. Stroke mortality was relatively unchanged for the third consecutive year in 1995. Between 1980 and 1990 stroke mortality had declined rapidly at an average rate of almost 4 percent per year.

- In 1995 age-adjusted death rates for Asian-American males and females were 37 percent lower than those for white males and white females. In 1995 the age-adjusted death rate for stroke among Asian-American males (31.2 deaths per 100,000 population) was 18 percent higher than the corresponding rate for white males. Stroke is the only leading cause of death for which mortality is higher for Asian-American males than for white males.

- Between 1990 and 1995 the age-adjusted death rate for cancer, the second leading cause of death, decreased nearly 4 percent to 129.9 deaths per 100,000 population, following an increase of 4 percent between 1970 and 1990. Between 1990 and 1995 the death rate for cancer declined more for those under 65 years of age than for older persons, more for men than women, and more for black persons than white persons. During this period among persons 55–64 years of age cancer mortality declined 12 percent for black males, 9 percent for white males, 8 percent for black females, and 4 percent for white females.

- In 1995 the age-adjusted death rate for lung cancer for males (55.3 deaths per 100,000 population) was double the rate for females. Between 1990 and 1995 the age-adjusted death rate for

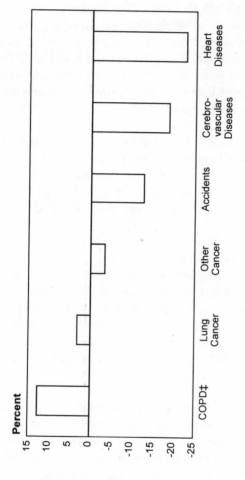

Change in Death Rates* for Leading Causes of Death, U.S., 1985-95†

Percent

15
10
5
0
-5
-10
-15
-20
-25

COPD‡ | Lung Cancer | Other Cancer | Accidents | Cerebro-vascular Diseases | Heart Diseases

Leading Cause of Death

* Age adjusted to the 1940 U.S. population.
† Provisional for 1995.
‡ Includes asthma. COPD increased 12 percent, and asthma increased 23 percent.
Source: Vital statistics of the U.S., NCHS.

Figure 2.3.

lung cancer for males decreased 9 percent while the corresponding rate for females increased 5 percent. Lung cancer death rates have continued to rise among older women while falling among younger women. Between 1990 and 1995 lung cancer death rates increased 26 percent for women 75–84 years of age while they decreased 15 percent for women 45–54 years of age.

- In 1995 the age-adjusted death rate for chronic obstructive pulmonary diseases (COPD), the fourth leading cause of death overall, was 54 percent higher for males than females (26.3 and 17.1 deaths per 100,000 population). Between 1980 and 1995 age-adjusted death rates for males were relatively stable while death rates for females nearly doubled. The COPD death rates are highest for the elderly and have been increasing most rapidly among females age 75 years and over.

- In 1994 and 1995 HIV infection was the leading cause of death for adults 25–44 years of age. Between 1994 and 1995 the HIV infection death rate remained stable in this age group after increasing at an average annual rate of 12 percent between 1990 and 1994. In 1995 among adults 25–44 years of age, the death rate for HIV infection for black females (54.5 deaths per 100,000 population) was 9 times the rate for white females and the rate for black males (182.0 per 100,000) was 4 times the rate for white males.

- Between 1993 and 1995 the homicide rate for young black males 15–24 years of age decreased at an average annual rate of 11 percent to 132.0 deaths per 100,000 population after increasing at an average annual rate of 12 percent between 1985 and 1993. Despite recent changes in homicide trends, substantial racial disparities in homicide rates remain. In 1995 the homicide rate for young black males was 8 times the rate for young white males.

- Overall mortality for black Americans continues to be about 60 percent higher than for white Americans. For most leading causes of death, mortality is higher for black Americans than for other racial and ethnic groups. In 1995 the age-adjusted homicide rate for black Americans was 6 times and the HIV infection death rate was nearly 5 times the corresponding rate for white Americans.

15

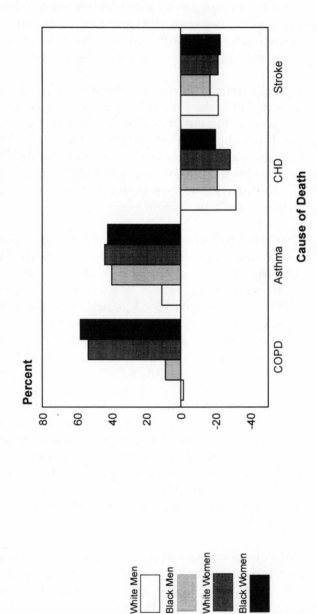

Change in Death Rates* for Selected Causes by Race and Gender, 1984-94

* Age adjusted to the 1940 U.S. population.
Source: Vital statistics of the U.S., NCHS.

Figure 2.4.

- Death rates for American Indians under 55 years of age are higher than those for white Americans. In 1993–95 for persons 25–34 years of age, the death rate for American Indian males was about 60 percent higher and the death rate for American Indian females was 85 percent higher than the corresponding rates for white males and white females, and the death rate for American Indian children 1–4 years of age was almost double that for white children.

- Overall mortality for Hispanic Americans was about 20 percent lower than for non-Hispanic white Americans in 1995. However for males 15–44 years of age death rates for Hispanic Americans were higher than those for non-Hispanic white Americans. In 1995 for Hispanic males 15–24 years of age the death rate was 53 percent higher and for Hispanic males 25–34 and 35–44 years of age, 30 and 24 percent higher than for non-Hispanic white males of similar ages.

- Between 1990 and 1992 the death rate for occupational injuries declined 11 percent to 4.1 deaths per 100,000 workers in the civilian work force. During this period, the occupational injury death rate declined 26 percent for the mining industry to 22.3 per 100,000 and 3 percent for the agriculture, forestry, and fishing industry to 17.5 per 100,000.

Hospitalization

- Hospital discharge rates for persons with a first-listed diagnosis of injury increase with age. Fractures, followed by poisonings, open wounds, intracranial injuries, sprains and strains, and internal injuries are the leading types of injuries resulting in hospitalization for injury.

- In 1993–94 at ages 15–24 years, the hospital discharge rate for injury among males was twice the rate for females, while at ages 75 years and over, the rate for males was about 30 percent lower than the rate for females.

- Discharge rates for open wounds and for internal injuries for all males were 3 times the rates for all females. At ages 15–24 years the discharge rate for open wounds for males was 4.5 times the rate for females. Discharge rates for poisoning for females ages

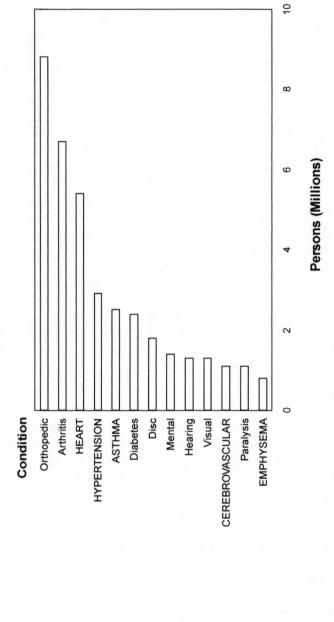

Prevalence of Leading Chronic Conditions Causing Limitation of Activity, U.S., 1990-92

Note: Capitalization indicates diseases addressed in Institute programs.
Source: National Health Interview Survey (NHIS), NCHS.

Figure 2.5.

15–24 years and 45–64 years, on the other hand, were 1.6 times the rates for males.

- In 1992–94, three out of five injury hospitalizations among elderly persons 75 years of age and over were for fractures, and more than one-half of the fractures were to the hip. Hip fracture rates for elderly females were twice the rates for males.

Emergency Department Utilization

- In 1993–94, 41 percent of all visits made to emergency departments were for injuries. Injury visit rates for males at ages 5–14 years, 15–24 years, and 25–44 years were 1.4 times the rates for females, while among those 75 years of age and over, the visit rate for females was 1.3 times the rate for males.

- In 1993–94, three causes of injury—falls, being struck by or against something, and motor vehicle traffic-related injuries—accounted for 18 percent of all emergency department visits, and for 43 percent of all emergency department visits due to injury.

- Open wounds and lacerations, superficial injuries, sprains and strains, and fractures were the four leading principal injury diagnoses in emergency departments in 1993–94, accounting for 63 percent of all first-listed principal injury diagnoses.

- Of the average annual 8 million emergency department visits for falls in 1993–94, 86 percent of the principal diagnoses were coded as injuries. Approximately one-fifth each were for fractures, superficial injury, open wounds and lacerations, and sprains and strains. Of the remaining 14 percent of the diagnoses, one-third were diseases of the musculoskeletal system and connective tissue disease.

- In 1994 the number of emergency department-treated injuries related to basketball, bicycle and accessories, football, baseball and softball, and playground equipment was greater than for injuries related to other sports and recreation products. Rates of injury vary by sport and by age. In 1994 the basketball-related injury rate was higher for persons 15–24 years of age than for younger or older persons and bicycle-related injuries were higher for children 5–14 years.

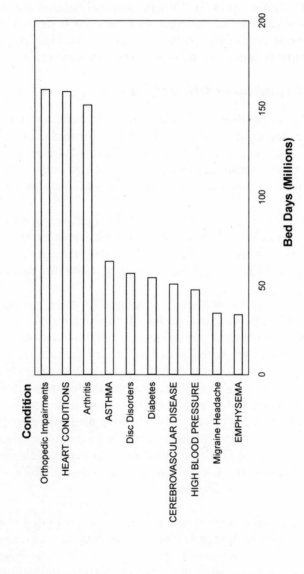

Leading Chronic Conditions Causing Bed Disability, U.S., 1990-92

Note: Capitalization indicates diseases addressed in Institute programs.
Source: NHIS, NCHS.

Figure 2.6.

- In 1992–93 the total number of people treated in emergency departments for nonfatal firearm injuries was about 2.6 times the number who died from firearm injuries. Among persons 15–24 years of age, however, the emergency department visit rate for nonfatal firearm injuries was about 4 times the fatality rate, while at age 45 years and over, the visit rate and the fatality rate were similar.

Poisoning Exposures

- In 1995 poison control centers managed more than 1 million potentially poisonous exposures among children under 6 years of age. In 94 percent of the cases, the site of the exposure was the child's home.

Victimization

- In 1994 in households where the annual family income was at least $25,000, there were no significant differences in criminal victimization rates between white persons and black persons. For family income less than $7,500 the victimization rate was higher for white than black persons because of the higher rate of simple assaults. When family income was between $15,000 and $24,999, the rate was higher for black than white persons because of the higher aggravated assault rate.

- Regardless of the type of violence (rape, other sexual assaults, robbery, or assault), women with lower income experience higher rates of violence perpetrated on them than women with higher income. In 1994 the victimization rate for women with annual income of less than $10,000 was twice the rate for women with annual income of at least $50,000.

- In 1994 an estimated 1 million children under the age of 19 years were victims of abuse and neglect.

Episodes of Injury

- In 1993–94 there were an estimated average annual 58 million reported episodes of injury occurring at a rate of 23 per 100 persons. The rate was higher for persons under 45 years of age than for older persons.

Table 2.2.

Direct and Indirect Economic Costs of Illness by Major Diagnosis, U.S., 1997

| | Amount (Dollars in Billions) | | | | Percent Distribution | | | |
| | | Indirect Costs | | | | Indirect Costs | | |
	Direct Costs*	Morbidity†	Mortality‡	Total	Direct Costs	Morbidity	Mortality	Total
Cardiovascular Disease§	$158.5	$24.6	$76.0	$259.1	14.8	15.7	23.6	16.7
(Including Blood Clotting)**	(37.2)	(5.8)	(21.3)	(64.3)	(3.5)	(3.7)	(6.6)	(4.1)
Lung Diseases††	78.3	20.4	16.0	114.7	7.3	13.0	5.0	7.4
Blood Diseases	7.6	0.6	1.5	9.6	0.7	0.4	0.5	0.6
Subtotal	244.4	45.6	93.5	383.4	22.8	29.1	29.0	24.7
Diseases of the Digestive System	111.8	8.0	13.1	132.9	10.4	5.1	4.1	8.6
Neoplasms	51.3	13.4	71.5	136.2	4.8	8.6	22.2	8.8
Mental Disorders	84.0	20.6	4.2	108.8	7.8	13.2	1.3	7.0
Diseases of the Nervous System	58.4	6.1	5.4	69.9	5.4	3.9	1.7	4.5
Diseases of the Musculoskeletal System	56.2	15.9	1.1	73.2	5.2	10.2	0.3	4.7
Diseases of the Genitourinary System	44.6	4.0	2.9	51.5	4.2	2.6	0.9	3.3
Endocrine, Nutritional, and Metabolic Diseases	39.5	5.1	9.0	53.6	3.7	3.2	2.8	3.4
Infectious and Parasitic Diseases	28.9	9.6	30.8	69.3	2.7	6.1	9.5	4.5
Diseases of the Skin	43.8	1.2	0.2	45.2	4.1	0.8	0.1	2.9
Other Respiratory Diseases	45.5	6.2	2.1	53.8	4.2	4.0	0.6	3.5
Other and Unallocable	263.9	20.9	88.8	373.6	24.6	13.3	27.5	24.1
Total	**$1,072.3**	**$156.6**	**$322.6**	**$1,551.5**	**100.0%**	**100.0%**	**100.0%**	**100.0%**

* Direct costs of CVD were estimated by NCHS. Direct costs are personal health care expenditures for hospital and nursing home care, drugs, home care, and physician and other professional services. Totals for these types of costs are estimated by the Health Care Financing Administration (HCFA). Allocation by diagnosis is based on statistics from the National Hospital Discharge Survey, the National Ambulatory Medical Care Survey, National Home and Hospice Survey, and the National Nursing Home Survey of the NCHS.

† Morbidity costs were estimated for 1997 by multiplying 1980 NCHS estimates by a 5 percent per year inflation factor.

‡ Mortality estimates are obtained by multiplying deaths in 1993 for these causes by the 1992 present value of lifetime earnings discounted at 6 percent times the 1992-97 inflation factor (assumed to be 5 percent per year).

§ Includes congenital cardiovascular disease.

** Based on NHLBI definition of blood-clotting diseases based primarily on proportions of morbidity and mortality statistics for acute myocardial infarction, cerebrovascular diseases, and diseases of arteries.

††Does not include lung cancer, leukemias, or pulmonary heart disease.

Note: Numbers may not add to total due to rounding.

Source: Estimates by the NHLBI; data from the NCHS, HCFA, and the Bureau of the Census.

Total Economic Costs, U.S., 1997

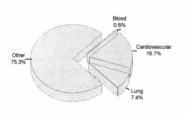

Economic Costs: Cardiovascular, Lung, and Blood Diseases, U.S., 1997

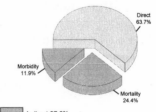

Determinants and Measures of Health.

- Large racial and ethnic differences continue in the rate of reported AIDS cases. For the 12 months ending June 30, 1996, the AIDS case rate for non-Hispanic black males 13 years of age and over (186 cases per 100,000 population) was nearly double that for Hispanic males and nearly 6 times that for non-Hispanic white males. Among females 13 years of age and over the AIDS case rate for non-Hispanic black females (62) was nearly triple that for Hispanic females and more than 16 times that for non-Hispanic white females.

- Cancer of the prostate is the most frequently diagnosed cancer in men. In 1994 the age-adjusted incidence rate for prostate cancer for black men was 73 percent higher than for white men (234 and 135 cases per 100,000 population). The 5-year relative survival rate for prostate cancer diagnosed during 1986–93 for black men was 15 percentage points lower than for white men (75 and 90 percent).

- Between 1990 and 1994 the age-adjusted prevalence of current cigarette smoking among persons 18 years of age or over has remained stable at 25–26 percent. In 1994 among white persons the age-adjusted prevalence of current smoking for males was slightly higher than for females (28 and 24 percent), and among black persons smoking prevalence was about 60 percent higher for males than females (34 and 21 percent).

- In 1994 the age-adjusted prevalence of current cigarette smoking among persons 25 years of age and over ranged from 12 percent for college graduates to 38 percent for persons with less than a high school education. Over the 20-year period 1974 to 1994 smoking levels declined for all educational groups with more rapid declines among persons with higher education levels. During this period the ratio of smoking prevalence for persons with less than 12 years education to that for college graduates doubled from 1.6 to 3.2.

- In 1996, 22 percent of high school seniors reported using marijuana in the past month, an increase of 84 percent since 1992. This increase follows a period of steady decline in marijuana use by twelfth graders, from 34 percent in 1980 to 12 percent in

1992. Between 1992 and 1996 the use of marijuana by eighth graders increased threefold to 11 percent.

- In 1995, 52 percent of the population 12 years of age and over reported using alcohol in the past month and 16 percent reported having five or more drinks on at least one occasion in the past month. Young people 18–25 years of age were more likely to binge on alcohol than were other age groups. Among 18–25 year olds, binge drinking was more than twice as likely for males as females (41 and 19 percent) and more than twice as likely for non-Hispanic white persons as for non-Hispanic black persons (34 and 16 percent).

- In 1994 and 1995 there were more than 142,000 cocaine-related emergency room episodes, the highest number ever reported since these events were tracked starting in 1978. Between 1988 and 1995 cocaine-related episodes among persons 35 years of age and over have almost tripled, reflecting an aging population of drug abusers being treated in emergency departments.

- Between 1976–80 and 1988–94 the age-adjusted prevalence of hypertension for adults 20–74 years declined from 39 to 23 percent. In 1988–94 the age-adjusted prevalence of hypertension for non-Hispanic black men (35 percent) was about 40 percent greater than for non-Hispanic white or Mexican-American men and hypertension prevalence for non-Hispanic black women (34 percent) was also substantially greater than for non-Hispanic white women (19 percent) or Mexican-American women (22 percent).

- Between 1960–62 and 1988–94 the age-adjusted mean serum total cholesterol level for adults 20–74 years declined from 220 to 203 mg/dL. During the same period the age-adjusted percent of adults with high serum cholesterol (greater than or equal to 240 mg/dL) declined from 32 to 19 percent.

- The age-adjusted percent of adults who were overweight increased from 25 percent in 1976–80 to 35 percent in 1988–94. Among adult women the age-adjusted prevalence of overweight in 1988–94 continued to be substantially higher for non-Hispanic black women (53 percent) and Mexican-American women (52 percent) than for non-Hispanic white women (33 percent).

- The age-adjusted percent of adolescents 12–17 years of age who were overweight increased from 6 percent in 1976–80 to 12 percent in 1988–94. During the same period the prevalence of overweight among 6–11 year old children also increased from 8 percent to 14 percent.

- An environmental health objective for the year 2000 is that at least 85 percent of the U.S. population should be living in counties that meet the Environmental Protection Agency's National Ambient Air Quality Standards (NAAQS). In 1994, 75 percent of Americans lived in counties that met the NAAQS for all pollutants, up from 50 percent in 1988. In 1994, 55–56 percent of the Hispanic and Asian-American population lived in counties that met NAAQS for all pollutants compared with 80 percent of the American Indian population. Disparities among racial and ethnic groups are attributable in part to different residence patterns. Data from the 1990 census indicate that higher proportions of Hispanics and Asian Americans than other racial and ethnic groups reside in metropolitan areas where air quality standards are more likely to be exceeded and higher proportions of American Indians reside in non-metropolitan areas where urban-based pollutants are less concentrated.

- Between 1990 and 1995 the injuries with lost workdays rate decreased 13 percent to 3.4 per 100 full-time equivalents (FTE's) in the private sector. The industries reporting the largest declines during this period (22–27 percent) were mining; agriculture, fishing, and forestry; and construction. The 1995 rate for the manufacturing industry (4.6 per 100 FTE's) was 13 percent lower than in 1990 and the rate for the transportation, communication, and public utilities industry (5.0 per 100 FTE's) was 7 percent lower than in 1990.

Chapter 3

Health Indicators: Why Do Men Die Seven Years Younger than Women?

Men live, on the average, about 7 less years than women do in the United States. Why? This report looks at some of the suspected causes of the disparity.

Health Indicators

Here are the major heath indicators. In short, here is a surprise. These indicators don't show a big difference between men and women in Hypertension, Cholesterol, and being overweight. The biggest difference is in frequency of doctor visits and in drinking.

Summary

These show:

- Women go to the doctor more often than men. Part of the difference is attributable to childbearing and birth control
- Men drink somewhat more.
- Hypertension is a little more prevalent in men
- Cholesterol is slightly higher in women
- Women are overweight slightly more often than men
- Men smoke slightly more than women

Web Document from Men's Health Network [http://www.vix.com/pub/men/health/stat/mort-factor.html] Friday 13 Oct 1995. (Ted W.). Reprinted with acknowledgement.

All data is from Health United States 1993, DHHS Pub No. (PHS) 94-1232

Table 3.1. Physician Contacts. Physician contacts by sex and age of patient: United States, 1992

age	5	5-14	15-44	45-64	65-74	75+
Male	7.1	3.5	3.7	6.1	9.2	12.2
Female	6.7	3.3	6.2	8.2	10.1	12.1

Table 3.2. Alcohol consumption by persons 18 years of age and over: United States, 1985 and 1990 [Data are based on household interviews of a sample of the civilian non-institutionalized population]

Alcohol consumption, age	Both sexes		Male		Female	
	1985	1990	1985	1990	1985	1990
Drinking status	Percent distribution					
All	100.0	100.0	100.0	100.0	100.0	100.0
Abstainer	26.9	29.7	14.4	16.6	38.0	41.5
Former drinker	7.5	9.6	9.2	11.6	6.1	7.8
Current drinker	65.6	60.7	76.4	71.8	55.9	50.7
Percent current drinkers among all persons All races:						
18-44 years	72.8	67.5	82.4	77.1	63.8	58.3
18-24 years	71.8	63.7	79.5	71.7	64.5	56.1
25-44 years	73.2	68.8	83.5	78.9	63.5	59.0
45 years and over	55.5	51.3	67.4	63.8	45.6	40.8
45-64 years	62.2	57.6	72.2	68.4	53.0	47.6
65 years and over	44.3	41.4	58.2	55.6	34.7	31.3

Table 3.3. Hypertension among persons 20 years of age and over: United States, [Data are based on physical examinations of a sample of the civilian non-institutionalized population]

	1960-62	1971-74	1976-80	1988-91
Both sexes*	36.9	38.3	39.0	23.4
Male	40.0	42.4	44.0	26.3
Female*	33.7	34.3	34.0	20.3
Male				
20-34 years	22.8	24.8	28.9	9.2
35-44 years	37.7	39.1	40.5	20.0
45-54 years	47.6	55.0	53.6	35.7
55-64 years	60.3	62.5	61.8	46.7
65-74 years	68.8	67.2	67.1	59.0
75 years and over	—	—	—	63.7
Female*				
20-34 years	9.3	11.2	11.1	3.0
35-44 years	24.0	28.2	28.8	12.3
45-54 years	43.4	43.6	47.1	23.2
55-64 years	66.4	62.5	61.1	46.5
65-74 years	81.5	78.3	71.8	57.8
75 years and over	—	—	—	75.2

Excludes pregnant women.

Table 3.4. Serum cholesterol levels among persons 20 years of age and over: United States, [Data are based on physical examinations of a sample of the civilian non-institutionalized population]

	Percent of population with high serum cholesterol				Mean serum cholesterol level, mg/dL			
	1960-62	1971-74	1976-80	1988-91	1960-62	1971-74	1976-80	1988-91
Both sexes	31.8	27.2	26.3	19.7	220	214	213	205
Male	28.7	25.8	24.6	19.0	217	213	211	205
Female	34.5	28.2	27.6	20.2	222	215	214	205
Male								
20-34 years	15.1	12.4	11.9	9.3	198	194	192	189
35-44 years	33.9	31.8	27.9	19.3	227	221	217	207
45-54 years	39.2	37.5	36.9	26.1	231	229	227	218
55-64 years	41.6	36.2	36.8	31.4	233	229	229	221
65-74 years	38.0	34.7	31.7	27.7	230	226	221	218
75 years +	—	—	—	19.9	—	—	—	205
Female								
20-34 years	12.4	10.9	9.8	8.3	194	191	189	185
35-44 years	23.1	19.3	20.7	11.7	214	207	207	195
45-54 years	46.9	38.7	40.5	25.2	237	232	232	217
55-64 years	70.1	53.1	52.9	40.4	262	245	249	237
65-74 years	68.5	57.7	51.6	43.2	266	250	246	234
75 years +	—	—	—	39.2	—	—	—	230

Table 3.5. Overweight persons 20 years of age and over, according to sex, age,: United States. [Data are based on physical examinations of a sample of the civilian non-institutionalized population]

	1960-62	1971-74	1976-80	1988-91
20-74 years, age adjusted	Percent of population			
Both sexes	24.4	24.9	25.4	33.3
Male	22.9	23.6	24.0	31.6
Female*	25.6	25.9	26.5	35.0
Male				
20-34 years	19.6	19.2	17.3	22.2
35-44 years	22.8	29.4	28.9	35.3
45-54 years	28.1	27.6	31.0	35.6
55-64 years	26.9	24.8	28.1	40.1
65-74 years	21.8	23.0	25.2	42.9
75 years and over	—	—	—	26.4
Female*				
20-34 years	13.2	14.8	16.8	25.1
35-44 years	24.1	27.3	27.0	36.9
45-54 years	30.7	32.3	32.5	41.6
55-64 years	43.2	38.5	37.0	48.5
65-74 years	42.9	38.0	38.4	39.8
75 years and over	—	—	—	30.9

*Excludes pregnant women.

Table 3.6. Current **cigarette smoking** by persons 18 years of age and over, according to sex, and age: United States, selected years 1965-92 [Data are based on household interviews of a sample of the civilian non-institutionalized population]

age	18-24 yrs		25-34 yrs		35-44 yrs		45-64 yrs		65 yrs+	
sex	m	f	m	f	m	f	m	f	m	f
1965	54.1	38.1	60.7	43.7	58.2	43.7	51.9	32.0	28.5	9.6
1974	42.1	34.1	50.5	38.8	51.0	39.8	42.6	33.4	24.8	12.0
1979	35.0	33.8	43.9	33.7	41.8	37.0	39.3	30.7	20.9	13.2
1983	32.9	35.5	38.8	32.6	41.0	33.8	35.9	31.0	22.0	13.1
1985	28.0	30.4	38.2	32.0	37.6	31.5	33.4	29.9	19.6	13.5
1987	28.2	26.1	34.8	31.8	36.6	29.6	33.5	28.6	17.2	13.7
1988	25.5	26.3	36.2	31.3	36.5	27.8	31.3	27.7	18.0	12.8
1990	26.6	22.5	31.6	28.2	34.5	24.8	29.3	24.8	14.6	11.5
1991	23.5	22.4	32.8	28.4	33.1	27.6	29.3	24.6	15.1	12.0
1992	28.0	24.9	32.8	30.1	32.9	27.3	28.6	26.1	16.1	2.4

Chapter 4

Gender and Health: Perceptions of Bias in Medical Research

These are troubled times for feminists who think their cause requires dramatic claims of women's oppression. In the August issue of *The Atlantic*, Dr. Andrew Kadar of the UCLA School of Medicine challenges another such claim: that women have been shortchanged by the health care system.

"*Medical research has mainly been done on men, largely to the benefit of men only*," cries a National Women's Health Network mailing. "[T]he often-cited study touting the benefits of aspirin in preventing heart attacks involved 22,071 men *and not one woman*."

Except that, Dr. Kadar points out, there was a similar study around the same time with 87,678 nurses, all women.

In response, NWHN board member Dr. Adriane Fugh-Berman pooh-poohed the nurses' study as less rigorous. Nonetheless, it is a respected study which followed its subjects a year longer than the one involving men. "To say that the benefits of aspirin in preventing heart attacks have been studied only in men," concludes Dr. David Gremillion of the Wake Medical Center in Raleigh, North Carolina, "would be completely false."

In 1990, Sen. Barbara Mikulski (D-Md.) cited the fact that the National Institutes for Health "spent less than 14 percent of their research budget on women's health projects" as "blatant discrimination." Yet the NIH spent *6.5 percent* of its budget on men's health projects; the rest went to research into diseases afflicting both sexes.

But wasn't that research done mainly on men? While fertile women have been excluded from some clinical trials because of concerns about reproductive damage and birth defects, a 1993 article by Drs. Judith LaRosa and Vivian Pinn of the Office of Research on Women's Health of the NIH concedes that the overall extent of this exclusion is unknown. Generally, Dr. Kadar says, health problems tend to be studied in the groups they affect most. Studies of eating disorders, osteoporosis, and nausea at the time of surgery have used primarily female subjects.

Aren't drugs tested only in men approved for general use? Not quite. Women have been excluded only from the early phases of testing dealing with basic safety; FDA surveys in 1983 and 1988 found that before drugs were released on the market, both sexes had been proportionately represented in the trials.

Some of the most passionate charges of sexism have had to do with breast cancer, which kills approximately 46,000 women a year. Yet prostate cancer kills about 35,000 men a year (though at a later age). Last year the National Cancer Institute spent $51.1 million on prostate cancer research and $213.7 million on breast cancer—about three times as much per death. This year, breast cancer research funding is scheduled to increase by 23 percent, partly due to women's activism; prostate research gets a 7.6 percent increase.

Feminist critics of the health care system have some valid points. Dr. Kadar and Dr. Gremillion agree that more women should be enrolled in medical research. Dr. Pinn of the NIH notes that even in clinical trials including both sexes, the results often haven't been analyzed for gender differences. She also stresses that our goal should be better care for all, not pitting the sexes against each other.

But that's not what happens when gender warfare is injected into medical debate. I asked Dr. Fugh-Berman (who believes that neglect of women's health reflects their status as "second-class citizens") about new research contradicting earlier studies which suggested that female heart patients received inferior care. She replied that she had "just skimmed" the new studies: "I guess I feel like we don't really need that evidence to show that women are treated badly in the medical system."

Charges of victimization can be a potent political weapon. Recently, advocates for the inclusion of abortion coverage in the national health plan ran ads saying, "Once again, women are not being treated equally. This time it's health care reform." Funny they should mention that. As a new activist group called the Men's Health Network points out, the Clinton plan covers Pap smears, pelvic exams, and mammograms for women—but not testicular or prostate cancer screening for men.

Part Two

Top Ten Causes of Death in Men

Chapter 5

Diseases of the Heart

Chapter Contents

Section 5.1

Facts about Major
Cardiovascular Diseases

Extracted from
NHLBI FY 1995 Fact Book, Chapter 4, Disease Statistics and
NHLBI FY 1996 Fact Book, Chapter 4, Disease Statistics.

Cardiovascular, lung, and blood diseases constitutes a large morbidity, mortality, and economic burden on individuals, families, and the Nation. Common forms are atherosclerosis, particularly coronary heart disease (CHD) (heart attack) and cerebrovascular disease (stroke); hypertension; chronic obstructive pulmonary disease (COPD);asthma; and the blood-clotting disorders: embolisms and thromboses. Because many of the diseases begin early in life, their early detection and control can reduce the risk of disability and delay death.

Together, all cardiovascular, lung, and blood diseases accounted for 1,188,000 deaths in 1995 and 51 percent of all deaths in the United States. The projected economic costs in 1997 are expected to be $383 billion, 25 percent of the total economic costs of illness, injuries, and death. Heart disease is the leading cause of death, cerebrovascular disease is third (behind cancer), and COPD ranks fourth. Cardiovascular and lung diseases account for 3 of the 10 leading causes of deaths, 6 of the 10 leading causes of infant deaths, and 5 of the 13 leading chronic conditions causing limitation of activity, and 5 of the leading chronic conditions causing bed-disability days.

From 1985 to 1995, the age-adjusted death rate declined 23 percent for heart disease (29 percent for the major form, CHD) and 18 percent for stroke, but there was a 12 percent increase in mortality from COPD and a 23 percent increase for asthma. Although improvement in mortality from cardiovascular diseases (CVD) has been extraordinarily great during the past 30 years, morbidity from these diseases remains high.

Cardiovascular Diseases

- Cardiovascular diseases caused 962,000 deaths in 1995, 42 percent of all deaths. Most were due to atherosclerosis.

- Heart disease is the leading cause of death; the main form is CHD, which caused 482,000 deaths in 1995.

- Heart disease is second only to all cancers combined in years of potential life lost.

- Cerebrovascular disease is the third leading cause of death. It caused 158,000 deaths in 1995.

- Among minority groups, heart disease ranks first and stroke ranks fifth or higher as the leading causes of death.

- Death rates decreased significantly for heart disease and stroke from 1985 to 1995 but increased for COPD and asthma during the same period.

- Between 1984 and 1994, the percent decline in death rates for CHD was greatest among white males and least among black females. For COPD and asthma, the percent increases were greater in females than in males.

- Because of the rapid decline in mortality from CHD since its peak in 1963, there were 594,000 fewer deaths from this cause in 1995 than would have occurred if there had been no decline.

- In 1994, among 36 industrialized countries, the United States ranked sixteenth in CVD mortality in both middle-aged men and middle-aged women.

- Declines in death rates for CVD contributed to 92 percent of the decline in total mortality between 1975 and 1995.

- Despite these improvements in mortality, almost one-fourth of persons ages 40 to 49 and 77 percent of persons ages 80 and older have some form of CVD.

- An estimated 57.5 million persons in the United States have some form of CVD; most (50 million) have hypertension, but nearly 14 million have CHD.

- Rates of hospitalization for congestive heart failure increased between 1971 and 1994.

- Heart disease, hypertension, and cerebrovascular disease rank among the leading chronic conditions causing limitation of activity and bed disability days.

- Except for an increase in the percent of the population who are overweight, the prevalence of high cholesterol, hypertension, and smoking declined appreciably.

- Hypertension is a highly prevalent condition that is more common in blacks than in whites.

- The percent of hospitalized CVD patients who were discharged dead declined markedly between 1974 and 1994.

- The estimated economic cost of CVD is expected to be $259 billion in 1997:

  —$158 billion in direct health expenditures.
  —$25 billion in indirect cost of morbidity.
  —$76 billion in indirect cost of mortality

Blood Diseases and Resources.

- An estimated 268,000 deaths, 12 percent of all deaths, were attributed to diseases of the blood in 1995. This includes:

  —259,000 due to blood-clotting disorders.
  —7,000 due to diseases of the red blood cell.
  —2,000 due to bleeding disorders.

- A large proportion of the deaths from acute myocardial infarction and cerebrovascular disease involve blood-clotting problems.

- In 1997, blood-clotting disorders will cost the Nation's economy $64 billion, and other blood diseases will cost $10 billion.

- In 1989, 13 million units of blood were collected from almost 9 million donors.

- In 1989, approximately 20 million units of blood products were transfused to 4 million patients.

Table 5.1.

Total Deaths and Deaths From Cardiovascular, Lung, and Blood Diseases, U.S., 1975 and 1995

Cause of Death	1975 Number of Deaths	1975 Percent of Total	1995 Number of Deaths	1995 Percent of Total
All Causes	1,893,000	100	2,312,000	100
All Cardiovascular, Lung, and Blood Diseases	1,133,000	60	1,188,000	51
Cardiovascular Diseases (CVD)	995,000	53	962,000	42
Blood	383,000*	20	268,000‡	12
Lung	146,000†	8	228,000†	10
All Other Causes	760,000	40	1,124,000	49

* Includes 378,000 CVD deaths involving blood clotting.

† Includes 13,000 CVD deaths due to pulmonary heart disease in 1975 and 12,000 in 1995.

‡ Includes 259,000 CVD deaths involving blood-clotting disease.

Source: Vital statistics of the U.S., National Center for Health Statistics (NCHS). Figures for 1995 are estimated by the NHLBI.

Total Deaths by Major Causes, U.S., 1995

Figure 5.1.

Other
48.6%

Blood
0.4%†

Lung
9.4%*

CVD
41.6%

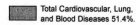
Total Cardiovascular, Lung, and Blood Diseases 51.4%.

* Excludes deaths from pulmonary heart disease.

† Excludes deaths from blood-clotting disorders and pulmonary embolism (12.3%).

Note: Numbers may not add to total due to rounding.

Cardiovascular, Lung, and Blood Disease Deaths, U.S., 1995

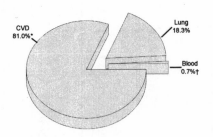

CVD
81.0%*

Lung
18.3%

Blood
0.7%†

Figure 5.2.

* CVD involving blood clotting (22.0%).

† Pulmonary heart disease included with CVD.

Table 5.2.

Estimated Number of Deaths From Specific Cardiovascular, Lung, and Blood Diseases, U.S., 1995

Cause of Death	Deaths (Thousands)		
	Cardiovascular	Lung	Blood
Acute Myocardial Infarction	219	—	149*
Other Coronary Heart Disease	263	—	—
Cerebrovascular Diseases (Stroke)	158	—	98*
Other Atherosclerosis	43	—	3*
Pulmonary Embolism	9	9*	9*
Other Cardiovascular Diseases	270	2*	—
Diseases of the Red Blood Cell	—	—	7
Bleeding Disorders	—	—	2
Chronic Obstructive Pulmonary Disease	—	99	—
Asthma	—	6	—
Other Airway Diseases	—	1	—
Pneumonia and Influenza	—	84	—
Neonatal Pulmonary Disorders	—	14	—
Interstitial and Inhalation Lung Diseases	—	8	—
Other Lung Diseases	—	5	—
Total†	**962**	**228**	**268**

* Deaths from clotting or pulmonary disorders also included as cardiovascular deaths.

† Numbers may not add to total due to rounding.

Note: Total, excluding overlap, is 1,188,000.

Source: Vital statistics of the U.S., NCHS. Figures shown are estimated by the NHLBI.

Deaths From Cardiovascular Diseases, U.S., 1995

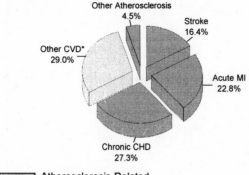

Other Atherosclerosis 4.5%

Stroke 16.4%

Other CVD* 29.0%

Acute MI 22.8%

Chronic CHD 27.3%

Atherosclerosis-Related Diseases 71%

Includes pulmonary embolism, cardiac failure, cardiac dysrhythmias, hypertensive disease, and other heart and blood vessel diseases.

Figure 5.3.

Deaths From Blood Diseases, U.S., 1995

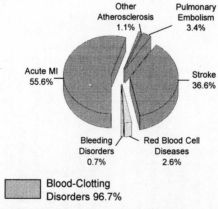

Other Atherosclerosis 1.1%

Pulmonary Embolism 3.4%

Acute MI 55.6%

Stroke 36.6%

Bleeding Disorders 0.7%

Red Blood Cell Diseases 2.6%

Blood-Clotting Disorders 96.7%

Source: Vital statistics of the U.S., NCHS. Figures shown are estimated by the NHLBI.

Figure 5.4.

Death Rates for Coronary Heart Disease, U.S., 1950-95
Actual Rate and Expected Rates if Rise Had Continued or Reached a Plateau

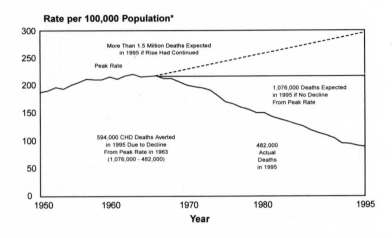

*   Age adjusted to 1940 U.S. population. (Comparability ratio applied to 1968-78 rates.)
Source: Vital statistics of the U.S., NCHS. Figures for 1995 are provisional.

Figure 5.5.

Deaths Due to Cardiovascular Diseases by Age, U.S., 1975 and 1995

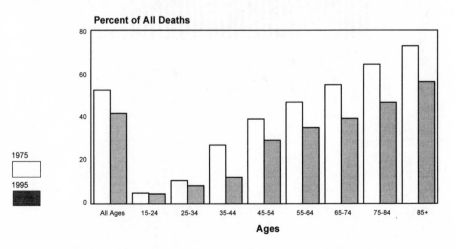

Source: Vital statistics of the U.S., NCHS. Data for 1995 are estimated by the NHLBI.

Figure 5.6.

45

Death Rates for All Causes and Cardiovascular Diseases* in Men Ages 35-74 Years, Selected Countries, 1994†

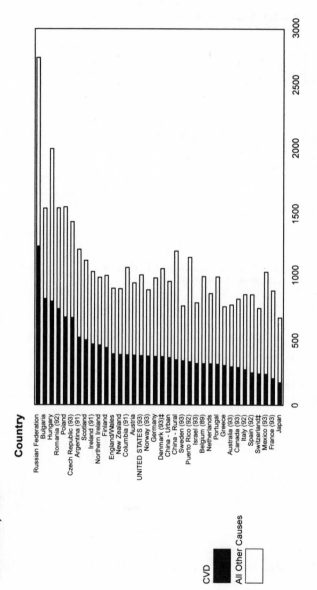

Figure 5.7. See notes with Figure 5.8 for an explanation of symbols used.

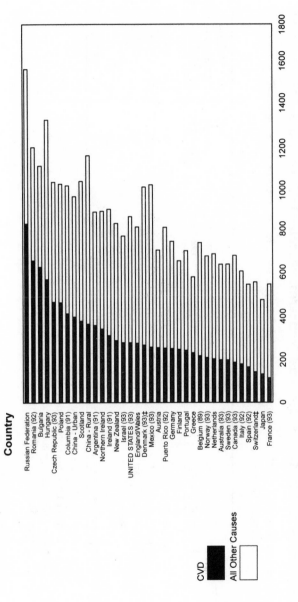

Death Rates for All Causes and Cardiovascular Diseases* in Women Ages 35-74 Years, Selected Countries, 1994†

* ICD/9 390-459 for CVD except as noted. Rates are age adjusted to the European standard population.

† Years may vary as indicated.

‡ ICD/8 390-458 for CVD.

Source: World Health Organization (WHO).

Figure 5.8.

47

Table 5.3.

Death Rates for Cardiovascular and Noncardiovascular Diseases, U.S., 1974 and 1994

Rates of Decline and Contributions to the Total Decline by Cardiovascular Diseases and Noncardiovascular Diseases

Cause of Death	Rate* 1974	Rate* 1994†	Rate Decline	Percent Decline	Percent Contribution to Total Decline
All Causes	660	508	151	23	100
Cardiovascular Diseases	313	178	136	43	90
Coronary Heart Disease	181	92	88	49	58
Stroke	59	27	33	55	22
Other	74	59	15	20	10
Noncardiovascular Diseases	346	331	16	5	10

* Age-adjusted rate per 100,000 population.
† Data for 1994 are provisional or estimated by the NHLBI.
Note: Numbers may not add to totals due to rounding.
Source: Vital statistics of the U.S., NCHS.

48

Figure 5.9.

Hospitalization Rates for Congestive Heart Failure, Ages 45-64 Years and 65+ Years, U.S., 1971-93

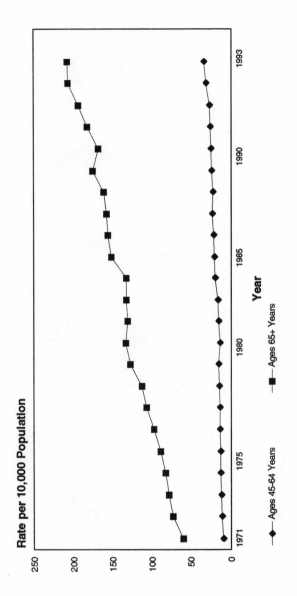

Source: National Hospital Discharge Survey, NCHS.

Figure 5.10.

Trends in Prevalence of Risk Factors, U.S., 1960-93

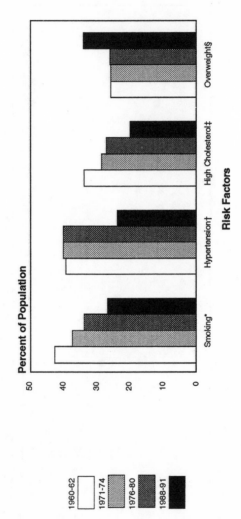

Figure 5.11.

Adult Population With Hypertension,* by Age, Gender, and Race, U.S., 1988-91

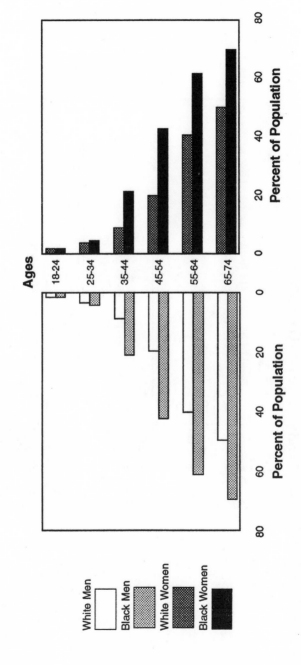

* Systolic blood pressure 140+ or diastolic 90+ or taking antihypertensive medication.
Source: NCHS, personal communication.

Figure 5.12.

Prevalence of Common Cardiovascular and Lung Diseases by Age, U.S., 1994

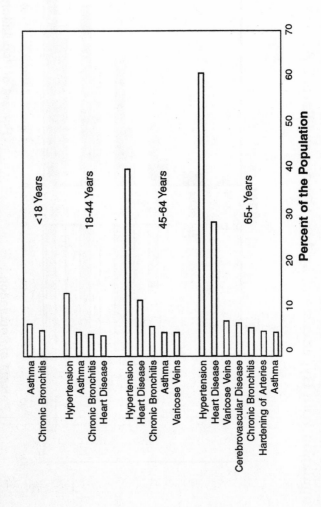

Each estimate for heart disease refers to the number of persons with one or more forms: coronary, arrhythmic, other. Numbers depicted in bars are not additive by disease because some persons have more than one disease.

Source: NHIS and, for hypertension, National Health and Nutrition Examination Survey, NCHS.

Figure 5.13.

Common Cardiovascular and Lung Diseases With High Percentage Discharged Dead From Hospitals, U.S., 1973, 1983, 1993

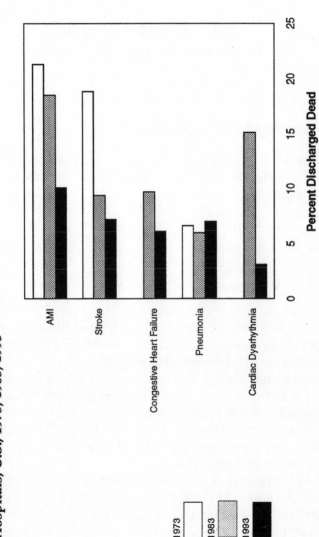

Source: National Hospital Discharge Survey, NCHS.

53

Section 5.2

High Blood Pressure: Controlling the Silent Killer

FDA Consumer, December 1991.

Who Has High Blood Pressure?

At age 18 to 74, hypertension affects more men than women and a third more blacks than whites, according to the National Center for Disease Statistics.

Men	**33%**
Women	**27%**
Blacks	**38%**
Whites	**29%**

More than 61 million people in the United States have high blood pressure, or hypertension, and nearly half don't even know they have it, according to the American Heart Association.

Because high blood pressure usually doesn't give early warning signs, it is known as the "silent killer." Nearly 33,000 Americans died of diseases related to high blood pressure in 1990 (the latest year for which figures are available), reports the National Center for Health Statistics, and that doesn't include deaths from heart attacks and strokes caused by hypertension.

High blood pressure increases the risk of stroke seven times, says Fletcher McDowell, M.D., of the National Stroke Association, but, "it is clearly the most major risk factor that can be controlled."

In fact, people diagnosed as hypertensive today have less chance of complications such as stroke than they did a decade ago, for physicians now know more about controlling high blood pressure with antihypertensive drugs and certain lifestyle changes.

Blood Pressure Basics

Arterial blood pressure is the pressure of blood within arteries as it's pumped through the body by the heart. Whether your blood pressure is high, low or normal depends mainly on several factors: the output from your heart, the resistance to blood flow by your blood vessels, the volume of your blood, and blood distribution to the various organs, says Victor Raczkowski, M.D., of the Food and Drug Administration's Center for Drug Evaluation and Research. "Your nervous system and some of your hormones can affect these factors," he says, "and thus play roles in regulating your blood pressure."

Everyone experiences hourly and even moment-by-moment blood pressure changes. For example, your blood pressure will temporarily rise with strong emotions such as anger and frustration, with water retention caused by too much salty food that day, and with heavy exertion, which makes your heart beat harder and faster, increasing its output by pushing more blood into your arteries. These transient elevations in blood pressure usually don't indicate disease or abnormality.

Blood pressure is spoken of as a fraction, such as 120/80 millimeters of mercury (mmHg). The numerator (120) is called the systolic pressure—the pressure of blood within arteries when the heart is pumping. The denominator (80) is called the diastolic pressure—the pressure in the arteries when the heart is resting between beats. A typical blood pressure for a young adult might be 120/80 mmHg. What is "normal," though, varies from person to person.

Defining Hypertension

While there's no clear dividing line between high blood pressure and normal blood pressure, most authorities define hypertension in adults as persistent elevation of the diastolic blood pressure above 90 mmHg. "When the diastolic pressure is less than this," Raczkowski says, "a person is considered to have borderline hypertension if the systolic pressure is between 140 and 159 mmHg and definite hypertension if the systolic pressure is 160 mmHg or greater." To be diagnosed as hypertensive, a person should have at least two to three readings performed on each of three separate visits, he says.

When persistently elevated blood pressure is due to a medical problem, such as hormonal abnormality or an inherited narrowing of the aorta (the largest artery leading from the heart), it's called "secondary hypertension." That is, the high blood pressure arises secondary to another condition. A person also may have secondary hypertension because:

- the blood vessels are chronically constricted or have lost elasticity from a buildup of fatty plaque on the inside walls of the vessel, a condition known as atherosclerosis. Narrowed or inelastic blood vessels exert a greater-than-normal resistance against the flow of blood, causing the blood pressure to rise.

- the heart pumps the blood at a greater rate. This increased rate of blood flow through the arteries will raise blood pressure.

- the kidneys function poorly, causing retention of excess sodium and fluid. The resulting increase in blood volume within the vessels causes high blood pressure. Kidneys may also elevate blood pressure by secreting substances that constrict the vessels.

The causes of most cases of hypertension are unknown, however. These cases are known as "essential hypertension." Because the cause remains a mystery, essential hypertension cannot be cured. But it can be controlled.

Who's at Risk?

Some risk factors for hypertension can't be changed—a family history of the disease, for instance. In addition, as reported in the Public Health Service's *Healthy People 2000: National Health Promotion and Disease Prevention Objectives*, hypertension affects more than half of people over age 65 and about a third more Afro-Americans than whites. Blacks at ages 24 to 44 are 18 times more prone than whites to kidney failure due to hypertension.

Men tend to develop hypertension more often than pre-menopausal women, though the risk for women increases when they take contraceptives or are pregnant. It's especially important that pregnant women have their blood pressure monitored frequently by their physicians, as untreated hypertension can suddenly progress to severe problems later in the pregnancy. People with hypertension who also have uncontrolled blood sugar from diabetes have an increased risk of a complication of high blood pressure such as heart attack or stroke.

Daily living habits can contribute to hypertension. Chronic stress, such as that produced by a job involving daily frustration, can cause blood pressure to become elevated. Overweight people have an increased risk of hypertension. Some people whose diet is high in salt may be at increased risk. Alcoholics appear to have an increased incidence of hypertension. Also, blood pressure can rise as a result of certain drugs, including cocaine, oral contraceptives, corticosteroids, sodium-containing antacids, some over-the-counter appetite suppressants and decongestants, and some nonsteroidal anti-inflammatory drugs.

Assessing Your Blood Pressure

Though giving you no sign of its presence, hypertension can be steadily damaging your heart and arteries. For this reason, it's important to have your blood pressure checked at least once a year. A doctor or nurse simply places a pressure cuff around your upper arm, pumps up the cuff, and listens with a stethoscope to measure the blood pressure.

Despite the simplicity of this procedure, some people react emotionally to it so that their blood pressure shoots up when they enter a doctor's office. This reaction is known as "white coat hypertension," says Gordon Johnson, M.D., director of health affairs at FDA's Center for Devices and Radiological Health, which regulates blood pressure monitors and other medical devices.

"When you have this problem," Johnson says, "make it a point to arrive at least 15 minutes early for your appointment. This will give you time to relax. As you sit there, breathe deeply and think soothing thoughts. Also, don't talk while the measurement is being taken. Talking seems to raise blood pressure."

You can team up with your physician in monitoring your blood pressure by using a home monitoring device. (See below.) "Daily readings help the doctor make a more accurate assessment of your blood pressure," Johnson says.

Living a Healthy Lifestyle

Adult patients with mild hypertension, such as 140/90, rarely need drugs and are often able to bring their blood pressure reading down with changes in diet and activity. Controlling even mild hypertension is vitally important, though, to stem its progression. At the University of Minnesota, patients are advised to lower their daily sodium intake to no more than the equivalent of one teaspoon (about 2,000 milligrams) of salt a day, lower and control their weight by obtaining no more than 30 percent of their calories from fat, and engage daily in a moderate form of exercise such as walking.

Some 80 million Americans have increased sensitivity to dietary sodium, according to Healthy People 2000. Whereas "salt-sensitive" people who eat a high-sodium diet develop hypertension, those who don't have this sensitivity can eat a great deal of sodium without a rise in blood pressure. Blacks in particular are prone to salt-sensitive hypertension.

There's no harm in moderate restriction (avoiding salty foods and not adding salt when preparing food), even for hypertensive patients who are not sensitive to salt, says Walter Glinsmann, M.D., associate director for clinical nutrition at FDA's Center for Food Safety and Applied Nutrition. "However," he says, "people with hypertension should not severely restrict their salt intake, as with a special diet, unless this is done under a physician's, care." Glinsmann says that when some people follow such a diet their kidneys don't adequately retain sodium, whose main role in the body is to maintain fluid balance.

Hypertensive patients often indirectly benefit from reducing dietary fat, "particularly when they're overweight or at increased risk for coronary heart disease and stroke because of an elevated blood cholesterol level," Glinsmann says. Cholesterol contributes to atherosclerosis, which in some people is aggravated by hypertension, he says.

The National Cholesterol Education Program of the National Heart, Lung and Blood Institute recommends a diet with no more than 30 percent fat, made up of equal amounts of saturated, polyunsaturated and monounsaturated fats. "Diets that contain polyunsaturated and monounsaturated fats may actually lower blood cholesterol levels when compared with diets with saturated fats," Glinsmann says. Polyunsaturated fats are found in sunflower, corn, soybean, cottonseed, and safflower oils; monounsaturated fats are in olive, canola, and peanut oils. Eating less red meat and more fish can help, too.

Stopping smoking is important. The nicotine in tobacco triggers the body to release adrenalin, which causes the blood vessels to constrict, which in turn raises blood pressure.

Learning to relax is good for your blood pressure. When you relax, your heart rate slows and tissues throughout your body demand less oxygen. As a result, your blood pressure decreases. Simple stretching and deep breathing exercises just a few minutes once or twice a day may provide this benefit.

Regular physical activity (at least three days a week for 20 minutes or more) cannot only help prevent or manage hypertension, it also may give your mental health a boost by countering stress and improving your mood and self-esteem.

Finally, it's wise to limit alcohol consumption and all drugs that can increase blood pressure. Some physicians believe that a daily drink, such as a 4-ounce glass of wine with dinner, benefits your heart. But not all experts agree. If you drink, it's a good idea to discuss this with your doctor, especially if you have high blood pressure.

Drug Therapy

While it's best to control hypertension without drugs, this is not always possible.

Anti-hypertensive drugs can reduce the risk of stroke, heart failure, and death. As reported in *The Lancet* in 1990, data on nearly 37,000 patients in 14 studies demonstrated that reducing blood pressure by just 5 or 6 points (for example, from 140/110 to 140/105) reduced the risk of stroke 42 percent and coronary disease 14 percent.

Some patients taking antihypertensive drugs experience side effects. These effects vary greatly among medications and from person to person. As hypertension tends to produce few, if any, symptoms, such people may feel worse during therapy and make the mistake of stopping the drugs without medical advice. If you are taking a medicine that has unwelcome side effects, tell your doctor. For there are now a large number and a wide variety of drugs available (see below), and it's likely that one or a combination of several can be found that will control your blood pressure without making you uncomfortable.

Monitoring your progress is essential to success in treating hypertension, especially when your therapy includes medication. To control your hypertension and reduce the risk of complications:

- Incorporate the lifestyle changes recommended by your doctor.

- Take your medication regularly and faithfully, as prescribed.

- Note any side effects from the drug therapy and report them to your doctor. Never stop taking the drug without first discussing it with your doctor.

- Weigh yourself weekly.

- Ask your doctor how often you should have your cholesterol checked.

- Consider measuring your blood pressure at home with one of the many self-monitoring systems.

Using Home Blood Pressure Monitoring Devices

People with hypertension may benefit from using home blood pressure monitoring devices. Measuring blood pressure at home on a regular schedule may:

- help identify people whose blood pressure is only high when taken during a medical visit

- enable patients to collaborate with their doctors in controlling their high blood pressure

- reduce the frequency with which a patient needs a doctor for blood pressure evaluation.

The mechanical gauge, or sphygmomanometer, is the type of blood pressure equipment most often used in physicians' offices. It consists of an instrument called a manometer to measure the pressure, an inflatable cuff (air bladder), and a pressure bulb with a release valve to pump up the cuff. Some gauges use mercury manometers (the height of a column of mercury indicates blood pressure), while others use aneroid manometers (the pressure is read on a gauge dial).

Mechanical gauges are much less expensive than electronic sets and give more accurate readings when they function properly. When taking your own blood pressure, however, you must pump up the cuff with one hand, read a dial, and listen with a stethoscope. In other words, these devices require dexterity, good eyesight, acute hearing, and some training.

Automated electronic gauges generally measure blood pressure by either the Korotkoff method or the oscillometric technique. Korotkoff devices use a microphone built into the cuff to detect arterial sounds related to blood pressure; they are subject to false readings caused by noises from the patient's surroundings or patient movement. Oscillometric devices measure and analyze the vibrations (oscillations) from the artery to determine blood pressure. Patient movement can cause false readings with these devices as well.

Finger cuff monitors typically are the oscillometric variety. Because they measure blood pressure at the fingers, they tend to have reduced accuracy and increased sensitivity to the effects of temperature and poor blood circulation.

For best results with automated gauges:

- Avoid eating, smoking or exercising for at least a half hour before measuring your blood pressure.

- Test daily at about the same time; plan ahead to give yourself time to get over feeling angry or anxious.

- When using a finger cuff device, be sure your body temperature is normal; a room colder than 60 degrees Fahrenheit can cause an inaccurate or unreliable reading.

- Sit quietly and eliminate extraneous noise.

- Follow the manufacturer's instructions carefully.

- Position your arm at heart level, palm up. Wrap the cuff just above the elbow—sleeve rolled above the cuff—and be sure it's not too tight. With a finger device, slip the finger fully into the cuff, keeping it level with the heart.

- Be sure the hoses from the cuff aren't tangled or pinched.

- Take care not to move the hoses during the reading.

- Wait at least five minutes with the cuff fully deflated before taking another reading.

- Bring the device along on medical visits once or more a year to check its accuracy against your doctor's measurements.

Also, the standard-size arm cuff on blood pressure monitors fits arms up to 13 inches in diameter. People with larger arms should order a larger cuff.

Drugs That Treat High Blood Pressure

Several classes of medications are used to treat hypertension. Here are some commonly prescribed brands from each class and a description of how they work:

Angiotensin-converting enzyme inhibitors appear to act in the body by inhibiting the production of angiotensin, a chemical that causes blood vessels to constrict, and by preserving the retention of chemicals that cause blood vessels to relax. They also inhibit production of substances that cause the kidneys to retain fluid:

- captopril (Capoten)
- enalapril (Vasotec)

- lisinopril (Prinivil, Zestril)
- ramipril (Altace)

Beta blockers block certain nerve signals to help slow the heartbeat and decrease the heart's workload and output:

- acebutolol (Sectral)
- atenolol (Tenormin)
- betaxolol (Kerlone)
- carteolol (Cartrol)
- labetalol (Normodyne, Trandate)
- metoprolol (Lopressor)
- nadolol (Corgard)
- penbutolol (Levatol)
- pindolol (Visken)
- propranolol (Inderal)
- timolol (Blocadren)

Calcium channel blockers act on the heart's muscles and nerve impulses to relax arteries throughout the body and decrease the heart's workload:

- diltiazem (Cardizem SR)
- nicardipine (Cardene)
- nifedipine (Adalat, Procardia XL)
- verapamil (Calan, Isoptin, Verelan)

Diuretics cause the kidneys to increase excretion of sodium and water, thus decreasing the volume the heart must pump through the vessels. There are several types of diuretics:

Thiazide Diuretics

- bendroflumethiazide (Naturetin)
- benzthiazide (Exna)
- chlorthalidone (Hygroton, Thalitone)
- chlorothiazide (Diuril)
- hydrochlorothiazide (Esidrix, HydroDIURIL, Oretic)
- hydroflumethiazide (Diucardin, Saluron)
- methyclothiazide (Aquatensen, Enduron)
- metolazone (Diulo, Mykrox, Zaroxolyn)
- quinethazone (Hydromox)
- polythiazide (Renese)

Potassium-Sparing Diuretics

- amiloride (Midamor)
- spironolactone (Aldactone)
- triamterene (Dyrenium)

Combination Diuretics

- amiloride/hydrochlorothiazide (Moduretic)
- spironolactone/hydrochlorothiazide (Aldactazide, Spirozide)
- triamterene/hydrochlorothiazide (Co-Triamterzide, Dyazide, Maxzide)

Loop Diuretics

- bumetanide (Bumex)
- ethacrynic acid (Edecrin)
- filrosemide (lasix)

Vasodilators relax the blood vessels:

- hydralazine (Apresoline)
- minoxidil (Loniten)

Centrally acting agents act on the control centers in the brain to lower blood pressure:

- methyldopa (Aldomet)
- clonidine (Catapres)
- guanfacine (Tenex)
- guanabenz (Wytensin)

Peripherally acting agents achieve their effect by acting on nerve substances throughout the body:

- guanadrel (Hylorel)
- guanethidine (Ismelin)
- mecamylamine (Inversine)
- prazosin (Minipress)
- rauwolfia alkaloids (Harmonyl, Raudixin, Rauzide, Serpasil)
- terazosin (Hytrin)

Chapter 6

Cancers

Chapter Contents

Section 6.1

Lung Cancer

NIH Pub No. 93-526.

Description and Function of the Lungs

The lungs, which are part of the respiratory system, are a pair of cone-shaped organs composed of soft, spongy, pinkish-gray tissue. They fill most of the thorax (chest) and are separated from each other by the mediastinum, a mass of tissues that includes the heart and major blood vessels, the trachea (windpipe), the esophagus, the thymus, and lymph nodes. The bronchi (air tubes), pulmonary blood vessels, and nerves enter and exit each lung through a slit called the hilus.

The right lung, which is divided into three sections, or lobes, is slightly larger than the left one, which has two lobes. Although fairly large, the lungs together weigh only about 2 pounds. They are filled with air and are enclosed and protected by a two-layer membrane called the pleura. The layer encasing the lungs is called the visceral pleura, and the layer lining the chest cavity is the parietal pleura. The space between these two membranes is called the pleural space.

The function of the lungs is to exchange gases between the body and the atmosphere. The lungs alternately take in oxygen, which is needed by the body's cells, and expel carbon dioxide, a cellular waste product. Air (which normally contains about 20 percent oxygen) enters the body through the nose and mouth and travels down the throat, or pharynx. From here, the air passes through the larynx and then into the chest through the tube-like structures of the tracheobronchial tree, which extend into the lungs.

The tracheobronchial system looks like a tree placed upside down in the chest. Its trunk, the trachea, descends from the throat into the chest and divides into the two primary bronchi. One bronchus leads to the right lung and the other to the left. In the lungs, each primary bronchus divides to form smaller bronchi, called the secondary bronchi. The secondary bronchi continue to branch, forming smaller and

66

smaller bronchi, which eventually divide into bronchioles. The bronchioles end in about 300 million tiny air sacs called alveoli.

The walls of the alveoli contain a network of tiny blood vessels called capillaries. Through the walls of these tiny blood vessels, red blood cells exchange carbon dioxide for the oxygen in the alveoli. The lungs expel the carbon dioxide, and red blood cells carry the oxygen to all the cells of the body.

As with all tissues and organs of the body, the lungs and the tracheobronchial tree are composed of individual cells. Several types of cells are found in the epithelium (lining) of the lungs and tracheobronchial tree. Some cells produce mucus, which covers the surface of the bronchial tubes and traps foreign particles that are breathed into the lungs. Other cells have tiny hairlike projections (cilia) on their surface; the cilia sweep mucus up toward the throat, helping to cleanse the lungs of impurities.

Normally, the cells lining the lungs and the tracheobronchial tree, like all cells of the body, divide and reproduce in an orderly way to repair worn-out or injured tissues and to allow for growth. If cells lose their ability to control division, excess growth takes place and tumors (masses of tissue) form. Tumors may be benign (noncancerous) or malignant (cancerous).

Because they can crowd nearby structures, benign tumors may interfere with normal functions and cause infection and bleeding, but they do not spread to other parts of the body and generally do not threaten a person's life.

Cancerous tumors, by contrast, not only crowd nearby structures but invade and destroy the normal tissues in which they arise and can extend into surrounding tissues. Cancer cells can also break away from the primary tumor and metastasize, or spread, through the blood and lymphatic system to other parts of the body, where they can form secondary (metastatic) tumors. When lung cancer spreads, it most commonly affects the lymph nodes, brain, bone, liver, or bone marrow, but it can spread to any organ of the body; in some patients, it spreads to more than one location at the same time. When examined under a microscope, the cells in secondary tumors appear similar to those of the primary cancer. As such, they retain many of the characteristics of the original lung cancer even though they are located in the brain, the liver, or elsewhere. These secondary tumors are referred to as metastatic lung cancer (rather than brain or liver cancer) to indicate that they are all part of a single disease and are not new cancers originating in these organs. (It is common for other types of cancer, such as breast or colon cancer, to metastasize to the lungs and form secondary tumors there. Cancer that spreads to the lungs from another organ is metastatic cancer and is named after the organ in which the cancer began.) Treatment for metastatic cancer depends on the site and type of the primary tumor, the location and extent of the secondary tumors, and other factors.

Types of Lung Cancer

Most lung cancers are classified as either non-small cell lung cancer (NSCLC) or small cell lung cancer (SCLC), based on the appearance of the tumor cells when viewed under a microscope. Because NSCLC and SCLC differ markedly in their pattern of spread and response to treatment, the identification of the cell type is extremely important. Sometimes, however, a single lung tumor contains a mixture of NSCLC and SCLC cells. When this is the case, the patient is usually given treatment that is appropriate for SCLC.

Non-Small Cell Lung Cancer

NSCLC is a general classification for three major types of lung cancer:

- **Squamous cell carcinoma** (also called epidermoid carcinoma),
- **Adenocarcinoma**, and
- **Large cell carcinoma**.

Viewed under a microscope, squamous cells resemble fish scales. Adenocarcinomas are composed of cube- or column-shaped cells that grow in patterns that are usually seen in glands. "Large cell carcinoma" describes lung cancers that do not readily fit into any other category; typically, the cells of these cancers are larger than those of other types of lung cancer.

Non-small cell lung cancers may be further subdivided according to the appearance of the individual tumor cells. Cells that are termed **"poorly differentiated"** bear little resemblance to normal cells; **"well-differentiated"** cells look more like normal ones. The degree of differentiation usually correlates with the rate of growth of cancer cells: Well-differentiated cancers generally grow more slowly than do poorly differentiated ones.

Squamous cell carcinoma. Squamous cell carcinoma often begins in the large bronchi. It tends to remain localized in the chest for longer periods than do other types of lung cancer. The most common form of lung cancer worldwide, squamous cell carcinoma, is diagnosed much more frequently in men than in women. It comprises about 25 to 30 percent of all lung cancer cases in the United States.

Adenocarcinoma. Adenocarcinomas often develop along the outer edges of the lungs and under the membranes lining the bronchi. Some produce mucin, the main component of mucus. **Bronchioloalveolar carcinoma** is an uncommon subtype of adenocarcinoma that arises from the bronchioles or alveoli and is sometimes found around scar tissue. It is not known whether these scars are a result or a cause of the cancerous growth.

An increase in the incidence of adenocarcinoma has been observed in some areas of the country over the past 20 years, with adenocarcinoma now accounting for 25 to 30 percent of all lung cancer cases in the United States. This change may be due in part to a rising incidence of lung cancer in women, who have a greater tendency than men to develop adenocarcinoma. In addition, improved methods of diagnosis may be revealing a greater number of adenocarcinomas than did earlier diagnostic methods.

Large cell carcinoma. A diagnosis of large cell carcinoma is made when the tumor cells cannot be classified as squamous cell carcinoma, adenocarcinoma, or SCLC. The incidence varies depending on how the other forms of NSCLC are classified, but large cell carcinoma probably comprises between 10 and 20 percent of all lung cancer cases. These tumors originate most frequently in the smaller bronchi.

Small Cell Lung Cancer

SCLC (sometimes called **oat cell carcinoma** because the cells occasionally resemble oats when viewed under a microscope) comprises approximately 20 percent of all lung cancer cases. It develops most often in the bronchial submucosa (a layer of tissue beneath the epithelium). This type of lung cancer spreads rapidly and is more likely than are other types of lung cancer to have metastasized at the time of diagnosis.

Scientists believe that SCLC arises in neuroendocrine cells in the lung. These cells can produce hormones that stimulate their own growth and the growth of neighboring cells. When neuroendocrine cells become cancerous (because of damage to their genetic material), the hormones may stimulate the growth of a tumor. In addition to

SCLC, other, less common types of lung cancer (such as slow-growing carcinoid tumors) may begin in neuroendocrine cells. Because such cancers are treated differently than SCLC, an accurate diagnosis is important.

Other Types of Lung Cancer

Although several other types of lung cancer have been identified, they are far less common than the types discussed in this Research Report. Information about uncommon lung cancers is available in the cancer textbooks listed in the reference section at the end of this chapter.

Causes

Lung cancer develops when the genetic material (DNA) of normal cells has been damaged, not once, but several times. Using methods to detect changes in DNA, scientists are beginning to identify and understand the alterations that lead to the development of lung cancer.

Scientists believe that the vast majority of all cases of lung cancer are caused by known carcinogens (agents that can cause cancer). Most lung cancers develop in the epithelium of the lungs and tracheobronchial tree, which is directly exposed to inhaled air and is a target for airborne carcinogens. Although several environmental agents are known to cause lung cancer, tobacco smoke is unquestionably the major culprit.

Tobacco Smoke

Smoking appears to cause all types of lung cancer (although it is most often associated with squamous cell carcinoma and SCLC). Between 85 and 90 percent of all cases of lung cancer are found in people who smoke. When researchers review the causes of death for smokers and for never-smokers, they find that lung cancer is mentioned at least 15 times more often for smokers. It is clear that the risk of developing lung cancer increases with the number of cigarettes smoked and the number of years of smoking. However, this risk begins to level off when a smoker quits and declines thereafter. After 15 to 20 years, the ex-smoker's risk of dying of lung cancer may approach that of an individual who has never smoked. People who smoke filtered low-tar cigarettes generally have a somewhat lower lung cancer risk than do those who smoke non-filtered high-tar cigarettes. Switching from non-filtered to filtered brands (or from high-tar to low-tar brands) reduces lung cancer risk. However, there is evidence that people may smoke more cigarettes if the nicotine content is reduced (as it is in low-tar cigarettes). Regardless of the type of cigarette smoked, it is clear that all smokers have a risk of developing lung cancer that is far greater than the risk for non-smokers.

Non-smokers' involuntary exposure to tobacco smoke also is associated with lung cancer. Non-smokers inhale environmental tobacco smoke, which consists of a combination of sidestream smoke (from the burning end of a cigarette as it smolders) and exhaled mainstream smoke (smoke that is breathed out by a smoker). Scientists believe that the risk for non-smokers of developing lung cancer increases by about 30 percent if they are married to a person who smokes and is even higher if the spouse is a heavy smoker. Significant exposure to environmental smoke during childhood and adolescence also may increase a non-smoker's risk of developing lung cancer. The Environmental Protection Agency's (EPA) 1992 report *Respiratory Health Effects of Passive Smoking: Lung Cancer and Other Disorders* discusses the health risks of exposure to environmental tobacco smoke.

Radon

Radon is a radioactive gas produced by the decay of uranium in soil and rocks. Radon and its radioactive decay products can be inhaled directly or can attach to air particles and be transported into the lungs, causing cell damage that may eventually lead to cancer. Uranium and fluorspar miners (especially those who smoke) are among those facing an increased risk of lung cancer from radon exposure.

Because uranium is found in virtually all soil and rock, the general public also may be exposed to radon. Radon is not dangerous in the low levels in which it is present in the outside air, but it can accumulate in closed structures. It moves through small spaces in soil and rock, seeping into buildings through dirt floors, cracks in concrete, and floor drains. Tight insulation and poor ventilation can increase household radon levels. Although most scientists agree that people who live in houses with a very high level of radon are at an increased risk of developing lung cancer, the lung cancer risk associated with lower levels of radon is less clear. Findings of studies conducted by NCI, EPA, the Department of Energy, and others to assess the risk have thus far been inconclusive. Additional study results, which should be available in the near future, may help clarify the health risks associated with exposure to radon in the home.

Asbestos

Asbestos is the name of a group of minerals that occur naturally as fibers. These fibers tend to break easily into particles that can float in the air and stick to clothes. When the particles are inhaled, they can lodge in the lungs, damaging cells and increasing the risk for lung cancer. The risk is highest among people who smoke.

Epidemiologic studies show that asbestos workers who have been exposed to large concentrations of asbestos have a risk of developing lung cancer that is three to four times greater than that for workers who have not been exposed to asbestos. Such exposure has been observed in industries such as shipbuilding, asbestos mining and manufacturing, insulation work, and brake repair. For asbestos workers who smoke cigarettes, the risk increases to 30 times that for non-smoking workers and 90 times that for people who neither smoke nor work with asbestos.

Other Occupational Exposures

Several other occupational carcinogens have been implicated as risk factors for lung cancer. Generally, the risk of lung cancer is much higher among workers in these occupations who also smoke cigarettes. Results of numerous studies conducted around the world indicate that the risk of lung cancer among workers exposed to bis-chloromethyl ether and chloromethyl methyl ether, chemicals used in the manufacture of a variety of other chemicals, is as much as 10 times higher than the risk in the general population. Similarly, an increased risk of developing lung cancer is seen for workers exposed to chromium compounds used in chromium plating and in the manufacture of chromate and chromate pigments. Recent evidence also suggests an association between occupational exposure to beryllium and the development of lung cancer. Beryllium is being used increasingly in aircraft, telecommunications, and other high-technology industries.

Epidemiologic studies of copper smelters in the western United States, Japan, and Sweden and of miners in China show an increased rate of lung cancer among those heavily exposed to arsenic, a byproduct of copper refining and a contaminant in many ores. A higher risk of lung cancer also has been observed among steel industry workers, who face exposure to a number of carcinogens.

Other Risk Factors

Certain genetic factors appear to increase a person's risk of developing lung cancer. Indoor air pollution also may play a role.

Genetic Factors. Lung cancer, like other cancers, arises after certain changes have occurred in a cell's chromosomes. These changes may occur in parts of chromosomes called genes, or they may affect an entire chromosome. One gene, known as p53, appears to be defective in virtually every small cell lung cancer and in half of non-small cell lung cancers. This gene normally functions as a tumor suppressor gene, one of the body's natural defenses against the cancer process. In its defective form, however, p53 allows lung cancer to develop, primarily when the lungs have been damaged by environmental factors. Mutations in other genes also have been associated with lung cancer.

Researchers at NCI recently discovered that people who have inherited a strong ability to metabolize the chemical debrisoquine (found in cigarette smoke) have a much higher risk of developing lung cancer than do people who do not metabolize it readily. The risk of lung cancer also is higher among people with chronic obstructive pulmonary disease, a condition that appears to have a familial association. Although heredity may be an important factor in the development of cancer, scientists believe that at least two independent events must occur to change a normal cell to a cancerous one. A genetic predisposition may be one such "event," but it is probably not enough to induce cancer by itself.

Indoor Air Pollution. Studies have been conducted to determine the reasons for the high rate of lung cancer in certain groups of women in China. Results suggest an association between the women's lung cancer risk and their exposure to indoor environmental pollutants formed by coal-burning stoves and by certain cooking practices, such as deep frying. However, the main cause of lung cancer in these women was found to be cigarette smoking.

Incidence and Mortality

One of the most common forms of cancer in the United States, lung cancer is the most common cause of cancer death. It accounts for about 15 percent of all cancer cases and 25 percent of all cancer deaths or about 168,000 new cases and 146,000 deaths annually. More than two-thirds of lung cancer cases and deaths occur in men; however, lung cancer has now surpassed breast cancer as the leading cause of cancer mortality in American women. The age at diagnosis for both sexes is usually over 45 years, with a peak during the seventies.

The number of new lung cancer cases and deaths in the United States has risen each year for many years. Recently, however, lung cancer incidence and mortality rates have begun to decrease slightly among white men; this decline is associated with a reduction in cigarette smoking since 1965. The prevalence of smoking among women, on the other hand, peaked at that time and has since shown only a moderate decline. Consequently, a decrease in lung cancer rates for this group is not expected until after the year 2000. Incidence and mortality rates have remained higher for black males than for white, a difference that is attributed to a higher prevalence of smoking among black males.

Lung cancer also is one of the most common types of cancer in many other countries. The incidence is highest in other parts of North America and in western Europe. Although the incidence of lung cancer is lower in certain Asian, African, and Latin American countries, the disease is still one of the three most common cancers in men in these countries. Current lung cancer rates in these areas of the world reflect the relatively limited use of tobacco over the lifetime of older men. However, cigarette smoking has become more prevalent with each succeeding generation in countries such as China, and the incidence of lung cancer is expected to rise dramatically as younger smokers age.

Scientists at NCI have analyzed and mapped lung cancer mortality rates in the United States. For white men, mortality rates in the 1950s were high in urban areas of the North and in certain coastal areas of the South, especially along the southeast Atlantic and gulf coasts. The geographic pattern appeared consistent with variations in smoking habits and with occupational exposures, including shipbuilding and ship repair, industries in which asbestos exposure is common. During the 1970s, the mortality for white men declined in the Northeast and increased in the South. This pattern of spread from the North to the South was similar for non-white men, except that clustering along seaboard areas was not observed. For women, the rate of increase rose sharply throughout the country in the 1970s. This increase corresponds with a rise in the prevalence of smoking among women during previous decades. There were high mortality rates for white women in Florida and along the mid-Atlantic and west coasts and for non-white women throughout the northern half of the United States. These patterns reflect geographic differences in smoking habits that vary by race and sex.

Prevention

Cigarette smoking is responsible for approximately 90 percent of male and 80 percent of female lung cancer deaths in the United States.

Lung cancer has now surpassed coronary heart disease as the leading cause of death attributable to smoking. One instrument in NCI's prevention efforts is the Smoking and Tobacco Control Program (STCP), which was established to reduce the incidence of and mortality from cancer caused by or related to smoking and the use of tobacco products. One of STCP's recent undertakings (in collaboration with the American Cancer Society) is the American Stop Smoking Intervention Study for cancer prevention (ASSIST), a large-scale demonstration project. In ASSIST, community-based coalitions have been established to develop and implement state-wide tobacco prevention and control activities. These activities are expected to affect more than 90 million Americans.

The NCI has intensified research in lung cancer prevention through studies of chemo-prevention and dietary intervention. Chemo-prevention is the use of natural and synthetic substances to reduce the incidence of cancer. Dietary intervention involves changes in the intake of specific nutrients, food groups, or non-nutritive factors that may inhibit the development of cancer. One goal of this research is to find ways to halt or reverse the development of cancer in people already exposed to cancer-causing agents, such as those found in cigarette smoke.

Several nutrients have been considered in dietary intervention studies for lung cancer. Results of a number of studies suggest that dietary vitamin A may reduce lung cancer risk among smokers. Preformed vitamin A, also called retinol, is found in animal foods such as milk, butter, egg yolks, and liver. In addition, substances known as carotenoids (beta carotene, for example) are converted by the body into vitamin A. Carotenoids are found in plant foods such as dark green, leafy vegetables and dark yellow fruits and vegetables. Whether the alleged protective effect of vitamin A is provided by the complete vitamin or by its precursors remains to be determined. It is not known whether this protection covers all types of lung cancer or is limited to certain subtypes.

The association between vitamin C and lung cancer risk also has been investigated, but results have been less consistent than those for vitamin A. Other nutrients that may offer some protection against lung cancer include vitamin E and selenium. The most consistent results of human studies suggest reduced risk with increased consumption of fruits and vegetables, although the precise components responsible for the apparent decrease are unknown. The association between dietary components and lung cancer risk continues to be studied.

Various chemo-prevention studies for lung cancer are under way. Several involve retinoids (natural and synthetic compounds that are chemically similar to vitamin A). In one, women who have an increased risk of developing lung cancer because of a long duration of smoking are receiving beta carotene and vitamin E. In another trial, the Carotene and Retinol Efficacy Trial (CARET), researchers are examining the usefulness of beta carotene and retinol in preventing lung cancer in two groups of people at high risk of developing the disease: heavy smokers and current or former workers who have been occupationally exposed to asbestos. In a study involving chronic smokers, 13-cis-retinoic acid (a synthetic derivative of vitamin A) is being evaluated for its effectiveness in reducing metaplasia and dysplasia, processes that may be intermediate steps in the development of lung cancer.

Other substances being studied in lung cancer chemo-prevention trials include Oltipraz, a substance that belongs to the class of compounds known as dithiolthiones (which are found in a number of cruciferous vegetables, such as broccoli, cauliflower, and other members of the cabbage family) and N-acetylcysteine, a drug used to treat chronic bronchitis. However, because conclusive data are not yet available on the effectiveness of these preventive approaches, NCI's highest lung cancer prevention priority is to reduce smoking.

Detection and Diagnosis

Early Detection

Early detection of lung cancer often is not possible. Current detection methods, using the most modern equipment, can disclose only about one-quarter of lung cancers at a localized stage, when treatment is likely to be most effective. The chest x-ray remains the most commonly used diagnostic tool for lung cancer.

Attempts to develop new methods of early lung cancer detection have thus far been frustrating. In the NCI-sponsored Early Lung Cancer Detection Study, scientists examined the usefulness of combining chest x-rays and sputum cytology (the microscopic examination of cells obtained from deep-cough sputum samples) to detect early lung cancer in people at high risk of developing the disease. Although some lung cancers were detected at an earlier stage than was previously possible, there was no reduction in lung cancer mortality for the participants in the study. Researchers concluded that screening using sputum cytology was not sufficiently sensitive to permit meaningful lung cancer detection.

A team of scientists from NCI and The Johns Hopkins Medical Institutions in Baltimore have been working on a new approach for detecting lung cancer before it can be found using x-rays or other screening tests. This technique involves the use of monoclonal antibodies. (Antibodies are proteins produced by certain cells of the immune system to help defend the body against foreign substances, or antigens. Monoclonal antibodies are pure, tailor-made antibodies that are produced in the laboratory and are capable of recognizing specific antigens.) In this technique, monoclonal antibodies that recognize certain antigens on lung cancer cells are applied to sputum specimens. Preliminary results show that antigen-producing cells can be detected 2 to 4 years before lung cancer becomes clinically evident. Although this test is more sensitive than other methods for early lung cancer detection, additional research on this technique is needed before it can be used on a large scale. A study to confirm the preliminary findings is under way.

Symptoms and Signs

Lung cancer often does not produce symptoms in its early stages. When symptoms occur, they can result from local tumor growth; invasion of and pressure on adjacent structures and nerves; regional growth, including spread to nearby lymph nodes; spread of the cancer to distant parts of the body; and paraneoplastic syndromes caused by hormones produced by lung cancer cells.

Lung cancers that originate and grow in the bronchi and spread to nearby lymph nodes can produce many symptoms, including pain, coughing, coughing up blood, shortness of breath, pneumonia, hoarseness (caused by pressure on a nerve), difficulty swallowing (because of obstruction of the esophagus), and swelling of the neck, face, and upper extremities (caused by pressure on blood vessels). Tumors that grow at the top (apex) of the lung may put pressure on the nerves that extend into the shoulder, arm, and hand, causing pain and weakness in these areas, a condition known as Pancoast's syndrome. Lung cancer cells that have broken away from the primary tumor and have spread to the brain, distant lymph nodes, the liver, or other parts of the body can cause a variety of symptoms, depending on the organ affected. Metastasis to the brain often causes headache and weakness and can affect behavior, memory, and speech. When the cancer spreads to other organs, symptoms may include pain, bone fractures, and jaundice.

Paraneoplastic syndromes occur most often in people with SCLC. These indirect effects of cancer occur "along with" (para) the tumor (neoplasm) and are caused by hormones or other substances produced by the cancer cells. Sometimes, paraneoplastic syndromes are the first sign of lung cancer. The wide range of paraneoplastic syndromes that occur in lung cancer patients includes disorders of hormone production, the nervous system, the blood, the kidneys, and the skin. For example, some lung cancer cells produce arginine vasopressin, which causes the body to lose sodium and the kidneys to retain water. The level of sodium in the body becomes very low, causing severe confusion and, in some cases, coma. Another paraneoplastic syndrome is caused by adrenocorticotropic hormone (ACTH), the hormone normally produced by the pituitary gland to act on the adrenal glands. Unrestrained ACTH production by lung cancer cells can cause an elevated blood sugar level, diabetes, decreased concentration of potassium in the blood, and an increase in body fat and hair growth. Hypercalcemia (an abnormally high concentration of calcium compounds in the blood), caused by production of a hormone-like substance called parahormone-related protein, occurs in about 5 percent of lung cancer patients, usually those with squamous cell or large cell carcinoma. Symptoms produced by hypercalcemia include loss of appetite, nausea, drowsiness, constipation, and mental confusion.

Diagnosis

If lung cancer is suspected or detected, the patient undergoes a series of tests designed to confirm the disease (diagnosis). The techniques used to diagnose lung cancer depend on the individual case. The first step for most patients is a thorough physical examination and chest x-rays. Following these procedures, it is important to obtain cells from any suspicious-looking area for microscopic examination (biopsy). These cells may be obtained by various techniques, including bronchoscopy, percutaneous needle biopsy, mediastinoscopy, and thoracotomy; in other cases, doctors will examine cells obtained from metastatic sites. For example, if the physician finds lymph nodes above the collarbone that feel abnormal, they are biopsied.

Bronchoscopy permits direct visual examination of the breathing tubes through a lighted tube (bronchoscope). This tube may be rigid or flexible, but with the advent of the flexible fiberglass bronchoscope, the use of a rigid bronchoscope is less common. The bronchoscope is inserted into the patient's nose or mouth and guided into the bronchi. Instruments can be passed through the bronchoscope to brush cells from the bronchial walls or snip tissue specimens for microscopic study. Bronchoscopy is generally done as an outpatient procedure at the hospital; the patient is given a local anesthetic and is awake during the procedure.

In percutaneous needle biopsy, a needle is inserted through the skin into the lung to withdraw tissue. One method of performing this type of biopsy is transthoracic fine-needle aspiration biopsy under fluoroscopic guidance. In this procedure, a needle is passed through the chest wall and directed to the abnormal tissue using fluoroscopy, an x-ray procedure in which an image is transmitted to a fluorescent screen rather than to a photographic plate. Fluoroscopy permits internal organs, such as the heart, to be observed while in motion. Ultrasonography (the use of sound waves to produce pictures of internal organs) also may be used to guide the needle during percutaneous biopsy.

To determine whether the cancer has spread to the lymph nodes in the mediastinum, mediastinoscopy may be employed. Because this test involves inserting an instrument called a mediastinoscope through an incision above the breastbone, it must be conducted under general anesthesia and therefore is not appropriate for all patients. Mediastinotomy is similar to mediastinoscopy, except the incision is made either to the right or to the left side of the breastbone.

Staging

Staging is the process of learning whether cancer has spread from its original location to another part of the body. It is important in determining the appropriate treatment for lung cancer. The stage is determined through physical exams, imaging procedures, laboratory tests, and pathologic studies of tissue and sputum samples.

Staging Techniques

Procedures that produce images of the organs inside the body are important in assessing the location and extent of the lung cancer. One such imaging technique is tomography, in which x-rays are focused on a specific plane (level) of the body. The x-rays record only what is in that plane, and areas above or below it are not recorded. In computed tomography (CT or CAT), a series of such x-rays is taken as an instrument called a scanner revolves around the patient. A computer receives the x-ray images and creates a cross-sectional picture of the area of the body being examined. These CT scans of the lungs, the mediastinum, the liver and upper abdomen, and the brain are usually helpful in staging lung cancer.

Radionuclide or nuclear medicine scans, such as bone scans or liver scans, can help the doctor determine whether the cancer has spread to other organs of the body. In these tests, a harmless amount of a radioactive substance is injected into the body. (Different organs take up different chemicals, so the choice of chemical depends on the organ being examined.) An instrument then scans the patient to measure radiation levels. In many instances, the radioactivity is visualized on a photographic plate or an x-ray plate. The results show the size and shape of the organ as well as any part of the organ that has an abnormal concentration of radio active material-an indication that metastatic cancer may be present. Other tests sometimes used in the staging of lung cancer include pulmonary angiography (an x-ray study in which material visible on x-rays is injected into the blood vessels leading to the lung) and bronchography (x-ray filming of the respiratory system after a substance is injected that makes the parts of the system visible on the x-ray). Ultrasonography also may be used to determine whether the lung cancer has spread to the abdomen. A sensitive technique known as magnetic resonance imaging (MRI) produces images of the internal organs of the body without exposing the patient to radiation. MRI uses a powerful electromagnet that excites the hydrogen molecules in water, the main component of all soft tissue. The hydrogen molecules, in turn, give off tiny electrical charges that are picked up by the scanner and transformed into an image of the tissue being examined. Researchers are conducting studies to evaluate this technique in staging lung cancer.

Staging Systems

Different staging systems are used for non-small cell lung cancer and small cell lung cancer. A complex "TNM" system, developed by the American Joint Committee on Cancer, is usually employed for NSCLC. In this classification, the stage depends on the characteristics of the primary tumor (T), the presence or absence of cancer cells in lymph nodes (N), and whether the cancer has metastasized to other parts of the body (M). NSCLC is classified as TX when the site of origin of the tumor cannot be determined but cancer cells are present in lung secretions, TO when there is no evidence of a primary tumor, Tis (tumor *in situ*) when the cancer is very small and confined to the bronchial mucosa, or T and a number from 1 to 4, reflecting the size, location, and invasiveness of the tumor. Lymph nodes are classified as NX when they cannot be assessed, NO when the nodes do not contain cancer, or N and a number from 1 to 3, indicating the extent and location of the nodes containing cancer. Distant metastases are classified as MX when the presence of metastases cannot be assessed, MO when there are no known metastases, or M1 when metastasis is found.

Doctors use this TNM system to divide NSCLC into stages. A simplified description of these stages follows.

Occult Stage: Cancer cells are present in lung secretions but no tumor has been found in the lung.

Stage 0: The tumor is found in a local area and in only a few layers of cells. It has not grown through the surface lining (epithelium) of the lung. Another term for this stage of lung cancer is carcinoma *in situ*.

Stage I: The tumor is confined to the lung and is surrounded by normal lung tissue.

Stage II: The tumor has spread to lymph nodes located near the hilus or bronchi.

Stage III: Cancer has spread to the chest wall, the diaphragm, or other organs or blood vessels near the lung, or the cancer has spread to the lymph nodes in the mediastinum or to those on the other side of the chest or in the neck. Stage III is further divided into **Stage IIIA** for cancer that can sometimes be treated with surgery and **Stage IIIB** for cancer that cannot.

Stage IV: The cancer has spread to other parts of the body.

The detailed TNM system is not commonly used to describe the stage of disease in patients with SCLC. Instead, physicians generally use a simple two-stage system developed by the Veterans' Administration Lung Cancer Study Group. In this system, SCLC is classified into two groups:

Limited Stage: The tumor is confined to the lung in which it originated, the mediastinum, and the lymph nodes immediately above the collarbone.

Extensive Stage: The tumor has spread beyond the sites defined for limited-stage disease.

Treatment

Standard treatments for patients with lung cancer are of limited effectiveness in all but the most localized tumors. For this reason, patients are encouraged to consider participating in clinical trials (research studies) designed to evaluate new approaches to therapy.

Types of Treatment

Many factors affect the choice of treatment for a person with lung cancer. These include the type and location of the primary tumor, the stage of the cancer, certain features of the cancer cells, the person's general health, and other considerations. In developing a treatment plan to meet individual patients' needs, doctors may recommend one or a combination of these treatment approaches:

- **Surgery**. An operation to remove the cancer;

- **Radiation therapy.** Using high-energy rays to damage or destroy cancer cells;

- **Chemotherapy.** Using drugs to kill cancer cells;

- **Biological therapy.** Using natural or synthetic substances to boost, direct, or restore the immune system, the body's normal defenses against the disease.

Surgical procedures that may be employed include **wedge or segmental resection** (removal of a portion of one lobe of the affected lung), **lobectomy** (removal of an entire lobe of the lung), or **pneumonectomy** (removal of the entire lung).

Radiation therapy is usually given by a machine (external beam radiation) that delivers x-rays or electrons to the location of the tumor. The radiation dose is based on the size and location of the tumor. Some patients first receive external beam radiation to a wide area that includes the primary tumor and surrounding tissue. After the initial treatments, progressively smaller areas are treated. In the final treatment, or **"boost,"** the treated area may be quite small. Another type of radiation therapy is known as internal radiation therapy, or brachytherapy. Instead of coming from a machine outside the body, radioactive material is placed directly into (or as close as possible to) the cancerous area. Like surgery, radiation therapy is a local treatment because it affects only the cells in the area being treated.

Chemotherapy is a systemic treatment; the anticancer drugs enter the bloodstream and travel to affect cancer cells throughout the body. Several types of drugs are used in cancer chemotherapy. Some are taken orally, but most are administered by injection. Although the drugs may act in different ways, they have the common ability to damage or destroy rapidly growing cells (such as cancer cells).

Biological therapy, also known as biotherapy or immunotherapy, is a relatively new form of cancer treatment that is being studied for its effectiveness against lung cancer. Based on the knowledge and tools of molecular biology, immunology, and genetics, biological therapy works in several ways. Acting indirectly against the cancer, it may boost the ability of a cancer patient's immune system to fight the growth of cancer cells; it also may eliminate or suppress body responses that permit cancer growth. In a direct mode of action, biological therapy may make cancer cells more vulnerable to destruction by the patient's immune system. Biological therapy also may increase the ability of the body to produce infection-fighting blood cells to recover from the damaging effects of anti-cancer drugs. Scientists have identified a number of substances called biological response modifiers (BRMs) that are used in biological therapy.

Photodynamic therapy (PDT) is a new technique that uses an interaction between light and a substance (photosensitizing agent) that makes cells more sensitive to light to destroy tumor tissue. The photosensitizing agent is injected into the body and is absorbed by all the cells. The substance rapidly leaves most cells, but it remains in or around cancer cells for a longer time. Light from a laser is then delivered through a bronchoscope and is absorbed by the photosensitizing agent in the cancer cells, causing a chemical reaction that destroys the cells. Light exposure must be carefully timed to correspond to the period when the agent has left most of the healthy cells but still remains in the cancer cells. PDT has several promising features:

- cancer cells can be selectively destroyed while most normal cells are spared;

- the damaging effect of the photosensitizing agent occurs only when it is exposed to light; and

- there appear to be relatively few side effects.

Because the laser light currently in use cannot pass through more than a centimeter of tissue (a little more than one-third of an inch), small tumors are treated most effectively. Researchers are evaluating different laser types and new photosensitizers that may increase the depth of effective treatment.

Non-Small Cell Lung Cancer Therapies

Occult Lung Cancer. Patients with occult lung cancer should have a thorough diagnostic evaluation to locate the primary tumor. Tests include chest x-rays (every month, if necessary), chest tomograms, and most importantly, bronchoscopy. CT scanning of the chest also may be performed. Cancers discovered in this fashion are usually localized and often can be cured by surgery.

Stage 0. Stage 0 non-small cell lung cancer, also called carcinoma *in situ*, is sometimes treated with surgery. Photodynamic therapy may be considered as an alternative to surgery for certain patients.

Stages I and II. Surgery is the usual primary treatment for patients with stage I or stage II NSCLC. The type of operation depends on the location and extent of the tumor. For patients who have medical problems that make surgery too risky, radiation therapy is used. Because patients with adenocarcinoma and large cell carcinoma often develop brain metastases, some physicians also recommend prophylactic (preventive) cranial irradiation (PCI). However, this treatment benefits only a small number of NSCLC patients, does not improve survival, and can produce significant side effects.

Stages III and IV. Treatment options for patients with stage IIIA NSCLC include radiation therapy, surgery, or combinations of the two. Patients with stage IIIB NSCLC do not benefit from surgery and are usually treated with radiation therapy. For patients whose lung cancer has spread to other parts of the body (stage IV), radiation therapy may be used to shrink the tumors (primary, or metastatic in locations such as the bone or brain) to relieve the symptoms they cause (palliative treatment).

Clinical Trials. Patients with NSCLC who are treated with surgery often have a recurrence of cancer even when treatment appears to have removed the primary tumor. For this reason, clinical trials are underway to evaluate the effectiveness of adjuvant therapy (the addition of anticancer drugs and/or radiation to the initial surgical treatment) to kill undetected cancer cells that may remain in the body. Clinical research also is being conducted to determine the value of preoperative chemotherapy (also called neoadjuvant therapy or induction chemotherapy) in patients whose cancer has spread to regional lymph nodes. In other clinical trials, investigators are examining the effectiveness of chemotherapy alone and in combination with radiation therapy. A number of new chemotherapeutic agents are under evaluation.

Two relatively new procedures, **endobronchial laser therapy** and **endobronchial brachytherapy**, are being evaluated by themselves and in combination with each other for the palliative treatment of lung tumors that obstruct patients' airways. In endobronchial laser therapy, laser beams, delivered through a rigid bronchoscope, are used to cut off the blood supply to the tumor. The tumor is then removed through the bronchoscope. Endobronchial brachytherapy involves direct irradiation of the tumor through a tube positioned in the lung by means of a bronchoscope. With endobronchial treatments, the external tissue damage that would occur with surgery or standard radiation therapy can be avoided. Other investigational approaches being evaluated in the treatment of NSCLC include different fractionation schedules of radiotherapy as well as the use of radiosensitizers, radio-immunotherapy, and particle beam therapy.

- Fractionation schedules are the doses and intervals at which radiation is given. In one new fractionation schedule, radiation is given in smaller doses but more frequently (such as twice a day) than is standard radiation therapy.

- Radiosensitizers are substances that make cancer cells more susceptible to radiation therapy.

- In radio-immunotherapy, radioactive substances are linked to antibodies in an attempt to selectively deliver radiation to cancer cells.

- Particle beam therapy is a type of radiation therapy. It involves the use of high-energy subatomic particles, such as protons and neutrons, to destroy tumor cells. The energy released by these particles is often more effective in killing the cells than is the energy of conventional radiation therapy. A very expensive and sophisticated machine is needed to produce and move the particles required for this treatment.

Various biological response modifiers are being evaluated in the treatment of non-small cell lung cancer, both alone and in combination with other forms of treatment. For example, colony-stimulating factors (CSFs) are BRMs that regulate the production of blood cells in the bone marrow, which are an important part of the immune system. Because many anticancer drugs damage the bone marrow and prevent normal production of these cells, large doses that might provide greater effectiveness against the cancer cannot be used. Researchers are trying to determine whether administration of CSFs will permit the use of higher, potentially more effective doses of anticancer drugs.

Other BRMs under evaluation include interferons and interleukin-2 (IL-2). These proteins are normally formed by human cells to help regulate certain cell processes, but they can be produced in large quantities in the laboratory. Also under study are monoclonal antibodies (substances that can locate and bind to cancer cells wherever they may be in the body). Monoclonal antibodies can be used alone, or they can be used to deliver radioactive material, drugs, or toxins to the tumor cells.

Small Cell Lung Cancer Therapies

Compared with other types of lung cancer, SCLC has a greater tendency to be widespread at the time of diagnosis. However, it is much more responsive to initial chemotherapy and radiation treatment. Local treatments (surgery or radiation therapy alone) are seldom effective in controlling SCLC, even in patients whose cancer does not appear to have spread outside the lung. However, the use of chemotherapy prolongs life for most patients and can produce a cure in 2 to 8 percent of patients, nearly all of whom have limited stage tumors. Nevertheless, the outlook for most patients with small cell lung cancer is unfavorable, even though improvements in diagnosis and therapy have been made over the past 10 to 15 years.

Limited Stage SCLC. Patients with limited stage SCLC are treated most effectively with a combination of two or more drugs. (A large number of potential combinations of drugs is available.) Radiation therapy plus combination chemotherapy is more effective than chemotherapy alone in controlling the primary tumor in the lung and has been shown in several studies to produce slightly longer survival. Because this combined therapy can cause significant side effects, proper treatment requires close coordination between the physician

86

administering the chemotherapy and the radiation oncologist. Many patients with SCLC, particularly those with prolonged survival, develop brain metastases. For this reason, doctors frequently recommend PCI (particularly for patients in whom the lung tumor has completely responded to treatment). This therapy does reduce the occurrence of brain metastases, but it has not been shown to improve survival. Because of growing numbers of reports of significant side effects from PCI, its benefits must be thoroughly weighed against its potential adverse effects. The value of PCI continues to be assessed in clinical studies.

Treatment options for limited stage SCLC include:

1. combination chemotherapy and chest radiation therapy;

2. combination chemotherapy alone; and

3. for certain patients, surgery to remove the tumor in the lung followed by combination chemotherapy.

Each of these therapies may be given with or without PCI. Many chemotherapy combinations have been used. The following combinations are representative of those that produce similar results:

- CAV: cyclophosphamide + doxorubicin + vincristine

- CAVP-16: cyclophosphamide + doxorubicin + etoposide

- VPP: etoposide + cisplatin, with or without such other drugs as vincristine, methotrexate, and doxorubicin

(The acronyms CAV, CAVP-16, and VPP represent the first initials of the trade names of the most commonly used drugs. Additional information about chemotherapy can be found in the chapter "Chemotherapy and You, A Guide to Self-Help During Treatment," in *The New Cancer Sourcebook* in this series.

Extensive Stage SCLC. As in limited stage SCLC, combination chemotherapy is the cornerstone of treatment for extensive disease. Unlike limited stage SCLC, however, combination chemotherapy plus chest radiation does not appear to increase survival over chemotherapy alone. However, radiation therapy can play an important role in relieving symptoms caused by the primary tumor and by metastatic tumors, particularly in the brain and bone. PCI, administered for the prevention of brain metastases, is generally reserved for patients whose lung tumor has completely responded to treatment.

Treatment options for extensive stage SCLC include:

1. Combination chemotherapy (using the same drugs that are used to treat limited stage disease), with or without PCI;

2. Combination chemotherapy and chest radiation, with or without PCI;

3. Radiation therapy to the brain, bone, and other sites of metastasis; and

4. Treatment with new drugs under evaluation in clinical trials.

Clinical Trials. In clinical trials for patients with SCLC, researchers are evaluating combinations of standard and new drugs and variations of doses for drug combinations already in use. In addition, investigators are looking at the possible benefits of combining chemotherapy with surgery to remove the tumor or radiation therapy to destroy it. New radiation therapy schedules also are being evaluated, both for the primary cancer and for metastatic tumors in the brain.

Scientists also are studying hormones, produced by SCLC cells, that act as growth factors for the cancer. (For example, certain SCLC cells produce a growth factor called gastrin-releasing peptide.) Information about growth factors may point to a new pathway for attacking cancer cells by developing agents that block the action of the growth factor.

Because basic research has yielded new knowledge about how lung cancer behaves, it is now possible to grow tumor cells outside the body (*in vitro*). Cells obtained by biopsy of a patient's tumor can be grown in test tube cultures and exposed to various anticancer drugs to see which ones kill the cancer cells. Scientists are investigating the usefulness of this technique in both SCLC and NSCLC, but as yet, no evidence exists to justify the routine use of this research tool for patients.

Some lung cancer patients do not respond well to chemotherapy because their tumor cells are resistant to the drugs that are usually effective against cancer. In an attempt to overcome this problem, researchers are trying to increase the effectiveness of chemotherapy by administering an anticancer agent together with one or more chemosensitizers. Chemosensitizers are drugs that increase the sensitivity of tumor cells to anticancer drugs.

Another new approach being examined in the treatment of SCLC and NSCLC is autologous bone marrow transplantation. The doses of chemotherapy and/or radiation used to treat cancers often must be limited because they damage the patient's bone marrow, making it unable to produce new blood cells. If the damaged marrow can be replaced by healthy marrow, higher-and potentially more effective-treatment doses can be used. In autologous bone marrow transplantation, part of the patient's marrow is removed and stored while the patient receives radiation or chemotherapy; the marrow, which may have been treated to destroy cancer cells, is then returned to the patient. Immature blood cells (stem cells) found in the patient's circulating blood may be used in addition to or instead of autologous bone marrow in a procedure known as peripheral blood stem cell transplantation. Further research is needed to evaluate transplantation approaches in the treatment of patients with lung cancer.

In other clinical trials, researchers are evaluating the usefulness of tumor markers in monitoring the effectiveness of treatment. Elevated levels of these substances are often present in the blood of lung cancer patients and may be useful for detecting a recurrence of lung cancer after treatment. Markers of particular interest include neuron-specific enolase and carcinoembryonic antigen.

For more information on clinical trials, see the chapter "What are Clinical Trials All About?" in *The New Cancer Sourcebook* in this series.

Side Effects of Treatment

Because treatment for lung cancer may involve major surgery, high doses of radiation, or potent drugs, healthy tissue as well as cancerous tissue can be affected. As a result, certain side effects are associated with each type of treatment.

Surgery

Patients whose lung cancer is surgically removed can generally expect to experience chest pain, coughing, weakness, and difficulty in breathing following surgery. Persistent weakness in the arm on the affected side may be prevented by exercising the arm after surgery. Because lung function is impaired by surgery, some patients benefit from the temporary support of an artificial respirator. Heart function also is frequently affected by lung cancer surgery; some patients develop complications ranging from an abnormal heartbeat to severely impaired cardiac function. For this reason, it is very important that a lung cancer patient's heart be tested for its ability to withstand surgery, particularly if the person has a history of heart disease.

Other complications may result from surgery, such as the accumulation of air or pus in the pleural space. These problems generally can be relieved by draining the pleural space with a tube and administering antibiotics.

Radiation

Radiation therapy commonly causes side effects that include dry, reddened skin and hair loss in the treated area, loss of appetite, and fatigue. Lung cancer patients may experience additional side effects. A non-productive cough is common and may persist throughout a patient's life. Treatment often causes dysphagia (difficulty in swallowing), a side effect that generally lasts 2 to 3 weeks after treatment ends. Esophagitis (inflammation of the esophagus) tends to occur during treatment, whereas pneumonitis (inflammation of the lungs) may occur 1 to 6 months after the treatment has been completed. Pneumonitis can sometimes lead to pulmonary fibrosis (the formation of fibrous tissue in the lungs), which in turn can cause shortness of breath. In many cases, radiation pneumonitis can be treated with corticosteroids.

Prophylactic cranial irradiation may produce additional side effects, such as involuntary trembling, loss of muscular coordination, and impairment of memory and thought processes. Vision and hearing also are affected in some cases.

Chemotherapy

Because chemotherapy targets rapidly growing cells, it can affect blood cells, cells lining the digestive tract, and cells in hair follicles. Treatment may cause several unpleasant side effects, including nausea, vomiting, and fatigue. Temporary loss of hair may also occur, and patients may be more susceptible to infection and bleeding; other side effects are specific to individual drugs. Most side effects disappear once treatment ends.

Biological Therapy

The side effects of biological therapy vary according to the biological response modifiers used. Side effects generally are temporary, ceasing when treatment ends. Common side effects include flu-like symptoms, such as fever, chills, fatigue, and weakness. Interferons also may affect liver function and may cause the body to become more susceptible to infection. Patients receiving IL-2 may have any of a number of symptoms, the most common of which is fluid retention. Colony-stimulating factors may cause bone pain and muscle aches.

Section 6.2

Colorectal Cancer

NIH Internet Publication. March 25, 1997, (http://www.hhs.gov/cvgi-bin/
waisgate?WAISdocID=7924222869+9+0+0+0&WAISaction=retrieve).

Cancers of the colon and rectum are some of the most common cancers in both men and women in the United States, with more than 131,000 new cases expected to be diagnosed in 1997. These cancers kill nearly 55,000 Americans each year, making them the second leading cause of cancer death.

Between 1973 and 1992, the annual rate of new colorectal cancer cases for all races dropped by 1 percent, and the death rate fell by 17 percent. The trend continued into the 1990s, with deaths falling 5.4 percent between 1991 and 1995.

Advances

Understanding Risk. Studies have shown that lifestyle factors may cause colon and rectum cancers. A diet high in fruits and vegetables and fiber and low in fat appears to reduce the risk of getting colorectal cancer. Exercise may also lower a person's risk for the disease.

Prevention. Increased use of flexible sigmoidoscopy and colonoscopy, procedures that use lighted tools that doctors insert into the rectum to look at the inside of the intestine, has made it simpler for doctors to remove abnormal growths before they turn into cancer.

Early Detection. Routine use of annual fecal occult blood tests has proven useful in identifying people who should have further tests to rule out colon cancer and other diseases.

New Drugs. Doctors have found new drugs that work with fluorouracil (5-FU) to treat colorectal cancer better than 5-FU alone. Until the mid-1970s, 5-FU was the mainstay of drug treatment for colorectal cancer patients.

Drugs With Surgery. After surgery, drug treatment has been found to improve the cure rate of certain patients at high risk by about one-third.

Quality of Life. New surgical techniques have reduced to a small fraction the number of colorectal cancer patients needing permanent colostomy bags.

Genetics. The discovery of four genes involved in hereditary nonpolyposis colon cancer (HNPCC) has provided crucial clues to the role of DNA repair in the development of colon and other cancers. Scientists have also identified genes involved in the more common, non-inherited form of colon cancer.

Opportunities

Diet. Scientists continue to pursue leads on how certain foods may cause colorectal cancer and how other foods may prevent it.

Early Detection. The National Cancer Institute's Prostate, Lung, Colorectal, and Ovarian Cancer Screening Trial may show whether screening tests can reduce deaths from cancers of the colon and rectum.

Genetics. Scientists are studying genes to find better ways of diagnosing and treating colon cancer. For example, a new gene test could eventually allow doctors to detect tumors by looking at stool samples rather than tissue removed through surgery.

Vaccines and Antibodies. Scientists are working on new vaccines and monoclonal antibodies that may improve the way patients' immune systems respond to cancers of the colon and rectum.

Computer Technologies. Researchers are working to develop "virtual colonoscopy," in which doctors use three-dimensional computer graphics to view the entire colon in less than two minutes without the need for inserting a sigmoidoscope or colonoscope.

Additional Reading

1. Cohen A.M., Minsky B.D., Schilsky R.L. "Colon Cancer," *Cancer: Principles and Practice of Oncology*; 4th ed., edited by Vincent T. DeVita, Jr., Samuel Hellman, and Steven A. Rosenberg. Philadelphia: J.B. Lippincott, 1993, pp. 929-977.

2. Greenwald P. "Colon Cancer Overview," *Cancer* (Supplement), 1992; 70(5), pp. 1206S-1215S.

Statistics are from the National Cancer Institute's *Surveillance, Epidemiology, and End Results (SEER)* database (January 1997) and from the American Cancer Society's *Cancer Facts and Figures: 1997*, which contains estimates based on SEER data.

Cancer Information Service

The Cancer Information Service (CIS), a national information and education network, is a free public service of the National Cancer Institute (NCI), the federal government's primary agency for cancer research. The CIS meets the information needs of patients, the public, and health professionals. Specially trained staff provide the latest scientific information in understandable language. CIS staff answer questions in English and Spanish and distribute NCI materials.

Toll-free phone number: 1-800-4-CANCER (1-800-422-6237)
TTY: 1-800-332-8615

For NCI information by fax, dial 301-402-5874 from the telephone on a fax machine and listen to recorded instructions.

For NCI information by computer:

CancerNet Mail Service (via E-mail). To obtain a contents list, send E-mail to cancernet@icicc.nci.nih.gov with the word "help" in the body of the message.
Internet. CancerNet is also accessible via the Internet through the World Wide Web (http://cancernet.nci.nih.gov) and Gopher (gopher://gopher.nih.gov) servers.

Section 6.3

Colorectal Cancer Screening: Summary

Agency for Health Care Policy and Research.
AHCPR Publication No. 97-0300.

The Agency for Health Care Policy and Research (AHCPR) is developing scientific information for other agencies and organization on which to base clinical guidelines, performance measures, and other quality improvement tools. Part of this effort includes evidence reports. This is the first summary of an evidence report to be published by AHCPR under the Agency's new Evidence-Based Practice Initiative, which was launched in the fall of 1996.

Background

Colorectal cancer is the third most commonly diagnosed cancer and the second leading cause of cancer death in the United States. In 1996, an estimated 133,500 new cases of colorectal cancer were diagnosed, and approximately 54,900 people died of the disease. In the United States, the incidence of colorectal cancer is increasing, while the mortality rate is decreasing. Incidence increases with age, beginning around 40 years of age, and it is higher in men than in women (60.4 in men versus 40.9 in women, per 100,000, per year).

Colorectal cancer survival is closely related to the clinical and pathological stage of the disease at diagnosis. Approximately 65 percent of patients present with advanced disease. Five-year survival for cancer limited to the bowel wall at the time of diagnosis approaches 90 percent. Survival at five years is 35 to 60 percent when lymph nodes are involved and less than 10 percent with metastatic disease.

Racial differences in colorectal cancer survival have been observed. The 1983 to 1989 5-year relative survival for colon cancer was 61 percent among white men, 59 percent among white women, 48 percent among black men, and 49 percent among black women. Analysis of the National Cancer Institute's Black/White Cancer

Survival Study found that black men and women with colorectal cancer had a 50 percent greater probability of dying of colon cancer than did white men and women. Colorectal cancer mortality is low in American Indians and high in Alaska Natives. Differences in stage of disease at diagnosis, aggressiveness of therapy, and sociodemographic and cultural characteristics are factors that have been postulated as contributors to the observed disparity in survival rates. However, none of these factors completely explains this observed disparity.

There are many risk factors for colorectal cancer, some of which are not amenable to change. These include older age, male sex, inflammatory bowel disease, certain hereditary conditions, and a family history of colorectal cancer or adenomatous polyps. Individuals with no predisposing factors are considered to be at average risk. About 75 percent of all colorectal cancer occurs in people with no known predisposing factors for the disease.

Preventing Colorectal Cancer Deaths

Evidence exists that reductions in colorectal cancer morbidity and mortality can be achieved through detection and treatment of early-stage colorectal cancers and the identification and removal of adenomatous polyps, the precursors of colorectal cancer. Colorectal cancer screening tests have been shown to achieve accurate detection of early stage cancer and its precursors.

Most Americans are not screened for colorectal cancer. Information from the National Health Interview Survey indicates that in 1992 only 17.3 percent of people 50 years of age or older had undergone fecal occult blood testing in the previous year, and 9.4 percent had undergone sigmoidoscopy in the previous three years. To estimate the prevalence of colorectal cancer screening practices, the Centers for Disease Control and Prevention analyzed data on use of colorectal cancer screening methods from the 1992 and 1993 Behavior Risk Factor Surveillance System. Low rates of use of colorectal cancer screening were documented nationwide, underscoring the need for efforts to increase screening.

There is a lack of consensus concerning the choice of screening and surveillance tests, the appropriate screening and surveillance intervals, and the cost-effectiveness of screening. AHCPR arranged for the development of an evidence report to summarize current scientific evidence on colorectal cancer screening and highlight areas for future research to improve screening.

Reporting the Evidence

Evidence Report No. 1: Colorectal Cancer Screening, is based on a systematic review of about 3,500 citations from the scientific literature published between 1966 and 1994.

The report provides a review of screening for colorectal cancer and adenomatous polyps in asymptomatic persons at average risk for colorectal cancer, subsequent diagnostic evaluation in those with positive screening tests, and surveillance of those with colorectal disease. Other populations addressed include persons who have:

- a family history of colorectal cancer,
- a family history of adenomatous polyps,
- inflammatory bowel disease,
- familial adenomatous polyposis or hereditary nonpolyposis colorectal cancer, or
- had adenomatous polyps removed.

There are several tests available as options for colorectal cancer screening, but the evidence supporting their use varies considerably. The screening tests reviewed for this evidence report include fecal occult blood testing (FOBT), 60 cm flexible sigmoidoscopy, FOBT combined with flexible sigmoidoscopy, double-contrast barium enema (DCBE), and colonoscopy. Evidence for each screening test is summarized for performance, effectiveness, possible screening frequency, test complications, and patient acceptance.

Methodology

Computer literature searches using *Medline* from 1966 to 1994 and *Cancerlit* from 1980 to 1994 were performed. Literature review was accomplished by:

1. establishing *a priori* criteria for relevant studies,
2. developing and completing abstract review forms for each study identified by computer searches and bibliography scans,
3. compiling and reviewing full articles,
4. developing and completing a 16-page data collection form for each article selected for inclusion in the evidence tables, and
5. compiling evidence tables summarizing these articles.

Summary Findings

The significant findings set forth in this evidence report can be summarized as follows:

- Colorectal cancer mortality can be reduced 15 to 33 percent by FOBT and diagnostic evaluation and treatment for positive tests. Annual FOBT screening leads to a greater reduction in colorectal cancer mortality than biennial screening.

- 60 cm flexible sigmoidoscopy identifies nearly all cancers and polyps greater than 1 cm in diameter and 75 to 80 percent of small polyps that are located in the portion of the bowel examined.

- Screening with flexible sigmoidoscopy can reduce colorectal cancer mortality risk. Sigmoidoscopy is associated with a 59 to 80 percent reduction in risk of death from cancer in the part of the colon examined by the rigid sigmoidoscope.

- There is indirect evidence that supports the use of DCBE in screening for colorectal cancer. DCBE can image the entire colon and detect cancers and large polyps.

- Screening colonoscopy offers the potential to both identify and remove cancers and premalignant lesions throughout the colon and rectum. No studies to date have been completed that show a mortality reduction associated with screening colonoscopy.

- There is evidence that detecting and removing polyps reduces the incidence of colorectal cancer and that detecting early cancers lowers mortality from colorectal cancer. Both DCBE and colonoscopy detect polyps and colorectal cancer, but they have not been studied as screening tests.

- Evidence suggests a low level of awareness about the risks of colorectal cancer and its symptoms among adults in the United States. However, methods to improve screening compliance have been identified. Patients who understand the nature of the disease are more likely to feel that they may be at risk, perceive fewer barriers to testing, and be more likely to participate in screening. In addition, good communication between health care providers and patients and effective use of educational materials can greatly enhance patient participation and satisfaction with screening.

Future Research Needs

Necessary evidence does not exist at this time to answer conclusively many important questions regarding colorectal cancer screening. To develop this evidence, research should be undertaken to:

- Investigate the optimal screening intervals for currently available screening test options.

- Translate findings from investigations of the molecular biology of colorectal cancer pathogenesis into clinically useful screening interventions.

- Examine the effect of colorectal cancer screening and subsequent diagnostic evaluation(s) on patient quality of life.

- Determine the effectiveness of screening flexible sigmoidoscopy, colonoscopy, and barium enema, ideally with randomized trials.

- Define more precisely the risk of colorectal cancer for people with small (less than 1 cm in diameter) adenomatous polyps as the sole finding identified on sigmoidoscopy.

- Characterize more precisely individual risk, according to such parameters as age, previous screening history, family history, and genetic background, in order to inform decisions on how best to tailor screening programs.

- Determine screening effectiveness in patients with inflammatory bowel disease.

- Determine the prevalence of genetic syndromes and the benefits of screening in patients found to have genetic syndromes.

- Define optimal methods to improve patient compliance with colorectal cancer screening.

- Identify the most effective strategies to raise public and patient awareness of the magnitude of the risk of colorectal cancer, its natural history, the importance of familial risk factors, and the available interventions for screening, diagnosis, and treatment.

For More Information

Printed copies of the *Executive Summary* (AHCPR Publication No. 97-0302), *Evidence Report No. 1: Colorectal Cancer Screening* (AHCPR Publication No. 97-0300), and the *Technical Appendix*

(AHCPR Publication No. 97-0301), which contains a complete bibliography and evidence tables, may be ordered from the AHCPR Publications Clearinghouse. Call the Clearinghouse at 800-358-9295 (410-381-3150 for callers outside the United States only; 888-586-6340 for toll-free TDD service for hearing-impaired callers only) or write to:

AHCPR Publications Clearinghouse
P.O. Box 8547
Silver Spring, MD 20907

For more information on AHCPR's Evidence-Based Practice Initiative or the development of this report, contact:

Office of the Forum, Agency for Health Care Policy and Research
6000 Executive Boulevard, Suite 310
Rockville, MD 20852

Phone (301) 594-4015; fax (301) 594-4027.

Section 6.4

Prostate Disorders

NIH, National Institute on Aging, *Age Page* 1994.

The prostate is a small organ about the size of a walnut. It lies below the bladder (where urine is stored) and surrounds the urethra (the tube that carries urine from the bladder). The prostate makes a fluid that becomes part of semen. Semen is the white fluid that contains sperm.

Prostate problems are common in men 50 and older. Most can be treated successfully without harming sexual function. A urologist (a specialist in diseases of the urinary system) is the kind of doctor most qualified to diagnose and treat many prostate problems.

Noncancerous Prostate Problems

Acute Prostatitis

Acute prostatitis is a bacterial infection of the prostate. It can occur in men at any age. Symptoms include fever, chills, and pain in the lower back and between the legs. This problem also can make it hard or painful to urinate. Doctors prescribe antibiotics for acute prostatitis and recommend that the patient drink more liquids. Treatment is usually successful.

Chronic Prostatitis

Chronic prostatitis is a prostate infection that comes back again and again. The symptoms are similar to those of acute prostatitis except that there is usually no fever. Also, the symptoms are usually milder in chronic prostatitis. However, they can last a long time.

Chronic prostatitis is hard to treat. Antibiotics often work when the infection is caused by bacteria. But sometimes no disease-causing bacteria can be found. In some cases, it helps to massage the prostate to release fluids. Warm baths also may bring relief. Chronic prostatitis clears up by itself in many cases.

Benign Prostatic Hypertrophy (BPH)

Benign prostatic hypertrophy is enlargement of the prostate. This condition is common in older men. More than half of men in their sixties have BPH. Among men in their seventies and eighties, the figure may go as high as 90 percent.

An enlarged prostate may eventually block the urethra and make it hard to urinate. Other common symptoms are dribbling after urination and the urge to urinate often, especially at night. In rare cases, the patient is unable to urinate.

A doctor usually can detect an enlarged prostate by rectal exam. The doctor also may examine the urethra, prostate, and bladder using a cystoscope, an instrument that is inserted through the penis.

BPH Treatment Choices. There are several different ways to treat BPH:

- **Watchful waiting** is often chosen by men who are not bothered by symptoms of BPH. They have no treatment but get regular checkups and wait to see whether or not the condition gets worse.

- **Alpha blockers** are drugs that help relax muscles near the prostate and may relieve symptoms. Side effects can include headaches. Also, these medicines sometimes make people feel dizzy, lightheaded, or tired. Alpha blockers are new drugs, so doctors do not know their long-term effects. Some common alpha blockers are doxazosin (Cardura), prazosin (Minipress), and terazosin (Hytrin).

- **Finasteride (Proscar)** is a drug that inhibits the action of the male hormone testosterone. It can shrink the prostate. Side effects of finasteride include declining interest in sex, problems getting an erection, and problems with ejaculation. Again, because it is new, doctors do not know its long-term effects.

- **Surgery** is the treatment most likely to relieve BPH symptoms. However, it also has the most complications. Doctors use three kinds of surgery for BPH:

1. **Transurethral resection of the prostate (TURP)** is the most common. After the patient is given anesthesia, the doctor inserts a special instrument into the urethra through the penis. With the instrument, the doctor then removes part of the prostate to lessen its obstruction.

2. **Transurethral incision of the prostate (TUIP)** may be used when the prostate is not too enlarged. In this procedure, the doctor passes an instrument through the urethra to make one or two small cuts in the prostate.

3. **Open surgery** is used when the prostate is very enlarged. In open surgery, the surgeon makes an incision in the abdomen or between the scrotum and the anus to remove prostate tissue.

Men should carefully weigh the risks and benefits of each of these options. The Agency for Health Care Policy and Research has designed a booklet to help in choosing a treatment; call 800-358-9295 and ask for their free patient guide on prostate enlargement.

Prostate Cancer

Prostate cancer is one of the most common forms of cancer among American men. About 80 percent of all cases occur in men over 65. For unknown reasons, prostate cancer is more common among African-American men than white men. In the early stages of prostate cancer, the disease stays in the prostate and is not life threatening. But without treatment, cancer can spread to other parts of the body and eventually cause death. Some 40,000 men die every year from prostate cancer that has spread.

Diagnosis

To find the cause of prostate symptoms, the doctor takes a careful medical history and performs a physical exam. The physical includes a digital rectal exam, in which the doctor feels the prostate through the rectum. Hard or lumpy areas may mean that cancer is present.

Some doctors also recommend a blood test for substance called prostate specific antigen (PSA). PSA levels may be high in men who have prostate cancer or BPH. However, the test is not always accurate. Researchers are studying changes in PSA levels over time to learn whether the test may someday be useful for early diagnosis of prostate cancer.

If a doctor suspects prostate cancer, he or she may recommend a biopsy. This is a simple surgical procedure in which a small piece of prostate tissue is removed with a needle and examined under a microscope. If the biopsy shows prostate cancer, other tests are done to determine the type of treatment needed.

Prostate Cancer Treatment

Doctors have several ways to treat prostate cancer. The choice depends on many factors, such as whether or not the cancer has spread beyond the prostate, the patient's age and general health, and how the patient feels about the treatment options and their side effects. Approaches to treatment include:

- **Watchful waiting.** Some men decide not to have treatment immediately if the cancer is growing slowly and not causing symptoms. Instead, they have regular checkups so they can be closely monitored by their doctor. Men who are older or have another serious illness may choose this option.

- **Radical prostatectomy surgery** usually removes the entire prostate and surrounding tissues. In the past, impotence was a side effect for nearly all men undergoing radical prostatectomy. But now, doctors can preserve the nerves going to the penis so that men can have erections after prostate removal.

  Incontinence, the inability to hold urine, is common for a time after radical surgery for cancer. Most men regain urinary control within several weeks. A few continue to have problems that require them to wear a device to collect urine.

- **Transurethral resection.** Another kind of surgery is a transurethral resection, which cuts cancer from the prostate but does not take out the entire prostate. This operation is sometimes done to relieve symptoms caused by the tumor before other treatment or in men who cannot have a radical prostatectomy.

- **Radiation therapy** uses high-energy rays to kill cancer cells and shrink tumors. It is often used when cancer cells are found in more than one area. Impotence may occur in men treated with radiation therapy.

- **Hormone therapy** uses various hormones to stop cancer cells from growing. It is used for prostate cancer that has spread to distant parts of the body. Growth of breast tissue is a common side effect of hormone therapy.

More detailed information on the pros and cons of these treatment options is available from the Cancer Information Service at 800-422-6237; ask for the prostate cancer "PDQ for Patients."

Protecting Yourself

The best protection against prostate problems is to have regular medical checkups that include a careful prostate exam. See a doctor promptly if symptoms occur such as:

- a frequent urge to urinate,
- difficulty in urinating, or
- dribbling of urine.

Regular checkups are important even for men who have had surgery for BPH. BPH surgery does not protect against prostate cancer because only part of the prostate is removed. In all cases, the sooner a doctor finds a problem, the better the chances that treatment will work.

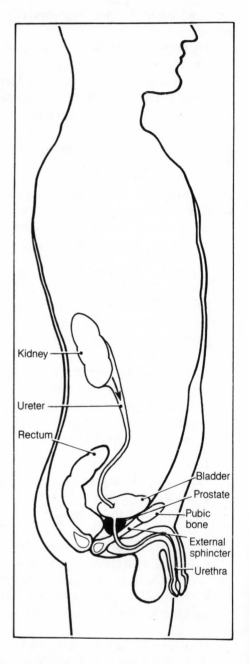

Figure 6.1. *Male Urinary System and Prostate*

104

Section 6.5

Treating Your Enlarged Prostate

Publication No. 94-0584. AHCPR Clinical Practice Guideline,
Consumer Version, Number 8.

What Is Your Prostate?

The prostate makes some of the milky fluid (semen) that carries sperm. The gland is the size of a walnut and is found just below the bladder, which stores urine. The prostate wraps around a tube (the urethra) that carries urine from the bladder out through the tip of the penis (Figure 6.1). During a man's orgasm (sexual climax), muscles squeeze the prostate's fluid into the urethra. Sperm, which are made in the testicles, also go into the urethra during orgasm. The milky fluid carries the sperm through the penis during orgasm.

Purpose of this Chapter Section

This chapter section can help you understand benign prostatic hyperplasia (BPH) and how it can be treated. BPH is an enlarged but otherwise normal prostate. It is common in older men and may cause no problems at all. If you want or need to choose a treatment, however, this chapter section describes both benefits and risks of all treatments.

Understanding the Problem

What Is BPH?

BPH (Benign Prostatic Hyperplasia) means that the prostate gland has grown larger than normal. BPH is not cancer and does not cause cancer. Benign means the cells are not cancerous. Hyperplasia means there are more cells than normal.

105

BPH results from growing older and cannot be prevented. Your chances of having prostate trouble increase as you age. BPH is common in men over age 50. More than half of all men over age 60 have BPH. By age 80, about 8 out of 10 men have it.

BPH does not always cause problems. Fewer than half of all men with BPH ever show any symptoms of the disease. And only some men with symptoms will need treatment.

What Are the Symptoms of BPH?

The most common symptom of BPH is trouble urinating. Many men with BPH have no bothersome symptoms. But BPH may cause some men to have problems urinating. Put a check next to the symptoms that you have:

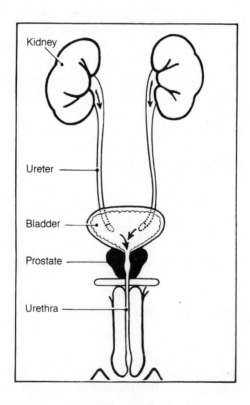

Figure 6.2. *Normal Urine Flow*

- I feel that I have not completely emptied my bladder after I stop urinating.

- I urinate often.

- I stop and start when I urinate.

- I have a strong and sudden desire to urinate that is hard to delay.

- My urine stream is weak. I need to push or strain to start the urine stream.

- I often wake up at night to urinate.

What Causes Symptoms?

As the prostate grows in BPH, it squeezes the urethra (urinary tube). This narrows the tube and can cause problems with urination. Sometimes with BPH you can also have urinary infection or bleeding.

In the early stages of BPH, the bladder muscle can still force urine through the narrowed urethra by squeezing harder. But if the blockage continues, the bladder muscle gets stronger, thicker, and more sensitive. The result is a stronger need to urinate.

In some cases, you may have trouble forcing urine through the urethra. This means the bladder cannot empty completely. Some men may find that they suddenly cannot urinate (a condition called acute urinary retention). Over time, a few men might have bladder or kidney problems or both.

Sometimes BPH causes infection of the urinary tract. This can cause burning or pain when you urinate. The urinary tract is the path that urine takes as it leaves the body. The tract includes the kidneys, ureters, bladder, and urethra (see Figure 6.1).

When Should You See a Doctor?

If you have symptoms that bother you, see a doctor. He or she can find out if BPH—or another disease—is the cause. If you do have BPH, your doctor can also see if it has caused other problems.

How Is BPH Diagnosed?

During your visit, the doctor will most likely:

- **Give you a list of questions** about your symptoms. These questions are important. Your answers will help the doctor decide if your symptoms are mild, moderate, or severe.

- **Take your medical history.** Your doctor will ask you about past and current medical problems.

- **Examine your prostate gland** by inserting a gloved, lubricated finger into your rectum.

- **Do a physical exam** to see if other medical problems may be causing your symptoms.

- **Check your urine for blood or signs of infection** (a urinalysis).

- **Test your blood** to see if the prostate has affected your kidneys. Your doctor may also recommend a blood test to help detect prostate cancer.

These tests are not painful or costly. They are done to help confirm that you have BPH and to find any problems it has caused. But tests used to diagnose your condition cannot predict if BPH will cause problems later if not treated now.

Your doctor may also recommend other tests. They may help find if BPH has affected your bladder or kidneys and make sure your problems are not caused by cancer. These tests may help some patients but not everyone:

- **Uroflowmetry** measures how fast your urine flows and how much you pass. This test can help find how much the urine is blocked.

- **Residual urine measurement** shows how much urine is left in your bladder after you urinate. This test can help find out how much your bladder has been affected by BPH. The test can be done several ways. You and your doctor should talk about the method used.

- **Pressure-flow studies** measure the pressure in your bladder as you urinate. Some doctors feel this test is the best way to find out how much your urine is blocked. The test can help most if results of other tests are confusing or if your doctor thinks you have bladder problems. In the test, a small tube called a catheter is inserted into the penis, through the urethra, and into the bladder. The test may cause discomfort for a short time. In a few men, it may cause a urinary tract infection.

- **Prostate-specific antigen (PSA)** is a blood test that can help find prostate cancer. BPH does not cause cancer. But some men do have BPH and cancer at the same time.

  The PSA test is not always accurate. PSA test results can suggest cancer in BPH patients who do not have prostate cancer. The results can also sometimes suggest no cancer in men who do have cancer.

  Not all doctors agree that being tested for PSA levels lowers a patient's chance of dying from prostate cancer. Each man with BPH is different. You and your doctor may want to discuss this test.

  Your doctor may also suggest other tests such as x-rays, cystoscopy, and ultrasound. Many men do not need these tests. They are costly and not very helpful for most men with BPH. Also, cystoscopy and x-rays can cause discomfort or problems for some men. But the tests can help patients with some BPH problems or men with other problems such as blood in the urine.

- **Cystoscopy** lets the doctor look directly at the prostate and bladder. This test helps the doctor find the best method in men who choose invasive treatments (such as surgery). In cystoscopy, a small tube is inserted into the penis, through the urethra, and into the bladder. Some men may have discomfort during and after the test. A few may get urinary infections or blood in the urine; a few may not be able to urinate for a short time after the test.

- An x-ray called a **urogram** lets the doctor see blockage in the urinary tract. A dye injected into a vein makes the urine show up on the x-ray. Some men are allergic to the dye.

- **Ultrasound** lets the doctor see the prostate, kidneys, and bladder without a catheter or x-rays. A probe put on the skin sends sound waves (ultrasound) into the body. The echoes result in pictures of the prostate, kidneys, or bladder on a television screen. This test is not harmful or painful. A special probe put in the rectum can give a better view of the prostate when the doctor wants to check for prostate cancer.

When Should BPH Be Treated?

BPH needs to be treated only if:

- The symptoms are severe enough to bother you.

- Your urinary tract is seriously affected.

- An enlarged prostate alone is not reason enough to get treatment. Your prostate may not get bigger than it is now, and your symptoms may not get worse.

Ask yourself how much your symptoms really bother you:

- Do they keep you from doing the things you enjoy, such as fishing or going to sports events?

- Would you be a lot happier or do more if the symptoms went away?

- Do you want treatment now?

- Are you willing to accept some risks to try to get rid of your symptoms?

- Do you understand the risks?

Your answers to these questions can help you choose a treatment that is right for you.

What Are Your Treatment Choices?

Currently, the five ways of treating BPH are:

- Watchful waiting.
- Alpha blocker drug treatment.
- Finasteride drug treatment.
- Balloon dilation.
- Surgery.

Surgery will do the best job of relieving your urinary symptoms, but it also has more risk than the other treatments. Unless you have a serious complication of BPH that makes surgery the only good choice, you can choose from a range of treatments. Which one you choose if any depends on how much your symptoms bother you. Your choice also depends on how much risk you are willing to take to improve your symptoms. You and your doctor will decide together.

Watchful waiting. If you have BPH but are not bothered by your symptoms, you and your doctor may decide on a program of watchful waiting. Watchful waiting is not an active treatment like taking medicine or having surgery. It means getting regular exams—about once a year—to see if your BPH is getting worse or causing problems. At these exams, your doctor will ask about any problems you have. He or she may also order some simple tests to see if your BPH is causing kidney or bladder problems.

A small number of men in watchful waiting become unable to urinate at all. Some also get infections or bleed, or their bladder or kidneys are damaged. But such major problems are uncommon.

Your doctor may suggest some tips to help control your symptoms. One is to drink fewer liquids before going to bed. Another is not to take over-the-counter cold and sinus medicines with decongestants, which can make a prostate condition worse.

Without treatment, BPH symptoms may get better, stay the same, or get worse. If your symptoms become a problem, talk to your doctor about treatment choices.

Alpha blocker drug treatment. Alpha blocker drugs are taken by mouth, usually once or twice a day. The drugs help relax muscles in the prostate, and some men will notice that their urinary symptoms get better.

During the first three or four weeks, the doctor may see you regularly to make sure everything is okay. The doctor will check your symptoms and see if the medicine's dosage (how much you take and how often) is right for you. After that, you will visit the doctor from time to time to have your symptoms checked and prescription refilled. There is no evidence that alpha blockers reduce the rate of BPH complications or the need for future surgery.

Side effects can include headaches or feeling dizzy, lightheaded, or tired. Low blood pressure is also possible. Because alpha blocker treatment for BPH is new, doctors do not know its long-term benefits and risks.

Alpha blockers include doxazosin (Cardura), prazosin (Minipress), and terazosin (Hytrin). Hytrin is the only alpha blocker now approved for BPH treatment by the Food and Drug Administration.

Finasteride drug treatment. Finasteride (Proscar) is taken by mouth once a day. It can cause the prostate to shrink, and some men will notice that their urinary symptoms get better. It may take six months or more before you notice the full benefit of finasteride. You still need to see your doctor on a regular basis while you take this drug. There is no evidence that finasteride reduces the rate of BPH complications or the need for future surgery.

Finasteride drug treatment is new, and doctors do not know its long-term benefits and risks. Also, finasteride lowers the blood level of prostate-specific antigen. Doctors do not know if this affects the ability of the PSA test to detect prostate cancer.

Side effects of finasteride include less interest in having sex, problems getting an erection, and problems with ejaculation.

Balloon dilation. Balloon dilation is done in the operating room in a hospital or doctor's office. After the patient gets anesthesia (medicine to reduce pain), the doctor inserts a catheter (plastic tube) into the penis. The catheter goes through the urethra and into the bladder. The catheter has a limp balloon at the end.

The doctor inflates the balloon to stretch the urethra where it has been squeezed by the prostate. In some patients, this can allow urine to flow more easily.

Balloon dilation can cause bleeding or infection. It can also make patients unable to urinate for a time. If there are no problems, you may go home the same day. Some patients have to stay overnight at the hospital.

Balloon dilation is a fairly new treatment for BPH, and doctors do not know all its long-term benefits and risks. In many patients, this treatment seems to work for only a short time.

Surgery. Because surgery has been used for many years to treat BPH, its benefits and risks are fairly well known. Compared with other treatments, surgery has the best chance for relief of BPH symptoms. Although surgery is also most likely to cause major problems, most men who undergo surgery have no major problems.

By itself, an enlarged prostate does not mean you need surgery. An enlarged prostate may not become larger. Also, no operation for BPH lowers the chance of getting prostate cancer in the future.

Surgery is almost always recommended for men with certain problems caused by BPH. These include:

- Not being able to urinate at all.
- Urine backup into the kidneys that damages the kidneys.
- Frequent urine infection.
- Major bleeding through the urethra caused by BPH.
- Stones in the bladder.

If you do not have any of these serious problems, but you are bothered by your BPH, you may still want to consider surgery.

There are three types of surgery for BPH:

1. Transurethral resection of the prostate (TURP).
2. Transurethral incision of the prostate (TUIP).
3. Open prostatectomy.

TURP is the most common. It is a proven way to treat BPH effectively. TURP relieves symptoms by reducing pressure on the urethra.

After the patient gets anesthesia, the doctor inserts a special instrument into the urethra through the penis. No skin needs to be cut. The doctor then removes part of the inside of the prostate.

After TURP, patients usually need to wear a catheter (a tube in the penis for draining urine) for 2-3 days and stay in the hospital for about three days. Most patients find that their symptoms improve quickly after TURP. These men do well for many years.

TUIP may be used when the prostate is not enlarged as much. In TUIP, tissue is not removed. Instead, an instrument is passed through the urethra to make one or two small cuts in the prostate. These cuts reduce the prostate's pressure on the urethra, making it easier to urinate. TUIP may have less risk than TURP in certain cases.

Open prostatectomy may be used if the prostate is very large. In this procedure, an incision is made in the lower abdomen to remove part of the inside of the prostate.

Surgery for BPH improves symptoms in most patients, but some symptoms may remain. For example, the bladder might be weak because of blockage. This means there still could be problems urinating even after prostate tissue is removed.

New Treatments

New treatments for BPH appear every year. Examples are:

- laser surgery,
- microwave thermal therapy,
- prostatic stents, and
- new drugs.

Use of a laser is still surgery, and doctors do not yet know if its benefits and risks are higher or lower than standard surgery.

There is not yet enough information about these treatments to include them in this chapter section. If your doctor suggests a treatment not discussed here, ask for the same type of information on risks and benefits given below for other treatments.

What Are the Benefits and Risks?

Each treatment may improve your symptoms. But each treatment has different chances of success. All treatments, even watchful waiting, have some risks. Ask your doctor these questions about each treatment:

- What is my chance of getting better?
- How much better will I get?
- What are the chances that the treatment will cause problems?
- How long will the treatment work?

Both benefits and risks are given below for each treatment. This can help you and your doctor make the best choice for you.

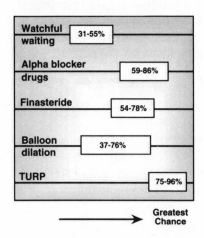

Figure 6.3. Chances symptoms will improve with treatment

Figure 6.3 shows that the chance your symptoms will improve after TURP surgery is greater than if you simply watch and wait.

But even with TURP, your chances for improvement are somewhat uncertain. This is because doctors do not know the exact chances that each patient's symptoms will improve. In general, the worse your symptoms are before treatment, the more they will improve if the treatment works. The success of TUIP and open prostatectomy is similar to TURP.

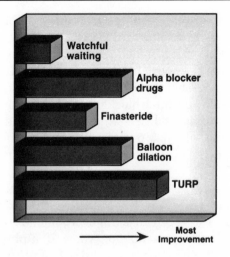

Figure 6.4. *Amount of Improvement. Note: Amount with watchful waiting is unknown but less than with other treatments.*

Figure 6.4 shows the amount of symptom improvement for each treatment. Again, TURP gives the greatest amount of improvement and watchful waiting gives the least.

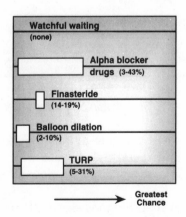

Figure 6.5.*Chance of Problems Right Away with Treatment.*

Figure 6.5 shows the chances of having problems during or soon after treatment.

Most of the time, treatments do not cause problems. Most problems are not serious, but some are. TURP can cause serious problems such as urinary infection, bleeding that requires transfusion, or blocked urine flow. Few patients have these serious problems after surgery (see Balance Sheet in Figure 6.10 for benefits and risks).

For patients taking alpha blocker drugs, the most common side effects are feeling dizzy and tired and having headaches.

With finasteride, about 5 out of 100 patients have some kind of sexual problem such as a lower sex drive or trouble getting an erection.

With watchful waiting, there is no active treatment and no added chance of problems right away. But over time, the BPH itself can cause symptoms to grow worse or cause other problems. Only TURP clearly reduces that risk. Doctors do not know if alpha blocker drugs, finasteride, or balloon dilation lower the risk of future BPH problems.

Treatment	Risk
Watchful waiting	No known added risk
Alpha blocker drugs	No known added risk
Finasteride	No known added risk
Balloon dilation	Not certain; probably less than TURP
TURP	Less than 2 out of 100 men; less than 1 out of 100 men if healthy

Figure 6.6. Chance of Dying Within 3 Months After Treatment.

Figure 6.6 shows the chance of dying from treatment. There are probably no added chances of dying from watchful waiting, alpha blocker drugs, and finasteride. There is now no information for balloon dilation.

The average age of men diagnosed with BPH is 67. The chances that a 67-year-old man might die from any cause are about 8 out of 1,000 in a three-month period. There is a greater chance (although small) of dying up to three months after TURP (about 15 out of every 1,000 patients). If you are healthy, your chance of dying after TURP is lower.

Some BPH treatments can make it hard to control urine, leading to leakage (urinary incontinence). Over time, BPH itself can cause incontinence. Also, men treated with alpha blocker drugs, finasteride, or balloon dilation may have some risk of incontinence from BPH in the future.

Treatment	Risk
Watchful waiting	None
Alpha blocker drugs	None
Finasteride	
Balloon dilation	None reported; possible
TURP	1 out of 100 men

Figure 6.7. Uncontrollable Urine Leakage after Treatment.

Although it is rare, some men have severe uncontrollable incontinence after treatment (Figure 6.7). About 7 to 14 out of 1,000 men have this problem after TURP. Men in a program of watchful waiting have no immediate risk of uncontrollable incontinence.

The chance of needing surgery in the future differs for each treatment. Some men who at first choose watchful waiting or nonsurgical treatment may later decide to have surgery to relieve bothersome symptoms. Also, some men who have surgery may need to have surgery again. One reason is that the prostate may grow back. Another is that a scar may form and block the urinary tract.

Within 8 years after TURP, 5 to 15 out of every 100 men will need another operation. Doctors are uncertain if treatment with alpha blocker drugs, finasteride, or balloon dilation lowers the chance that surgery will be needed in the future.

Treatment	Risk
Watchful waiting	Probably no added risk
Alpha blocker drugs	
Finasteride	4 out of 100 men. Impotence may end when drug is stopped.
Balloon dilation	Unknown
TURP	For most, 5-10 out of 100 men; may be higher in men with sexual problems before surgery.

Figure 6.8. *Chance of Impotence (Loss of Erection)*

Figure 6.8 shows the chance of becoming impotent (not being able to get an erection) because of BPH treatment. Each year, about 2 out of every 100 men 67 years old will become impotent without BPH treatment.

There is probably no added risk of impotence with watchful waiting and alpha blocker drugs. Finasteride has a small added risk of impotence, but the problem should stop when the drug is stopped. The risk with balloon dilation is unknown, but probably low. With TURP, the risk of impotence ranges from 3 to 35 out of 100 patients. If your erections are normal before surgery, however, the risk of impotence after surgery may be no higher than with watchful waiting.

Figure 6.9 shows about how many days you can expect to lose from work or from what you normally do over the first year. Time at the doctor's office and in the hospital is included.

One other problem—retrograde ejaculation—can result. It is common with surgery and rare with alpha blocker drug treatment. Retrograde ejaculation means that during sexual climax, semen flows back into the bladder rather than out of the penis.

Treatment	Days
Watchful waiting*	1
Alpha blocker drugs*	3.5
Finasteride*	2
Balloon dilation	4
TURP	7-21

Figure 6.9. Loss of Work and Activity Time, First Year (*Mainly from visits to doctor's office.)

Men with this problem may not be able to father children. But it does not affect the ability to get an erection or have sex, and it does not cause any other problems. You may want to talk to your doctor about retrograde ejaculation.

Between 40 and 70 out of 100 patients have this problem after surgery. About 7 out of 100 patients have the problem while taking alpha blocker drugs. Retrograde ejaculation does not occur with watchful waiting or finasteride. Some men who take finasteride do notice that they make less semen.

The Balance Sheet shown in Figure 6.10 lists the benefits and risks for each treatment. You can use this table to compare treatments. For example, treatment with either alpha blocker drugs or TURP can result in problems, but some are minor and others are serious.

What Is the Next Step?

Before choosing a treatment, ask yourself these two important questions:

- If my BPH is not likely to cause me serious harm, do I want any treatment other than watchful waiting?

- If I do want treatment, which is best for me based on the benefits and risks of each?

No matter what you decide, talk it over with your doctor. Take this chapter with you to your visits. Ask questions. Together, you and your doctor can choose the treatment best for you.

For More Information

The information in this chapter section was based on the *Benign Prostatic Hyperplasia: Diagnosis and Treatment. Clinical Practice Guideline*. The guideline was developed by an expert panel sponsored by the Agency for Health Care Policy and Research (AHCPR), an agency of the U.S. Public Health Service. Other guidelines on common health problems are available, and more are being developed to be released in the near future.

For more information on guidelines and to receive additional copies of this chapter section, call toll free (800) 358-9295 or write to:

AHCPR Publications Clearinghouse
P.O. Box 8547
Silver Spring, MD 20907

Figure 6.10. Balance Sheet: Outcomes of BPH Treatments

Direct treatment outcomes	Balloon dilation	Surgical Options			Watchful waiting	Nonsurgical Options	
		TUIP	Open surgery	TURP		Alpha blockers	Finasteride
Chance for improvement of symptoms (90% confidence interval)	37-76%	78-83%	94-99.8%	75-96%	31-55%	59-86%	54-78%
Degree of symptom improvement (percent reduction in symptom score)	51%	73%	79%	85%	Unknown	51%	31%
Morbidity/complications associated with surgical or medical treatment (90% from BPH confidence interval), progression about 20% of all complications assumed to be significant	1.78-9.86%	2.2-33.3%	6.98-42.7%	5.2-30.7%	1-5% complications from BPH progression	2.9-43.3%	13.6-18.8%
Chance of dying within 30-90 days of treatment (90% confidence interval)	0.72-9.78% (high-risk/elderly patients)	0.2-1.5%	0.99-4.56%	0.53-3.31%	0.8%	chance of death <= 90 days for 67-year-old man	
Risk of total urinary incontinence (90% confidence interval)	Unknown	0.06-1.1%	0.34-0.74%	0.68-1.4%	Incontinence associated with aging		
Need for operative treatment for surgical complications in future (90% confidence interval)	Unknown	1.34-2.65%	0.6-14.1%	0.65-10.1%		0	
Risk of impotence (90% confidence interval)	No long-term followup available	3.9-24.5%	4.7-39.2%	3.3-34.8%	About 2% of men age 67 become impotent per year. Long-term data on alpha blockers are not available.		2.5-5.3% (also decreased volume of ejaculate)
Risk of retrograde ejaculation (percent of patients)	Unknown	6-55%	36-95%	25-99%	0	4-11%	0
Loss of work time (days)	4	7-21	21-28	7-21	1	3.5	1.5
Hospital stay (days)	1	1-3	5-10	3-5	0	0	0

Section 6.6

Prostatitis

Introduction

Prostatitis is an inflammation of the prostate. It affects a great majority of men and can become a chronic problem with debilitating recurrent symptoms. As a major disease of the prostate, the prostate center contains all the latest diagnostic and treatment modalities for the care of the male patient with prostatitis. The center is equipped to provide a complete and thorough evaluation of all forms of infectious and noninfectious prostatitis, and conducts many studies involving the accurate diagnosis of the chronic prostatitis patients. With correct diagnosis, successful treatment is the goal. The prostate center facilities include a thorough microbial evaluation of the urinary tract including seminal fluid specimens, prostate ultrasound facilities, endoscopic facilities and a computerized videourodynamic laboratory.

The following information will answer general questions concerning prostatitis and about the prostate itself, where it is and what is does.

What Is the Prostate and What Does it Do?

The prostate is a gland of the male reproductive system that is located in front of the rectum and just below the bladder. The prostate is small and weighs about 15 to 25 grams. It is about the same size and shape as a walnut. The prostate is wrapped around a tube called the urethra, which carries urine from the bladder out through the tip of the penis.

The prostate is made up largely of muscular and glandular tissues. Its main function is to produce fluid for semen, which transports sperm. During the male orgasm (climax), muscular contractions squeeze the prostate's fluid into the urethra. Sperm, which are produced in the testicles, are also propelled into the urethra during orgasm. The sperm-containing semen leaves the penis during ejaculation.

Prostatitis: Definition and Classification

By definition, prostatitis is an inflammation of the prostate gland. Inflammation in tissue can be sudden and acute or long standing, recurrent, and therefore, chronic. Processes of inflammation can have many causes. They can be infectious and caused by bacteria, fungus or viruses. They can be caused by processes of trauma either mechanical or even chemical, and can involve a voiding abnormality. They can even be caused by autoimmune processes that have the body's own immune system attack the body's own cells. Because of these various potential causes, prostatitis has been classified to its various types based on these presumed causes. This classification aims to provide a systematic approach to study and treat this disease.

Types of Prostatitis

There are three types of prostatitis:

- acute infectious prostatitis
- chronic infectious prostatitis
- noninfectious prostatitis

Acute infectious prostatitis is usually caused by bacteria and is treated with antimicrobial medication or antibiotic. Acute infectious prostatitis comes on suddenly, and its symptoms such as frequency, urgency, lower abdominal pain and pressure, burning on urination, and including chills and fever can be severe and life threatening. In these situations, a visit to your doctor's office or the emergency room is essential, and hospitalization is frequently required.

Chronic infectious prostatitis is also caused by bacteria and also requires antimicrobial medication or antibiotic. Unlike an acute prostate infection, the only symptoms of chronic infectious prostatitis may be recurring infectious cystitis (bladder infection). While its chronic symptoms may not be as severe as acute infectious prostatis, it is as potentially debilitating due to it chronic recurrent nature and it can impact on one's quality of life significantly.

Noninfectious prostatitis is reserved for prostatitis that after a thorough evaluation to eliminate infectious causes are found to be not caused by bacteria. This class of prostatitis, that is, chronic non-infectious prostatitis, has been the subject of much research and had been a problem that has been most difficult to treat successfully. It is generally a chronic recurrent process that can wax and wane in severity. In addition, its cause is not well known, and this class or type of prostatitis represents a majority of chronic prostatitis patients with or without an infectious etiology. Antimicrobial medications or antibiotics are not effective for this type of prostatitis. These patients may probably have underlying or coexisting urologic problems that predispose them to prostatitis. These patients can also comprise a group whose symptoms resemble "prostatism," misdiagnosed with prostatitis and have been consequently accurately diagnosed and treated successfully. In is this type or class of "prostatitis" that a rigorous and thorough evaluation is sought for an appropriate diagnosis.

How Does Prostatitis Develop?

Acute and chronic infectious prostatitis are not usually considered sexually transmitted diseases. The way in which the prostate becomes infected is not well understood and is the subject of many research endeavors. Bacteria that cause prostatitis probably get into the prostate from the urethra by backward flow of infected urine into the prostate ducts or from rectal bacteria. Certain conditions or medical procedures increase the risk of contracting prostatitis. You are at higher risk for getting prostatitis if you recently have had a medical instrument, such as a urinary catheter or tube, inserted during a medical procedure, engage in rectal intercourse or oral sex, have an abnormal urinary tract, have had a recent bladder infection, have an enlarged prostate or have a voiding dysfunction.

What Are the Symptoms of Prostatitis?

The symptoms of prostatitis are nonspecific and mimic many other urologic and non-urologic diseases. You may experience no symptoms or symptoms so sudden and severe that they cause you to seek emergency medical care. Symptoms, when present, can include any of the following: fever, chills, urinary frequency, frequent urination at night, difficulty urinating, burning or painful urination, perineal (referring to the perineum, the area between the scrotum and the anus) and low-back pain, joint or muscle pain, tender or swollen prostate, blood in the urine, or painful ejaculation.

Are the Symptoms of Prostatitis Unique?

The symptoms of prostatitis resemble those of other infections or prostate diseases. Thus, even if the symptoms disappear, you should have your prostate checked. For example, benign prostatic hyperplasia (BPH), a noncancerous enlargement of the prostate that is common in men over age 40, may produce urinary tract symptoms similar to those experienced with prostatitis. Often, lower urinary tract symptoms (LUTS) are generally attributed to BPH, but this chronic condition can be misdiagnosed as chronic noninfectious prostatitis. Similarly, urethritis, an inflammation of the urethra (often caused by an infection), may also give rise to many of the symptoms associated with prostatitis. Another condition that mimics the symptoms of prostatitis—when prostatitis is not present (no inflammation)—is prostatodynia (painful prostate). This problem is not well understood, but may be related to a voiding dysfunction involving the spasm of muscles involved with the voiding process. Patients with prostatodynia have pain in the pelvis or in the perineum. Such pain may result from a prostate problem, but the pain can have a variety of different causes including muscle spasms from other musculoskeletal conditions. Because of the connections between the urethra, the bladder, and the prostate, conditions affecting one or the other organ have similar or overlapping symptoms. In addition, these conditions may occur concurrently in the same patient complicating diagnosis and treatment. A thorough evaluation and accurate diagnosis is important in establishing treatment in these situations.

How Is Prostatitis Diagnosed?

To help make an accurate diagnosis, several types of examinations are useful to establishing a diagnosis. Since the prostate is an internal organ, the physician cannot look at it directly. However, the prostate lies in front of the rectum and the doctor can feel it by inserting a gloved, lubricated finger into the rectum. This simple procedure, called a digital rectal examination. The physician can estimate whether the prostate is enlarged or has lumps or other areas of abnormal texture and tenderness. This examination can provide an accurate diagnosis in acute and chronic bacterial prostatitis that are responsive to antibiotics.

This examination is also essential in detecting early prostate cancer, which is often without symptoms. The American Urological Association recommends a yearly prostate examination for every man over age 40 and an immediate examination for any man who develops persistent urinary symptoms. This examination is also utilized in the assessment of men with BPH.

One test that may be performed when chronic prostatitis is suspected is prostate massage, during which prostatic fluid is collected. While performing the digital rectal examination, your doctor may vigorously massage the prostate to force prostatic fluid out of the gland and into the urethra. One may feel some discomfort depending on the sensitivity of your prostate.

The prostatic fluid is then analyzed under a microscope for signs of inflammation and infection. The three-glass urine collection method is used to measure the presence of white blood cells and bacteria in the urine and prostatic fluid. You will be asked to collect two urine samples separately: the first ounce of the urine you void (urine from your urethra) and then another sample of flowing, midstream urine (urine from your bladder). You will then almost empty your bladder by urinating into the toilet. At this point, your doctor will massage your prostate and collect on a slide any secretions that appear. You will then collect in a third container the first ounce of urine that remains in your bladder.

Examination of these samples will help your physician determine whether your problem is an inflammation or an infection and whether the problem is in your urethra, bladder, or prostate. If an infection is present, your doctor will also be able to identify the type of bacteria involved so that the most effective antimicrobial medication can be prescribed.

In cases where there is a history of chronic prostatitis, obtaining an accurate diagnosis may involve diagnostic procedures to evaluate potential contributing factors or underlying causes. Videourodynamics, a special examination that analyzes bladder function and the physiology of the voiding process, for example, has been instrumental in our institution in rediagnosing patients with chronic prostatitis with anatomical blockage of their urinary tract at the bladder neck. It has also been instrumental in revealing a group of young men with "prostatitis" who have an underlying voiding dysfunction. One a diagnosis is made that reveals an underlying abnormality, correct treatment can be initiated. In fact, treatment may range from medication to surgery and may even involve behavioral therapies such as biofeedback to correct certain voiding dysfunctions that can predispose to "prostatitis" symptoms.

How Do I Know Which Type of Prostatitis I Have?

Acute infectious prostatitis is the easiest of the three conditions to diagnose because it comes on suddenly and the symptoms require quick medical attention. Not only will you have urinary problems, but you may also have a fever and pain and, frequently, blood in your urine.

Chronic infectious prostatitis is associated with repeated urinary tract infections, while noninfectious prostatitis is not. In fact, if you do not have a urinary tract infection or a history of one, you probably do not have chronic infectious prostatitis. Other symptoms, if any, may include urinary problems such as the need to urinate frequently, a sense of urgency, burning or painful urination, and possibly perineal and low-back pain.

Noninfectious prostatitis is more common than infectious prostatitis. It may cause no symptoms, or its symptoms may mimic those of chronic infectious prostatitis. If you have noninfectious prostatitis, it is unlikely that you have a urinary tract infection.

Why Is a Complete and Accurate Diagnosis So Important?

Because the treatment is different for the three types of prostatitis, the correct diagnosis is very important. Noninfectious prostatitis will not clear up with antimicrobial treatment, and infectious prostatitis will not go away without such treatment.

In addition, it is important to make sure that your symptoms are not caused by urethritis or some other condition that may lead to permanent bladder or kidney damage.

How Is Prostatitis Treated?

Your treatment depends on the type of prostatitis you have. If you have acute infectious prostatitis, you will usually need to take antimicrobial medication for 7 to 14 days. Almost all acute infections can be cured with this treatment. Analgesic drugs to relieve pain or discomfort and, at times, hospitalization may also be required.

If you have chronic infectious prostatitis, you will require antimicrobial medication for a longer period of time—usually 4 to 12 weeks. About 60 percent of all cases of chronic infectious prostatitis clear up with this treatment. For cases that don't respond to this treatment, long-term, low-dose anti-microbial therapy may be recommended to relieve the symptoms. In some cases, surgical removal of the infected portions of the prostate may be advised.

If you have noninfectious prostatitis, you do not need antimicrobial medication. Depending on your symptoms, you may receive one of a variety of treatments. These may range from medication to surgery, and may even involve behavioral therapies such as biofeedback to correct certain voiding dysfunctions associated with prostatitis.

In addition, it is common to find patients who have recurrent episodes of infectious and noninfectious prostatitis over a long period of time. These patients may actually be suffering from an underlying voiding abnormality that may be functional or structural that predisposes them to these episodes of prostatitis. Correcting these abnormalities may cure or at least decrease the episodes of these recurrent events.

You may find that tub baths or changes in your diet may help to alleviate your symptoms. While there is no scientific evidence proving that these "home remedies" are effective, they are not harmful and some people experience relief from symptoms while using them.

Will Prostatitis Affect Me or My Lifestyle?

Prostatitis is a treatable disease. Even if the problem cannot be cured, you can usually get relief from your symptoms by following the recommended treatment.

Prostatitis is not a contagious disease. You can live your life normally and continue sexual relations without passing it on.

You should keep in mind the following ideas:

- Correct diagnosis is key to management of prostatitis.
- Treatment should be followed even if you have no symptoms.

Having prostatitis does not increase your risk of getting any other prostate disease. But remember, even if your prostatitis is cured, there are other prostate conditions, such as prostate cancer, that require prostate checkups at least once a year after age 40.

Section 6.7

Prostate Cancer: New Tests Create Treatment Dilemmas

FDA Consumer, July 1997. Publication No. (FDA) 97-1220.

The names are familiar: actors Don Ameche, Bill Bixby, and Telly Savalas, entertainment mogul Steve Ross, rock musician Frank Zappa. Though show business links these men, they share another connection. Each has died of prostate cancer.

If there's a silver lining to be found amid the clouds of these tragic deaths, it is that the fame of these men has helped spotlight a disease that now ranks as the second most common cancer men get—after skin cancer. The American Cancer Society says prostate cancer will strike 334,500 U.S. men in 1997, twice the number of male lung cancer cases. Some 41,800 will die. One out of every five American men will develop prostate cancer in their lifetime.

Public notice is something new to prostate cancer. For years, men didn't worry much about the disease. They typically thought of it as a slow-moving condition that affects men well past retirement, when they are likely to die of something else before succumbing to cancer. In many cases, that's still true. Most cases are in men 65 and older. But like Bixby, who was 59 when he died, and Zappa, who was 52, younger men also can fall victim.

Experts say the recent increase in reported cases can be attributed to new tests that make detection easier. Longer male life-spans also may play a part. With today's methods, men who otherwise would be unaware of their cancer are learning sooner they have the disease. Thus, reported cases rise. Still undetermined, however, is whether improved early detection will reduce prostate cancer's mortality rate.

A walnut-sized gland tucked away under the bladder and adjacent to the rectum, the prostate provides about a third of the fluid that propels sperm through the urethra and out of the penis during sex. Many males are what one cancer survivor called "abysmally ignorant"

129

about where the prostate is and what it does. Also, health officials say, men tend to dismiss troubles related to their sex organs, so they may shy away from seeing a doctor, even after disease symptoms appear.

Though prostate cancer historically has kept a low profile, its visibility is rapidly changing. Like breast cancer a decade ago, prostate cancer suddenly is a topic on talk shows and in newspaper and magazine articles. Support groups now number over 300 nationwide. Screening booths are popping up at state fairs and shopping malls. Famous people are going public. Sen. Jesse Helms, and former Sen. Bob Dole have openly discussed their prostate cancer treatments. Others who have publicly fought the disease include retired Gen. H. Norman Schwarzkopf, Supreme Court Justice John Paul Stevens, comedian Jerry Lewis, and former financier Michael Milken.

Early Detection

All the attention, along with new scientific information, is contributing to a growing quandary for doctors and patients over how best to manage the disease. A relatively new blood test called the prostate specific antigen (PSA) test has increased early detection odds considerably. But the test alone cannot determine if a man has prostate cancer.

The PSA test measures a protein made only by the prostate. In all healthy men, a small amount of PSA protein passes into the bloodstream from the prostate. If a man's prostate becomes enlarged, it may secrete increased amounts of PSA, creating higher blood levels of the protein. This also may occur when infection damages the prostate lining and allows more than normal PSA amounts to be released. Prostate cancer itself may produce increased PSA levels. Though the PSA test may be the first step toward a cancer diagnosis, elevated PSA levels may signal conditions other than cancer. These include benign prostatic hyperplasia (BPH) and an infection called prostatitis.

"What the PSA test does is alert the physician that a man may have something wrong with his prostate,"says Max Robinowitz, M.D., medical officer in FDA's Center for Devices and Radiological Health. "The doctor then must decide if more testing is needed to identify the problem."

Since 1985, FDA has approved several PSA tests for monitoring possible recurrence of prostate cancer in men being treated for the disease. The PSA method is not intended for mass screening of men with no symptoms.

Digital Rectal Examination (DRE)

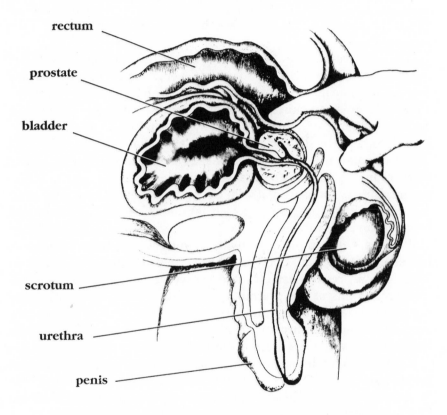

rectum

prostate

bladder

scrotum

urethra

penis

One important way doctors check for prostate abnormalities is by inserting a rubber-gloved finger into the rectum, where the prostate can be explored by touch. The exam is performed with the patient in a bent-over position.

Figure 6.11. *Digital Rectal Examination (DRE)*

First Approval

In August 1994, FDA approved the Hybritech Tandem PSA Assay, the first test the agency has sanctioned to help doctors detect prostate tumors in patients with or without symptoms who are suspected prostate cancer risks. FDA specifies that the Hybritech test be used with the traditional test for screening prostate cancer, the digital rectal exam (DRE). Physicians perform the DRE by inserting a lubricated, rubber-gloved finger into the rectum, where they can probe the prostate for lumps or enlargements that may indicate prostate or even rectal tumors.

The American Cancer Society and American Urological Association recommend annual PSA tests for men over 50 and for high-risk men over 40. Men at increased risk include African Americans, whose incidence of prostate cancer is about 30 percent higher than that of whites, and those with urinary tract symptoms or who are genetically predisposed to the disease. Study data show that if a man's brother and father had prostate cancer, he may have as much as an 11-fold increase in risk and may be stricken before age 50. The National Cancer Institute is sponsoring a trial to find out whether extensive prostate cancer screening, as well as earlier detection and treatment, can improve survival rates.

PSA tests are simple, non-invasive, and cost $30 to $70. They are, however, not perfect. Doctors interpret cancer potential based on whether PSA results are elevated, a level usually defined as above four nanograms of the protein per milliliter of blood (ng/mL). But noncancerous conditions can increase this level. Also, a certain percentage of men with prostate cancer, such as those taking drugs for BPH, will show low or "normal" PSA amounts.

"A patient may have an elevated PSA test, but this doesn't mean he has prostate cancer," says Peter Maxim, Ph.D., who heads FDA's immunology branch. He adds that it's always best to use the DRE and PSA tests together to achieve maximum benefit. Despite drawbacks with both techniques, more than 50 percent of men referred for further testing have prostate tumors, says the American Cancer Society.

Making Sure

Doctors follow up an elevated PSA or positive DRE with more definitive testing. Some physicians employ transrectal ultrasound (TRUS), which uses a rectal probe that creates a video image of the prostate using harmless sound waves collected by a computer. TRUS helps the physician "map" uneven areas of firmness in the prostate, and it can help a doctor decide if a biopsy is needed. If so, the doctor will take tiny prostate tissue samples with a small-gauge needle, injected typically through the rectum. Another physician, a pathologist, then examines the samples under a microscope.

"No surgery or other anti-cancer therapy is done without first ensuring with a biopsy that a patient has cancer and not some other condition that can cause symptoms and other suspicious signs," says FDA's Robinowitz. Once cancer is diagnosed, other tests such as computerized tomography, lymph-node biopsies, and bone scans can determine if tumors have spread beyond the prostate.

For cancer confined to the prostate, opinions are split over what to do. Orthodox wisdom holds that cancer should be treated aggressively. With prostate cancer, this means removing the gland (radical prostatectomy) or bombarding it with radiation. Experts say these options may offer good prospects for curing the disease if exercised early enough. Treatment choice usually depends on what specialist the patient consults. Urologists tend to recommend surgery while oncologists generally advise radiation therapy.

Surgery may cause unpleasant adverse effects. Because radical prostatectomy can result in severing nerves and blood vessels related to sexual or bladder function, the operation in the past has left virtually all patients impotent, incontinent, or both. That is changing, however, thanks to pioneering research done in the 1980s by Patrick Walsh, M.D., urology chairman at Johns Hopkins University Hospital. His "nerve-sparing" surgical technique, which increasing numbers of doctors are adopting, now allows many men to preserve erectile functions. Walsh says his patients under age 50 have about a 90 percent chance of regaining potency, but that number drops to 25 percent for patients in their 70s.

Radiation therapy also has adverse effects, including impotence in about 40 to 50 percent of patients.

For older men with early-stage prostate cancer, a number of physicians are dispensing a different kind of advice: Wait and see.

Doctors clearly are divided on its merits, but this "watchful waiting" philosophy got a boost by a 1994 report in the *New England Journal of Medicine*. The study analyzed case records of 828 prostate cancer patients treated conservatively (watchful waiting or hormone treatments but no surgery or radiation therapy). It found that 10 years after diagnosis, 87 percent of those with slow-growing, localized prostate tumors still were alive. Of those diagnosed with more aggressive cancer, 34 percent remained alive at the 10-year mark. Supporters say watchful waiting is a practical alternative for men in their late 60s or older, whose lifespans may be limited by advanced age and serious ailments such as heart disease. If treated, these men could suffer the trauma and adverse effects of cancer therapy with little or no benefit.

Not all prostate cancer is equal. One type of tumor may lie dormant for years while another is virulent and deadly. Deciding whether to wait or act can be difficult because physicians often can't judge conclusively which tumors might spread. Size can give some indication. Another gauge, the Gleason system, identifies a tumor's growth potential based on its appearance under the microscope. The system distinguishes progressive grades of prostate cancer on a scale of 2 to 10. Clumped-together cancer cells with well-defined edges are less likely to grow rapidly and are given a low Gleason number. Cells distributed randomly with uneven edges are more apt to spread and receive a high Gleason number.

Also important is "staging"—a predictor of how extensively the disease has grown within or beyond the prostate. This ranges from stage A, where the tumor is still microscopic and confined, to stage D, where cancer has spread to the lymph nodes or to other organs outside the prostate. The lower the staging, the more likely the cancer can be cured. Stage D tumors are rarely curable. The ideal watchful waiting candidate is a man with a low Gleason score and a stage A or B tumor.

Prostate tumors are fueled by male hormones called androgens. Advanced prostate cancer is usually treated with therapy that reduces androgen levels—such as testicle removal or drug/hormone therapy.

Though prostate cancer research has yielded significant advancements in the last decade, there's still a long way to go, says FDA's Robinowitz. "The dilemmas [of treatment] are due to the power of the cancer and the limits to our current knowledge and therapies," he says. "New tests [such as PSA] may be only partial solutions, but they are the best we can do for now."

—John Henkel

John Henkel is a staff writer for FDA Consumer.

For More Information on Prostate Disorders

Information on BPH and Its Treatment

Agency for Health Care Policy and Research (AHCPR)
Publications Clearinghouse
P.O. Box 8547
Silver Spring, MD 20907
800-358-9295

Ask for the free booklet called *Treating Your Enlarged Prostate*. It contains detailed information on the pros and cons of different treatments for BPH.

Prostate Health Council
American Foundation for Urologic Disease, Inc.
300 West Pratt Street
Baltimore, MD 21201
(800) 242-2383

National Kidney and Urologic Diseases
Information Clearinghouse
Box NKUDIC
Bethesda, MD 20892
301-468-6345

Ask for free materials on BPH.

Prostate Cancer Information and Support

American Cancer Society
1599 Clifton Road, NE
Atlanta, GA 30329
800-227-2345
(http://www.cancer.org/)

Offers the free brochure "Facts on Prostate Cancer" and other information.

American Foundation for Urologic Diseases
1-800-242-2383

Has a free booklet, "Prostate Cancer: What Every Man Over 40 Should Know," and other materials on cancer and other noncancerous prostate conditions.

Cancer Information Service (CIS)
National Cancer Institute
Building 31, Room 10A24
Bethesda, MD 20892
800-4-CANCER

CIS staff can answer questions and mail free booklets about prostate cancer. The prostate cancer "PDQ for Patients" contains detailed information on diagnosis and treatment. Spanish-speaking CIS staff are available during daytime hours.

Mathews Foundation for Prostate Cancer Research
(http://www.mathews.org/)
1-800-234-6284

Trained persons will answer questions and send prostate cancer information.

National Cancer Institute
http://www.nci.nih.gov/
1-800-422-6237

Can give information on clinical trials, as well as send "Cancer Facts" and other materials.

Us Too
(http://www.ustoo.com/)
1-800-808-7866

Publishes a monthly newsletter for prostate cancer survivors and has local chapters throughout North America.

Other Resources:

Prostate Health Council
The American Foundation for Urologic Disease, Inc.
300 West Pratt Street,
Suite 401
Baltimore, MD 21201
800-242-2383

Ask for free brochures in English and Spanish on prostate disease and prostate cancer.

For more information about health and aging, contact:

National Institute on Aging
Information Center
P.O. Box 8057
Gaithersburg, MD 20898-8057
800-222-2225
800-222-4225 (TTY)

The NIA distributes free *Age Pages* on a number of topics, including *Cancer Facts for People Over 50, Urinary Incontinence,* and *Considering Surgery.*

Section 6.8

Testicular Cancer

FDA Consumer, January 1996.

Glenn Knies wasn't thinking the worst when he felt the abnormality in his groin area 11 years ago. It was probably a hernia, he guessed.

He had just finished working out. In the shower, he noticed his right testicle seemed enlarged.

"I thought I had strained something," says Knies, an insurance adjuster in Schwenksville, PA. He was 23 and barely out of college at the time.

"I wasn't having any discomfort or symptoms to speak of," he says. "I was strong as ever, and there was nothing else to indicate a problem."

He mentioned the condition to his mother, a nurse, who urged him to see a urologist quickly. She suspected something more serious than a hernia was bothering her son.

His doctor determined the enlargement was cancer, and he removed Knies' right testicle, the standard first-line treatment for testicular tumors. Later, after tests showed that cancer may have spread to the lymph nodes deep within the abdomen where the testicles drain, doctors also removed the nodes.

But the lymph nodes were "clean," free of cancer, Knies says. It was the first sign that he probably was going to be OK, that his doctor likely had gotten all the cancer after removing the testicle. To make sure, a regimen of regular examinations followed—monthly at first, tapering off to annually after five years. Eleven years later, he still has a yearly exam but considers himself a cancer survivor.

Most Common Cancer in Young Men

Cancer of the testicles—egg-shaped sex glands in the scrotum that secrete male hormones and produce sperm—accounts for only about 1 percent of all cancers in men, according to the National Cancer Institute. About 7,000 Americans were expected to get the disease in 1995, with an estimated 325 deaths. Compared with prostate cancer, estimated to kill 40,400 of its 244,000 victims in 1995, testicular cancer is relatively rare. However, in men aged 15 to 34, it ranks as the most common cancer. For unknown reasons, the disease is about four times more common in white men than in black men.

Only 15 years ago, a diagnosis of testicular cancer was grim news. Ten times as many patients died then as now. But dramatic advances in therapeutic drugs in the last two decades, along with improved diagnostics and better tests to gauge the extent of the disease, have boosted survival rates remarkably. Now, testicular cancer often is completely curable, especially if found and treated early.

The Food and Drug Administration has approved several drugs to treat testicular cancer, including Ifex (ifosamide), Vepesid (etoposide), Velban (vinblastine sulfate), Blenoxane (bleomycin sulfate), and Platinol (cisplatin).

Many medical professionals regard Platinol as the "magic bullet" for treating certain forms of testicular cancer. FDA approved the platinum-based drug for use after surgery or radiation. Platinol almost always is used in combination with other chemotherapy drugs.

"[Platinum-based treatment] is truly the great success story for solid-tumor chemotherapy," says S. Bruce Malkowicz, M.D., co-director of urologic oncology at the University of Pennsylvania Medical Center. These drugs have helped cut testicular cancer's death rate and bolster its cure rate, he says, adding that many patients "respond very nicely" to platinum-based drug treatments, which are effective even when cancer has spread beyond the testicle.

"That is not a death sentence," Malkowicz says. About 70 percent of men with advanced testicular cancer can be cured, according to the National Cancer Institute.

Detection and Diagnosis

Most testicular tumors are discovered by patients themselves, either by accident, as Knies did, or while performing a self-examination on each testicle. "The usual presentation is of an enlarged, painless lump," says Malkowicz. "Occasionally there can be pain." The lump typically is pea-sized, but sometimes it might be as big as a marble or even an egg.

Besides lumps, if a man notices any other abnormality (an enlarged testicle, a feeling of heaviness or sudden collection of fluid in the scrotum, a dull ache in the lower abdomen or groin, or enlargement or tenderness of the breasts), he should discuss it with a physician right away. These symptoms can be caused by conditions other than cancer. But only a doctor can tell for sure, and it is critical to seek attention promptly.

Physicians have various methods to help diagnose testicular cancer. Often a physical exam can rule out disorders other than cancer. Imaging techniques can help indicate possible tumors. One such method is ultrasound, which creates a picture from echoes of high-frequency sound waves bounced off internal organs. Malkowicz calls this method "a painless, non-invasive way to check for a mass."

But the only positive way to identify a tumor is for a pathologist to examine a tissue sample under a microscope. Doctors obtain the tissue by removing the entire affected testicle through the groin. This procedure is called an inguinal orchiectomy. Surgeons do not cut through the scrotum or remove just a part of the testicle, because if cancer is present, a cut through the outer layer of the testicle may cause the disease to spread locally. Besides enabling diagnosis, testicle removal also can prevent further growth of the primary tumor.

Nearly all testicular tumors stem from germ cells, the special sperm-forming cells within the testicles. These tumors fall into one of two types, seminomas or non-seminomas. Other forms of testicular cancer, such as sarcomas or lymphomas, are extremely rare.

Seminomas account for about 40 percent of all testicular cancer and are made up of immature germ cells. Usually, seminomas are slow growing and tend to stay localized in the testicle for long periods. It was a seminoma that struck former Philadelphia Phillies first baseman John Kruk at age 33 in 1994. His right testicle was removed, and doctors say his prognosis is good.

Non-seminomas are a group of cancers that sometimes occur in combination, including choriocarcinoma, embryonal carcinoma, and yolk sac tumors. Non-seminomas arise from more mature, specialized germ cells and tend to be more aggressive than seminomas. According to the American Cancer Society, 60 to 70 percent of patients with non-seminomas have cancer that has spread to the lymph nodes.

Cancer Stages

Physicians measure the extent of the disease by conducting tests that allow the doctor to categorize, or "stage," the disease. These staging tests include blood analyses, imaging techniques, and sometimes additional surgery. Staging allows the doctor to plan the most appropriate treatment for each patient.

There are three stages of testicular cancer:

- Stage 1: Cancer confined to the testicle.

- Stage 2: Disease spread to retroperitoneal lymph nodes, located in the rear of the body below the diaphragm, a muscular wall separating the chest cavity from the abdomen.

- Stage 3: Cancer spread beyond the lymph nodes to remote sites in the body.

Through blood tests, doctors can check for tumor-associated markers, substances often present in abnormal amounts in cancer patients. Comparing levels of markers before and after surgical treatment helps doctors determine if cancer has spread beyond the testicles. Likewise, measuring marker levels before and after chemotherapy treatment can help show how well the chemotherapeutic drugs are working.

FDA has approved a test that checks blood levels of alpha-fetoprotein (AFP) as a tumor-associated marker. Other tests, such as those that gauge levels of beta-human chorionic gonadotropin (bHCG) or lactate dehydrogenase (LDH), are widely used as tumor-associated markers, but FDA has insufficient data to approve these tests.

Imaging techniques provide doctors with pictures of internal organs, giving visual clues to cancer staging. Chest x-rays can tell doctors if disease has spread to the lungs. Lymphangiography allows the lymph nodes to be visualized on an x-ray. CT scans create detailed views of cross sections of the body and can indicate possible tumors at various body sites.

Surgery to remove the retroperitoneal lymph nodes, into which the testicles drain, often is necessary for testicular cancer patients. Doctors examine lymph tissue microscopically to help determine the stage of the disease. Also, removing the tissue helps control further cancer spread.

Cancer Treatment

No one treatment works for all testicular cancers. Seminomas and non-seminomas differ in their tendency to spread, their patterns of spread, and response to radiation therapy. Thus, they often require different treatment strategies, which doctors choose based on the type of tumor and the stage of disease.

Because they are slow growing and tend to stay localized, seminomas generally are diagnosed in stage 1 or 2. Treatment might be a combination of testicle removal, radiation, or chemotherapy. But surgical removal of lymph nodes usually is not necessary for seminoma patients because this type of tumor is what the University of Pennsylvania's Malkowicz calls "exquisitely sensitive" to radiation. Normally directed to the retroperitoneal lymph nodes but sometimes to other lymph nodes, radiation can effectively remove cancer cells there. Stage 3 seminomas are usually treated with multi-drug chemotherapy.

Though most non-seminomas are not diagnosed at an early stage, cases confined to the testicle may need no further treatment other than testicle removal. These men must have careful follow-up for at least two years because about 10 percent of stage 1 patients have recurrences, which then are treated with chemotherapy. Stage 2 non-seminoma patients who have had testicle and lymph node removal may also need no further therapy. Some doctors opt for a short course of multi-drug chemotherapy for stage 2 patients to reduce the risk of recurrence. Most stage 3 non-seminomas can be cured with drug combinations.

Side Effects

Any kind of cancer treatment can cause undesirable side effects. But not all patients react the same way or to the same degree. One of the main concerns of young men is how treatment might affect their sexual or reproductive capabilities.

Removing one testicle does not impair fertility or sexual function. The remaining testicle can produce sperm and hormones adequate for reproduction. Removal of the retroperitoneal lymph nodes usually does not affect the ability to have erections or orgasms. It can, however, disrupt the nerve pathways that control ejaculation, causing infertility.

Modern "nerve-sparing" surgical techniques have increased the odds of retaining fertility. Many surgeons are abandoning a "total scorched-earth policy where you take out every single lymph node," Malkowicz says.

"We now can limit the amount of dissection necessary to get a good therapeutic cure, but not over dissect to disrupt every bit of nerves," he says, adding that "ejaculation can be preserved" in as many as 80 percent of cases.

Testicular cancer patient Knies points to his twin sons as proof that though his reproductive capacity was temporarily lost, it was restored.

Chemotherapy can cause increased risk of infection, nausea or vomiting, and hair loss. Not all patients experience these. Some drugs may cause infertility, but studies have shown that many men recover fertility two to three years after therapy ends. Radiation patients may experience fatigue or lowered blood counts. Infertility may also occur, but this usually is temporary.

Doctors emphasize that even though the cure rate is very high for all types and stages of testicular cancer, many of the drastic measures taken to cure later-stage disease can be avoided if the tumor is caught early enough. The best way to do this is through regular self-examination, a message that Knies says might be difficult to convey to the prime risk group.

"You have a real sense when you're in your late teens and early 20s of invincibility," he says. "The last thing you're thinking then is that something can stop you. But as I know, it can."

How to Examine the Testicles

"I never examined myself."

Pennsylvania resident Glenn Knies, 34, says he wasn't consciously looking for possible cancer 11 years ago. He calls it "pure luck" that he noticed an abnormality in the shower and sought medical attention.

Now a survivor of testicular cancer, Knies strongly urges men to examine their testicles regularly.

Medical professionals say men can greatly increase their chances of finding testicular tumors by testicular self-examination, or TSE. Locating a tumor this way can boost the odds of early intervention and total cure.

"Diagnosis of testicular cancer usually starts with self-discovery," says S. Bruce Malkowicz, co-director of urologic oncology at the University of Pennsylvania Medical Center. He advises men of all ages to do TSEs, not just those in the prime risk group of ages 15 to 34.

TSE is best performed after a warm bath or shower. Heat relaxes the scrotum, making it easier to spot anything abnormal. The National Cancer Institute recommends following these steps every month:

1. Stand in front of a mirror. Check for any swelling on the scrotum skin.

2. Examine each testicle with both hands. Place the index and middle fingers under the testicle with the thumbs placed on top. Roll the testicle gently between the thumbs and fingers. Don't be alarmed if one testicle seems slightly larger than the other. That's normal.

3. Find the epididymis, the soft, tube-like structure behind the testicle that collects and carries sperm. If you are familiar with this structure, you won't mistake it for a suspicious lump. Cancerous lumps usually are found on the sides of the testicle but can also show up on the front.

If you find a lump, see a doctor right away. The abnormality may not be cancer, but if it is, the chances are great it can spread if not stopped by treatment. Only a physician can make a positive diagnosis.

Knies says fear shouldn't keep men from doing the TSE. "And men need not feel self-conscious about touching themselves there. It only takes a few seconds for them to tell if everything's fine. If they find something, they shouldn't be afraid to say something. Wishing it away isn't going to make it go away."

—John Henkel

John Henkel is a staff writer for FDA Consumer.

Chapter 7

Stroke

Chapter Contents

Section 7.1

Brain Attack: Warning Signs of Stroke

NIH Publication Web Document. Last updated May 20, 1997.
National Institute of Neurological Disorders and Stroke. Web Document,
URL: (http//www.ninds.nih.gov/healinfo/disorder/stroke/strkmini.HTM).

If you observe one or more of these signs of a stroke or "brain attack,"
don't wait, call a doctor or 911 right away.

- Sudden **weakness or numbness** of the face, arm, or leg on one
  side of the body.

- Sudden **dimness or loss of vision**, particularly in one eye.

- Sudden **difficulty speaking or trouble understanding
  speech**.

- Sudden **severe headache** with no known cause.

- Unexplained **dizziness, unsteadiness, or sudden falls**, especially with any of the other signs.

Warning signs may last a few moments and then disappear. They are
signs of a serious condition that won't go away without medical help.

Risk Factors for a Stroke

Stroke prevention is still the best medicine. The most important treatable conditions linked to stroke are:

- **High blood pressure.** Eat a balanced diet, maintain a healthy
  weight, and exercise to reduce blood pressure. Drugs are also
  available.

- **Cigarette smoking.** Medical help is available to help quit.

- **Heart disease.** Your doctor will treat your heart disease and
  may also prescribe medication to help prevent the formation of

clots. If you are over 50, NINDS scientists believe you and your doctor should make a decision about aspirin therapy.

• **Diabetes.** Treatment can delay complications that increase the risk of stroke.

• **Transient ischemic attacks.** These are brief episodes of stroke's warning signs and can be treated with drugs or surgery.

Section 7.2

What You Should Know about Stroke Prevention

Agency for Health Care Policy and Research.
AHCPR Publication No. 95-0090.

A stroke occurs when blood flow to the brain is blocked, either by narrowed blood vessels or blood clots or when there is bleeding in the brain. Deprived of nutrients, brain nerve cells begin to die within a few minutes. As a result, stroke can cause vision and sensory loss, problems with walking and talking, or difficulty in thinking clearly. In many cases, the effects of stroke are irreversible.

Some people are more at risk for stroke than others. Chronic health conditions such as high blood pressure and diabetes can increase your risk, as well as lifestyle choices such as smoking cigarettes, being overweight, or drinking excessively. Men, African Americans, and people with a family history of stroke have a higher risk as well. If you have already had a stroke or a transient ischemic attack (referred to as a TIA or "mini-stroke"), you are at highest risk. Warning signs include sudden unexplained numbness or tingling (especially on one side), slurred speech, blurred vision, stumbling, or clumsiness.

Preventing Stroke

Experts now believe that stroke is as preventable as heart attack. In addition to primary prevention tactics such as quitting smoking, drinking only in moderation, and exercising, there are medical interventions that can decrease your risk of stroke if you are in a high-risk group. Recent studies, including those supported by the Agency for Health Care Policy and Research (AHCPR), show that if you have conditions known as atrial fibrillation or carotid artery disease, there are interventions that can dramatically lower your risk of stroke.

Atrial Fibrillation

If you have atrial fibrillation, the upper left chamber of your heart beats rapidly and unpredictably, making it hard for all the blood in the chamber to empty. The remaining blood tends to form clots that can travel to any part of your body. If they travel to the brain, these clots can cause a stroke. Treatment with anticoagulants (or blood-thinners) such as warfarin can prevent these clots from forming. Aspirin also is used to reduce the risk of stroke, but the most recent clinical studies have shown that warfarin is superior to aspirin in preventing stroke. Current studies show that treatment with warfarin can prevent over half of the 80,000 strokes that are caused annually by atrial fibrillation.

If you have atrial fibrillation, your health care provider may recommend that you take warfarin. If you do, you need to know:

- Warfarin may increase the risk of bleeding. Careful regular monitoring of blood levels and proper dosage should keep this risk in check. Your health care provider will tell you where to go for monitoring.

- When properly administered, warfarin prevents 20 strokes for every major bleeding complication caused by the medicine.

- Most bleeding incidents are preventable and treatable.

- Certain drugs can interfere with proper anticoagulation. Antibiotics and anticonvulsants (for example, phenobarbital and Tegretol) are examples of drugs that can cause problems. Talk to your physician or pharmacist for complete information.

Carotid Artery Disease

The carotid arteries run through the neck and supply blood to the brain. When the walls of the carotid arteries are narrowed by fatty deposits known as plaque, small clots in the blood can cut off blood supply to the brain and cause a stroke. A surgical procedure known as a carotid endarterectomy clears arteries of plaque. If you have had a minor stroke or symptoms that suggest you are at high risk for a stroke, and there is evidence of severe blockage in your carotid arteries, your health care provider may suggest you consider carotid endarterectomy as a preventive procedure.

If you are considering this surgery, you should know:

- Certain tests may be required to confirm the diagnosis of carotid artery disease. With angiography, a dye is injected into the artery, followed by an x-ray to check for blockage. Magnetic resonance imaging (MRI) and ultrasonic scans also can test for blockage without entering the arteries.

- Carotid endarterectomy carries some risks. There can be complications if parts of the plaque break away during the procedure and block an artery to the brain or if artery incisions leak.

- Complication rates vary greatly by hospital and surgeon. Ask if your hospital monitors its complication rates for carotid endarterectomy and ask your surgeon how many times he or she has performed the procedure. Evidence shows that surgeons who have performed more procedures have higher success rates.

AHCPR Research

This information is based on research by the Stroke Prevention Patient Outcomes Research Team (PORT) headed by David B. Matchar, MD, of Duke University's Center for Health Policy Research and Education. PORTs are multi-disciplinary research studies, sponsored by AHCPR, that are focused on common and costly clinical conditions. PORTs examine the outcomes of treatments provided to typical patients by typical practitioners in typical health care settings.

Like other AHCPR medical effectiveness research studies, PORTs address three core questions about available treatments:

- Are they effective?
- For which patients are they most effective?
- Are they cost-effective?

Printed copies of *What You Should Know About Stroke Prevention* are available by writing or calling:

AHCPR Publications Clearinghouse
P.O. Box 8547
Silver Spring, MD 20907
800-358-9295 (24 hours a day)

Recovering After a Stroke, the Consumer Version of a Clinical Practice Guideline, is available from the AHCPR Publications Clearinghouse (AHCPR Pub. No. 95-0664) and is printed as the next section of this chapter. The booklet is on the Internet at URL:

(http://text.nlm.nih.gov/ftrs/dbaccess/psrp)

Fax copies of these materials are available by calling AHCPR InstantFAX at 301/594-2800 using a fax machine with a telephone handset.

Section 7.3

Recovering from a Stroke

Agency for Health Care Policy and Research. AHCPR Publication No. 95-0664. URL: (http://text.nlm.nih.gov/ftrs/dbaccess/psrp).

What Is a Stroke?

A stroke is a type of brain injury. Symptoms depend on the part of the brain that is affected. People who survive a stroke often have weakness on one side of the body or trouble with moving, talking, or thinking.

Most strokes are ischemic (is-KEE-mic) strokes. These are caused by reduced blood flow to the brain when blood vessels are blocked by a clot or become too narrow for blood to get through. Brain cells in the area die of lack of oxygen. In another type of stroke, called hemorrhagic (hem-or-AJ-ic) stroke, the blood vessel isn't blocked; it bursts, and blood leaks into the brain, causing damage.

Strokes are more common in older people. Almost three-fourths of all strokes occur in people 65 years of age or over. However, a person of any age can have a stroke.

A person may also have a transient ischemic attack (TIA). This has the same symptoms as a stroke, but only lasts for a few hours or a day and does not cause permanent brain damage. A TIA is not a stroke but it is an important warning signal. The person needs treatment to help prevent an actual stroke in the future.

A stroke may be frightening to both the patient and family. It helps to remember that stroke survivors usually have at least some spontaneous recovery or natural healing and often recover further with rehabilitation.

This section is about stroke rehabilitation. Its goal is to help the person who has had a stroke achieve the best possible recovery. Its purpose is to help people who have had strokes and their families get the most out of rehabilitation.

Note that this section sometimes uses the terms "stroke survivor" and "person" instead of "patient" to refer to someone who has had a stroke. This is because people who have had a stroke are patients for only a short time, first in the acute care hospital and then perhaps in a rehabilitation program. For the rest of their lives, they are people who happen to have had a stroke. The section also uses the word "family" to include those people who are closest to the stroke survivor, whether or not they are relatives.

Rehabilitation works best when stroke survivors and their families work together as a team. For this reason, both stroke survivors and family members are encouraged to read all parts of the section.

Recovering from Stroke

The process of recovering from a stroke usually includes treatment, spontaneous recovery, rehabilitation, and the return to community living. Because stroke survivors often have complex rehabilitation needs, progress and recovery are different for each person.

Treatment for stroke begins in a hospital with "acute care." This first step includes helping the patient survive, preventing another stroke, and taking care of any other medical problems.

Spontaneous recovery happens naturally to most people. Soon after the stroke, some abilities that have been lost usually start to come back. This process is quickest during the first few weeks, but it sometimes continues for a long time.

Rehabilitation is another part of treatment. It helps the person keep abilities and gain back lost abilities to become more independent. It usually begins while the patient is still in acute care. For many patients, it continues afterward, either as a formal rehabilitation program or as individual rehabilitation services. Many decisions about rehabilitation are made by the patient, family, and hospital staff before discharge from acute care.

The last stage in stroke recovery begins with the person's return to community living after acute care or rehabilitation. This stage can last for a lifetime as the stroke survivor and family learn to live with the effects of the stroke. This may include doing common tasks in new ways or making up for damage to or limits of one part of the body by greater activity of another. For example, a stroke survivor can wear shoes with Velcro closures instead of laces or may learn to write with the opposite hand.

How Stroke Affects People

Effects on the Body, Mind, and Feelings

Each stroke is different depending on the part of the brain injured, how bad the injury is, and the person's general health. Some of the effects of stroke are:

Weakness (hemiparesis—hem-ee-par-EE-sis) or paralysis (hemiplegia—hem-ee-PLEE-ja) on one side of the body. This may affect the whole side or just the arm or the leg. The weakness or paralysis is on the side of the body opposite the side of the brain injured by the stroke. For example, if the stroke injured the left side of the brain, the weakness or paralysis will be on the right side of the body.

Problems with balance or coordination. These can make it hard for the person to sit, stand, or walk, even if muscles are strong enough.

Problems using language (aphasia and dysarthria). A person with aphasia (a-FAY-zha) may have trouble understanding speech or writing. Or, the person may understand but may not be able to think of the words to speak or write. A person with dysarthria (dis-AR-three-a) knows the right words but has trouble saying them clearly.

Being unaware of or ignoring things on one side of the body (bodily neglect or inattention). Often, the person will not turn to look toward the weaker side or even eat food from the half of the plate on that side.

Pain, numbness, or odd sensations. These can make it hard for the person to relax and feel comfortable.

Problems with memory, thinking, attention, or learning (cognitive problems). A person may have trouble with many mental activities or just a few. For example, the person may have trouble following directions, may get confused if something in a room is moved, or may not be able to keep track of the date or time.

Being unaware of the effects of the stroke. The person may show poor judgment by trying to do things that are unsafe as a result of the stroke.

Trouble swallowing (dysphagia—dis-FAY-ja). This can make it hard for the person to get enough food. Also, care must sometimes be taken to prevent the person from breathing in food (aspiration—as-per-AY-shun) while trying to swallow it.

Problems with bowel or bladder control. These problems can be helped with the use of portable urinals, bedpans, and other toileting devices.

Getting tired very quickly. Becoming tired very quickly may limit the person's participation and performance in a rehabilitation program.

Sudden bursts of emotion, such as laughing, crying, or anger. These emotions may indicate that the person needs help, understanding, and support in adjusting to the effects of the stroke.

Depression. This is common in people who have had strokes. It can begin soon after the stroke or many weeks later, and family members often notice it first.

Depression after Stroke

It is normal for a stroke survivor to feel sad over the problems caused by stroke. However, some people experience a major depressive disorder, which should be diagnosed and treated as soon as possible. A person with a major depressive disorder has a number of symptoms nearly every day, all day, for at least two weeks. These always include at least one of the following:

- Feeling sad, blue, or down in the dumps.
- Loss of interest in things that the person used to enjoy.

A person may also have other physical or psychological symptoms, including:

- Feeling slowed down or restless and unable to sit still,
- Feeling worthless or guilty,
- Increase or decrease in appetite or weight,
- Problems concentrating, thinking, remembering, or making decisions,
- Trouble sleeping or sleeping too much,
- Loss of energy or feeling tired all of the time,
- Headaches,
- Other aches and pains,
- Digestive problems,
- Sexual problems,

- Feeling pessimistic or hopeless,
- Being anxious or worried, or
- Thoughts of death or suicide.

If a stroke survivor has symptoms of depression, *especially thoughts of death or suicide,* professional help is needed right away. Once the depression is properly treated, these thoughts will go away. Depression can be treated with medication, psychotherapy, or both. If it is not treated, it can cause needless suffering and also makes it harder to recover from the stroke.

Disabilities after Stroke

A "disability" is difficulty doing something that is a normal part of daily life. People who have had a stroke may have trouble with many activities that were easy before, such as walking, talking, and taking care of "activities of daily living" (ADLs). These include basic tasks such as bathing, dressing, eating, and using the toilet, as well as more complex tasks called "instrumental activities of daily living" (IADLs), such as housekeeping, using the telephone, driving, and writing checks.

Some disabilities are obvious right after the stroke. Others may not be noticed until the person is back home and is trying to do something for the first time since the stroke.

What Happens During Acute Care?

The main purposes of acute care are to:

- Make sure the patient's condition is caused by a stroke and not by some other medical problem.

- Determine the type and location of the stroke and how serious it is.

- Prevent or treat complications such as bowel or bladder problems or pressure ulcers (bed sores).

- Prevent another stroke.

- Encourage the patient to move and perform self-care tasks, such as eating and getting out of bed, as early as medically possible. This is the first step in rehabilitation.

Stroke survivors and family members may find the hospital experience confusing. Hospital staffs are there to help, and it is important to ask questions and talk about concerns.

Before acute care ends, the patient and family with the hospital staff decide what the next step will be. For many patients, the next step will be to continue rehabilitation.

Preventing Another Stroke

People who have had a stroke have an increased risk of another stroke, especially during the first year after the original stroke. The risk of another stroke goes up with older age, high blood pressure (hypertension), high cholesterol, diabetes, obesity, having had a transient ischemic attack (TIA), heart disease, cigarette smoking, heavy alcohol use, and drug abuse. While some risk factors for stroke (such as age) cannot be changed, the risk factors for the others can be reduced through use of medicines or changes in lifestyle.

Patients and families should ask for guidance from their doctor or nurse about preventing another stroke. They need to work together to make healthy changes in the patient's lifestyle. Patients and families should also learn the warning signs of a TIA (such as weakness on one side of the body and slurred speech) and see a doctor immediately if these happen.

Deciding about Rehabilitation

Some people do not need rehabilitation after a stroke because the stroke was mild or they have fully recovered. Others may be too disabled to participate. However, many patients can be helped by rehabilitation. Hospital staff will help the patient and family decide about rehabilitation and choose the right services or program.

Types of Rehabilitation Programs

There are several kinds of rehabilitation programs:

Hospital programs. These programs can be provided by special rehabilitation hospitals or by rehabilitation units in acute care hospitals. Complete rehabilitation services are available. The patient stays in the hospital during rehabilitation. An organized team of specially trained professionals provides the therapy. Hospital programs are usually more intense than other programs and require more effort from the patient.

Nursing facility (nursing home) programs. As in hospital programs, the person stays at the facility during rehabilitation. Nursing facility programs are very different from each other, so it is important to get specific information about each one. Some provide a complete range of rehabilitation services; others provide only limited services.

Outpatient programs. Outpatient programs allow a patient who lives at home to get a full range of services by visiting a hospital outpatient department, outpatient rehabilitation facility, or day hospital program.

Home-based programs. The patient can live at home and receive rehabilitation services from visiting professionals. An important advantage of home programs is that patients learn skills in the same place where they will use them.

Individual Rehabilitation Services

Many stroke survivors do not need a complete range of rehabilitation services. Instead, they may need an individual type of service, such as regular physical therapy or speech therapy. These services are available from outpatient and home care programs.

Paying for Rehabilitation

Medicare and many health insurance policies will help pay for rehabilitation. Medicare is the Federal health insurance program for Americans 65 years of age or over and for certain Americans with disabilities. It has two parts: hospital insurance (known as Part A) and supplementary medical insurance (known as Part B). Part A helps pay for home health care, hospice care, inpatient hospital care, and inpatient care in a skilled nursing facility. Part B helps pay for doctors' services, outpatient hospital services, durable medical equipment, and a number of other medical services and supplies not covered by Part A. Social Security Administration offices across the country take applications for Medicare and provide general information about the program.

In some cases, **Medicare** will help pay for outpatient services from a Medicare-participating comprehensive outpatient rehabilitation facility. Covered services include physicians'services; physical, speech, occupational, and respiratory therapies; counseling; and other related services. A stroke survivor must be referred by a physician who certifies that skilled rehabilitation services are needed.

Medicaid is a Federal program that is operated by the States, and each State decides who is eligible and the scope of health services offered. Medicaid provides health care coverage for some low-income people who cannot afford it. This includes people who are eligible because they are older, blind, or disabled, or certain people in families with dependent children.

These programs have certain restrictions and limitations, and coverage may stop as soon as the patient stops making progress. Therefore, it is important for patients and families to find out exactly what their insurance will cover. The hospital's social service department can answer questions about insurance coverage and can help with financial planning.

Choosing a Rehabilitation Program

The doctor and other hospital staff will provide information and advice about rehabilitation programs, but the patient and family make the final choice. Hospital staffs know the patient's disabilities and medical condition. They should also be familiar with the rehabilitation programs in the community and should be able to answer questions about them. The patient and family may have a preference about whether the patient lives at home or at a rehabilitation facility. They may have reasons for preferring one program to another. Their concerns are important and should be discussed with hospital staff.

Things to Consider When Choosing a Rehabilitation Program

- Does the program provide the services the patient needs?

- Does it match the patient's abilities or is it too demanding or not demanding enough?

- What kind of standing does it have in the community for the quality of the program?

- Is it certified and does its staff have good credentials?

- Is it located where family members can easily visit?

- Does it actively involve the patient and family members in rehabilitation decisions?

- Does it encourage family members to participate in some rehabilitation sessions and practice with the patient?

- How well are its costs covered by insurance or Medicare?

- If it is an outpatient or home program, is there someone living at home who can provide care?

- If it is an outpatient program, is transportation available?

A person may start rehabilitation in one program and later transfer to another. For example, some patients who get tired quickly may start out in a less intense rehabilitation program. After they build up their strength, they are able to transfer to a more intense program.

When Rehabilitation Is Not Recommended

Some families and patients may be disappointed if the doctor does not recommend rehabilitation. However, a person may be unconscious or too disabled to benefit. For example, a person who is unable to learn may be better helped by maintenance care at home or in a nursing facility. A person who is, at first, too weak for rehabilitation may benefit from a gradual recovery period at home or in a nursing facility. This person can consider rehabilitation at a later time. It is important to remember that:

- Hospital staffs are responsible for helping plan the best way to care for the patient after discharge from acute care. They can also provide or arrange for needed social services and family education.

- This is not the only chance to participate in rehabilitation. People who are too disabled at first may recover enough to enter rehabilitation later.

What Happens During Rehabilitation

In hospital or nursing facility rehabilitation programs, the patient may spend several hours a day in activities such as physical therapy, occupational therapy, speech therapy, recreational therapy, group activities, and patient and family education. It is important to maintain skills that help recovery. Part of the time is spent relearning skills (such as walking and speaking) that the person had before the stroke. Part of it is spent learning new ways to do things that can no longer be done the old way (for example, using one hand for tasks that usually need both hands).

159

Setting Rehabilitation Goals

The goals of rehabilitation depend on the effects of the stroke, what the patient was able to do before the stroke, and the patient's wishes. Working together, goals are set by the patient, family, and rehabilitation program staff. Sometimes, a person may need to repeat steps in striving to reach goals.

If goals are too high, the patient will not be able to reach them. If they are too low, the patient may not get all the services that would help. If they do not match the patient's interests, the patient may not want to work at them. Therefore, it is important for goals to be realistic. To help achieve realistic goals, the patient and family should tell program staff about things that the patient wants to be able to do.

Rehabilitation Goals

- Being able to walk, at least with a walker or cane, is a realistic goal for most stroke survivors.

- Being able to take care of oneself with some special equipment is a realistic goal for most.

- Being able to drive a car is a realistic goal for some.

- Having a job can be a realistic goal for some people who were working before the stroke. For some, the old job may not be possible but another job or a volunteer activity may be.

Reaching treatment goals does not mean the end of recovery. It just means that the stroke survivor and family are ready to continue recovery on their own.

Rehabilitation Specialists

Because every stroke is different, treatment will be different for each person. Rehabilitation is provided by several types of specially trained professionals. A person may work with any or all of these:

Physician. All patients in stroke rehabilitation have a physician in charge of their care. Several kinds of doctors with rehabilitation experience may have this role. These include family physicians and internists (primary care doctors), geriatricians (specialists in working with older patients), neurologists (specialists in the brain and nervous system), and physiatrists (specialists in physical medicine and rehabilitation).

Rehabilitation nurse. Rehabilitation nurses specialize in nursing care for people with disabilities. They provide direct care, educate patients and families, and help the doctor to coordinate care.

Physical therapist. Physical therapists evaluate and treat problems with moving, balance, and coordination. They provide training and exercises to improve walking, getting in and out of a bed or chair, and moving around without losing balance. They teach family members how to help with exercises for the patient and how to help the patient move or walk, if needed.

Occupational therapist. Occupational therapists provide exercises and practice to help patients do things they could do before the stroke such as eating, bathing, dressing, writing, or cooking. The old way of doing an activity sometimes is no longer possible, so the therapist teaches a new technique.

Speech-language pathologist. Speech-language pathologists help patients get back language skills and learn other ways to communicate. Teaching families how to improve communication is very important. Speech-language pathologists also work with patients who have swallowing problems (dysphagia).

Social worker. Social workers help patients and families make decisions about rehabilitation and plan the return to the home or a new living place. They help the family answer questions about insurance and other financial issues and can arrange for a variety of support services. They may also provide or arrange for patient and family counseling to help cope with any emotional problems.

Psychologist. Psychologists are concerned with the mental and emotional health of patients. They use interviews and tests to identify and understand problems. They may also treat thinking or memory problems or may provide advice to other professionals about patients with these problems.

Therapeutic recreation specialist. These therapists help patients return to activities that they enjoyed before the stroke such as playing cards, gardening, bowling, or community activities. Recreational therapy helps the rehabilitation process and encourages the patient to practice skills.

Other professionals. Other professionals may also help with the patient's treatment. An orthotist may make special braces to support weak ankles and feet. A urologist may help with bladder problems. Other physician specialists may help with medical or emotional problems. Dietitians make sure that the patient has a healthy diet during rehabilitation. They also educate the family about proper diet after the patient leaves the program. Vocational counselors may help patients go back to work or school.

Rehabilitation Team

Rehabilitation professionals, the patient, and the family are vitally important partners in rehabilitation. They must all work together for rehabilitation to succeed.

In many programs, a special rehabilitation team with a team leader is organized for each patient. The patient, family, and rehabilitation professionals are all members. The team has regular meetings to discuss the progress of treatment. Using a team approach often helps everyone work together to meet goals.

Getting the Most out of Rehabilitation

What the Patient Can Do

If you are a stroke survivor in rehabilitation, keep in mind that you are the most important person in your treatment. You should have a major say in decisions about your care. This is hard for many stroke patients. You may sometimes feel tempted to sit back and let the program staff take charge. If you need extra time to think or have trouble talking, you may find that others are going ahead and making decisions without waiting. Try not to let this happen.

- Make sure others understand that you want to help make decisions about your care.
- Bring your questions and concerns to program staff.
- State your wishes and opinions on matters that affect you.
- Speak up if you feel that anyone is "talking down" to you; or, if people start talking about you as if you are not there.
- Remember that you have the right to see your medical records.

To be a partner in your care, you need to be well informed about your treatment and how well you are doing. It may help to record important information about your treatment and progress and write down any questions you have.

If you have speech problems, making your wishes known is hard. The speech-language pathologist can help you to communicate with other staff members, and family members may also help to communicate your ideas and needs.

Most patients find that rehabilitation is hard work. They need to maintain abilities at the same time they are working to regain abilities. It is normal to feel tired and discouraged at times because things that used to be easy before the stroke are now difficult. The important thing is to notice the progress you make and take pride in each achievement.

How the Family Can Help

If you are a family member of a stroke survivor, here are some things you can do:

- Support the patient's efforts to participate in rehabilitation decisions.

- Visit and talk with the patient. You can relax together while playing cards, watching television, listening to the radio, or playing a board game.

- If the patient has trouble communicating (aphasia), ask the speech-language pathologist how you can help.

- Participate in education offered for stroke survivors and their families. Learn as much as you can and how you can help.

- Ask to attend some of the rehabilitation sessions. This is a good way to learn how rehabilitation works and how to help.

- Encourage and help the patient to practice skills learned in rehabilitation.

- Make sure that the program staff suggests activities that fit the patient's needs and interests.

- Find out what the patient can do alone, what the patient can do with help, and what the patient can't do. Then avoid doing things for the patient that the patient is able to do. Each time the patient does them, his or her ability and confidence will grow.

- Take care of yourself by eating well, getting enough rest, and taking time to do things that you enjoy.

To gain more control over the rehabilitation process, keep important information where you can find it. One suggestion is to keep a notebook with the patient. Some things to include are provided in the sample that follows.

Discharge Planning

Discharge planning begins early during rehabilitation. It involves the patient, family, and rehabilitation staff. The purpose of discharge planning is to help maintain the benefits of rehabilitation after the patient has been discharged from the program. Patients are usually discharged from rehabilitation soon after their goals have been reached.

Some of the things discharge planning can include are to:

- Make sure that the stroke survivor has a safe place to live after discharge.

- Decide what care, assistance, or special equipment will be needed.

- Arrange for more rehabilitation services or for other services in the home (such as visits by a home health aide).

- Choose the health-care provider who will monitor the person's health and medical needs.

- Determine the caregivers who will work as a partner with the patient to provide daily care and assistance at home, and teach them the skills they will need.

- Help the stroke survivor explore employment opportunities, volunteer activities, and driving a car (if able and interested).

- Discuss any sexual concerns the stroke survivor or husband/wife may have. Many people who have had strokes enjoy active sex lives.

Preparing a Living Place

Many stroke survivors can return to their own homes after rehabilitation. Others need to live in a place with professional staff such as a nursing home or assisted living facility. An assisted living facility can provide residential living with a full range of services and staff. The choice usually depends on the person's needs for care and whether caregivers are available in the home. The stroke survivor needs a living place that supports continuing recovery.

It is important to choose a living place that is safe. If the person needs a new place to live, a social worker can help find the best place.

During discharge planning, program staff will ask about the home and may also visit it. They may suggest changes to make it safer. These might include changing rooms around so that a stroke survivor can stay on one floor, moving scatter rugs or small pieces of furniture that could cause falls, and putting grab bars and seats in tubs and showers.

It is a good idea for the stroke survivor to go home for a trial visit before discharge. This will help identify problems that need to be discussed or corrected before the patient returns.

Deciding about Special Equipment

Even after rehabilitation, some stroke survivors have trouble walking, balancing, or performing certain activities of daily living. Special equipment can sometimes help. Here are some examples:

Cane. Many people who have had strokes use a cane when walking. For people with balancing problems, special canes with three or four "feet" are available.

Walker. A walker provides more support than a cane. Several designs are available for people who can only use one hand and for different problems with walking or balance.

Ankle-foot orthotic devices (braces). Braces help a person to walk by keeping the ankle and foot in the correct position and providing support for the knee.

Wheelchair. Some people will need a wheelchair. Wheelchairs come in many different designs. They can be customized to fit the user's needs and abilities. Find out which features are most important for the stroke survivor.

Aids for bathing, dressing, and eating. Some of these are safety devices such as grab bars and nonskid tub and floor mats. Others make it easier to do things with one hand. Examples are velcro fasteners on clothes and placemats that won't slide on the table.

Communication aids. These range from small computers to homemade communication boards. The stroke survivor, family, and rehabilitation program staff should decide together what special equipment is needed. Program staff can help in making the best choices. Medicare or health insurance will often help pay for the equipment.

Preparing Caregivers

Caregivers who help stroke survivors at home are usually family members such as a husband or wife or an adult son or daughter. They may also be friends or even professional home health aides. Usually, one person is the main caregiver, while others help from time to time. An important part of discharge planning is to make sure that caregivers understand the safety, physical, and emotional needs of the stroke survivor, and that they will be available to provide needed care.

Since every stroke is different, people have different needs for help from caregivers. Here are some of the things caregivers may do:

- Keep notes on discharge plans and instructions and ask about anything that is not clear.

- Help to make sure that the stroke survivor takes all prescribed medicines and follows suggestions from program staff about diet, exercise, rest, and other health practices.

- Encourage and help the person to practice skills learned in rehabilitation.

- Help the person solve problems and discover new ways to do things.

- Help the person with activities performed before the stroke. These could include using tools, buttoning a shirt, household tasks, and leisure or social activities.

- Help with personal care, if the person cannot manage alone.

- Help with communication, if the person has speech problems. Include the stroke survivor in conversations even when the person cannot actively participate.

- Arrange for needed community services.

- Stand up for the rights of the stroke survivor.

If you expect to be a caregiver, think carefully about this role ahead of time. Are you prepared to work with the patient on stroke recovery?

Talk it over with other people who will share the caregiving job with you. What are the stroke survivor's needs? Who can best help meet each of them? Who will be the main caregiver? Does caregiving need to be scheduled around the caregivers' jobs or other activities? There is time during discharge planning to talk with program staff about caregiving and to develop a workable plan.

Going Home

Adjusting to the Change

Going home to the old home or a new one is a big adjustment. For the stroke survivor, it may be hard to transfer the skills learned during rehabilitation to a new location. Also, more problems caused by the stroke may appear as the person tries to go back to old activities. During this time, the stroke survivor and family learn how the stroke will affect daily life and can make the necessary adjustments.

These adjustments are a physical and emotional challenge for the main caregiver as well as the stroke survivor. The caregiver has many new responsibilities and may not have time for some favorite activities. The caregiver needs support, understanding, and some time to rest. Caregiving that falls too heavily on one person can be very stressful. Even when family members and friends are nearby and willing to help, conflicts over caregiving can cause stress.

A stroke is always stressful for the family, but it is especially hard if one family member is the only caregiver. Much time may be required to meet the needs of the stroke survivor. Therefore, the caregiver needs as much support as possible from others. Working together eases the stress on everyone.

Tips for Reducing Stress

The following tips for reducing stress are for both caregivers and stroke survivors:

- Take stroke recovery and caregiving one day at a time and be hopeful.

- Remember that adjusting to the effects of stroke takes time. Appreciate each small gain as you discover better ways of doing things.

- Caregiving is learned. Expect that knowledge and skills will grow with experience.

- Experiment. Until you find what works for you, try new ways of doing activities of daily living, communicating with each other, scheduling the day, and organizing your social life.

- Plan for "breaks" so that you are not together all the time. This is a good way for family and friends to help on occasion. You can also plan activities that get both of you out of the house.

- Ask family members and friends to help in specific ways and commit to certain times to help. This gives others a chance to help in useful ways.

- Read about the experiences of other people in similar situations. Your public library has life stories by people who have had a stroke as well as books for caregivers.

- Join or start a support group for stroke survivors or caregivers. You can work on problems together and develop new friendships.

- Be kind to each other. If you sometimes feel irritated, this is natural and you don't need to blame yourself. But don't "take it out" on the other person. It often helps to talk about these feelings with a friend, rehabilitation professional, or support group.

- Plan and enjoy new experiences and don't look back. Avoid comparing life as it is now with how it was before the stroke.

Followup Appointments

After a stroke survivor returns to the community, regular followup appointments are usually scheduled with the doctor and sometimes with rehabilitation professionals. The purpose of followup is to check on the stroke survivor's medical condition and ability to use the skills learned in rehabilitation. It is also important to check on how well the stroke survivor and family are adjusting. The stroke survivor and caregiver can be prepared for these visits with a list of questions or concerns.

Where to Get Help

Many kinds of help are available for people who have had strokes and their families and caregivers. Some of the most important are:

Information about stroke. A good place to start is with the books and pamphlets available from national organizations that provide information on this subject. Many of their materials are available free of charge. A list of these organizations is included at the end of this section.

Local stroke clubs or other support groups. These are groups where stroke survivors and family members can share their experiences, help each other solve problems, and expand their social lives.

Home health services. These are available from the Visiting Nurses Association (VNA), public health departments, hospital home care departments, and private home health agencies. Services may include nursing care, rehabilitation therapies, personal care (for example, help with bathing or dressing), respite care (staying with the stroke survivor so that the caregiver can take a vacation or short break), homemaker services, and other kinds of help.

Meals on Wheels. Hot meals are delivered to the homes of people who cannot easily shop and cook.

Adult day care. People who cannot be completely independent sometimes spend the day at an adult day care center. There they get meals, participate in social activities, and may also get some health care and rehabilitation services.

Friendly Visitor (or other companion services). A paid or volunteer companion makes regular visits or phone calls to a person with disabilities.

Transportation services. Most public transportation systems have buses that a person in a wheelchair can board. Some organizations and communities provide vans to take wheelchair users and others on errands such as shopping or doctor's visits.

Many communities have service organizations that can help. Some free services may be available or fees may be on a "sliding scale" based on income. It takes some work to find out what services and payment arrangements are available. A good way to start is to ask the social workers in the hospital or rehabilitation program where the stroke survivor was treated. Also, talk to the local United Way or places of worship. Another good place to look is the Yellow Pages of the telephone book, under "Health Services," "Home Health Care," "Senior Citizen Services," or "Social Service Organizations." Just asking friends may turn up useful information. The more you ask, the more you will learn.

Additional Resources

ACTION
1100 Vermont Avenue, NW
Washington, D.C. 20525
(202) 606-4855 (call for telephone number of regional office)

Sponsors older American volunteer programs.

Administration on Aging
330 Independence Avenue, SW
Washington, D.C. 20201
Toll-free (800) 677-1116 (call for list of community services for older Americans in your area)

AHA Stroke Connection (formerly the Courage Stroke Network)
American Heart Association
7272 Greenville Avenue
Dallas, TX 75231
Toll-free (800) 553-6321 (or check telephone book for local AHA office)

Provides prevention, diagnosis, treatment, and rehabilitation information to stroke survivors and their families.

American Dietetic Association/
National Center for Nutrition and Dietetics
216 West Jackson Boulevard
Chicago, IL 60606
Toll-free (800) 366-1655 (Consumer Nutrition Hotline)

Consumers may speak to a registered dietitian for answers to nutrition questions, or obtain a referral to a local registered dietitian.

American Self-Help Clearinghouse
St. Clares-Riverside Medical Center
Denville, NJ 07834
(201) 625-7101 (call for name and telephone number of State or local clearinghouse)

Provides information and assistance on local self-help groups.

National Aphasia Association

P.O. Box 1887
Murray Hill Station
New York, NY 10156
Toll-free (800) 922-4622

Provides information on the partial or total loss of the ability to speak or comprehend speech, resulting from stroke or other causes.

National Easter Seal Society

230 West Monroe Street, Suite 1800
Chicago, IL 60606
(312) 726-6200 (or check telephone book for local Easter Seal Society)

Provides information and services to help people with disabilities.

National Stroke Association

8480 East Orchard Road, Suite 1000
Englewood, CO 80111
(303) 771-1700
Toll-free (800) STROKES (787-6537)

Serves as an information referral clearinghouse on stroke. Offers guidance on forming stroke support groups and clubs.

Rosalynn Carter Institute

Georgia Southwestern College
600 Simmons Street
Americus, GA 31709

Provides information on caregiving. Reading lists, video products, and other caregive resources are available by writing to the address listed above.

Stroke Clubs International

805 12th Street
Galveston, TX 77550
(409) 762-1022 (call for the name of a stroke club located in your area)

Maintains list of over 800 stroke clubs throughout the United States.

The Well Spouse Foundation
P.O. Box 801
New York, NY 10023
(212) 724-7209
Toll-free (800) 838-0879

Provides support for the husbands, wives, and partners of people who are chronically ill or disabled.

For Medicare Information:
Consumer Information Center
Department 59
Pueblo, CO 81009

By writing to this address, you can receive a free copy of *The Medicare Handbook* (updated and published annually). This handbook provides information about Medicare benefits, health insurance to supplement Medicare, and limits to Medicare coverage. It is also available in Spanish.

For Further Information

Information in this section is based on *Post-Stroke Rehabilitation. Clinical Practice Guideline, Number 16.* It was developed by a non-Federal panel sponsored by the Agency for Health Care Policy and Research (AHCPR), an agency of the Public Health Service. Other guidelines on common health problems are available, and more are being developed.

Four other patient guides are available from AHCPR that may be of interest to stroke survivors and their caregivers:

- *Preventing Pressure Ulcers: Patient Guide* gives detailed information about how to prevent pressure sores (AHCPR Publication No. 92-0048).

- *Treating Pressure Sores: Patient Guide* gives detailed information about treating pressure sores (AHCPR Publication No. 95-0654).

- *Urinary Incontinence in Adults: Patient Guide* describes why people lose urine when they don't want to and how that can be treated (AHCPR Publication No. 92-0040).

- *Depression Is a Treatable Illness: Patient Guide* discusses major depressive disorder, which most often can be successfully treated with the help of a health professional (AHCPR Publication No. 93-0053).

For more information about these and other guidelines, or to get more copies of this section, call toll-free: 800-358-9295 or write to:

Agency for Health Care Policy and Research
Publications Clearinghouse
P.O. Box 8547
Silver Spring, MD 20907

Chapter 8

Unintentional Injuries

Chapter Contents

Section 8.1

Mortality

Extracted from NIH Publication No. 97-1232.
Health United States 1996-97 and Injury Chartbook.

Age and Sex

The age distribution of injury deaths can be described as having three separate ranges. The first one includes the population under 15 years of age. Injury death rates are lowest at these ages. Within this group, the injury death rate for infants in 1995 (29 per 100,000 population) was about 2-3 times the rate for children 1-4 years, 5-9 years, and 10-14 years of age. The next age group is comprised of persons 15-74 years of age. Injury death rates ranged from 49 per 100,000 at 55-64 years to 80 per 100,000 at 20-24 years. Persons 75 years of age and over comprise the third group. Injury death rates were highest in this group. The rates for persons 75-84 years and 85 years of age and over were 116 and 281 per 100,000 persons. Injury death rates were higher for males than for females in each age group except for infancy where the rates were similar. In 1995 for children 1-9 years of age, injury death rates for males were about 1.5 times the rates for females, and the difference increases with age. Beginning with ages 10-14 years, injury mortality increases more rapidly for males than for females. The death rate for males aged 20-24 years was 6.8 times the rate at 10-14 years of age, while for females, the rate at ages 20-24 years was 3.1 times the rate at ages 10-14 years. Accordingly, the mortality sex ratio (the ratio of death rate for males to that for females) jumped from 2.1 at ages 10-14 years to 4.6:1 at 20-24 years.

From ages 20-24 years to ages 55-64 years, injury death rates for males declined, decreasing almost by a factor of 2, while rates for females remained relatively constant for the same ages. Injury death rates for males and females 85 years and over were 4.7 and 6.0 times the rates for males and females 65-74 years. The mortality sex ratio for persons 65 years and over was about 2:1, less than half of what it was at ages 20-24 years.

The percent of all deaths that were caused by an injury was greater for males (9 percent) than for females (4 percent). Among males ages 15-19 years and 20-24 years, 83 and 80 percent respectively of all deaths were caused by injuries compared with 69 and 56 percent among females. With increasing age, the percents decrease for both males and females. For persons 65 years and over only about 2 percent of all deaths were caused by injuries.

Intent

Unintentional injury. Unintentional injury comprised the largest portion of fatal injuries, about 61 percent, ranging from 50 percent at ages 20-24 years and 25-34 years to 79-91 percent for persons 1-9 years of age and 75 years and over. In 1995, 90,402 persons died as a result of an unintentional injury, at a crude rate of 34.4 per 100,000.

Age-specific unintentional injury death rates follow a pattern similar to that of all injury—relatively higher in infancy than for young children, rising through the early to mid-twenties, then declining through middle age, and rising again among the elderly. The rate for persons 85 years of age and over was 8 times the rate for persons aged 55-64 years. The mortality sex ratios were higher among persons ages 20-54 years (averaging 3:1) than among younger or older persons.

Suicide. Suicide accounted for 21 percent of injury mortality, ranging from about 8 percent of all injury among those aged 85 years and over to 28 percent at 45-54 years. In 1995, 31,284 suicides were completed at a crude rate of 11.9 per 100,000 population.

Age-specific suicide rates rise rapidly from ages 10-14 years to 15-19 years. From ages 20-24 years to 65-74 years the rates were relatively constant (13-16 per 100,000 population), and then rose among those 75 years and over. Among those aged 15-74 years suicide rates for males were about 3-6 times the rates for females. Among the elderly 75-84 years of age and 85 years and over, the mortality sex ratio increased to 8:1 and nearly 12:1.

Homicide. Homicide accounted for 15 percent of all injury deaths, about 23-28 percent of injury deaths for infants and for teens and young adults 15-34 years of age. In 1995, 22,552 persons were victims of homicide, at a crude rate of 8.6 per 100,000 population.

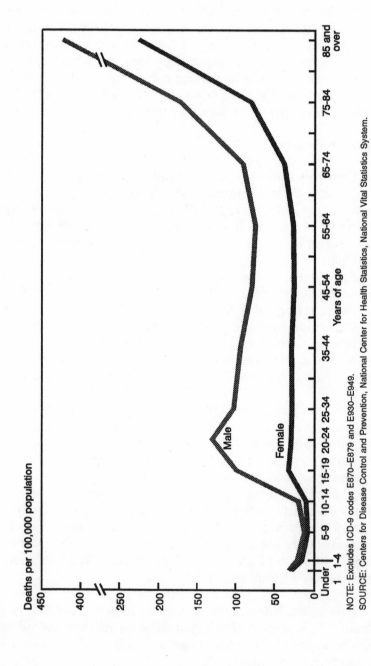

Figure 8.1. Injury death rates by age and sex: United States, 1995. NOTE: Excludes ICD-9 codes E870-E879 and E930-E949. SOURCE: Centers for Disease Control and Prevention, National Center for Health Statistics, National Vital Statistics System.

NOTE: Excludes ICD-9 codes E870–E879 and E930–E949.

SOURCE: Centers for Disease Control and Prevention, National Center for Health Statistics, National Vital Statistics System.

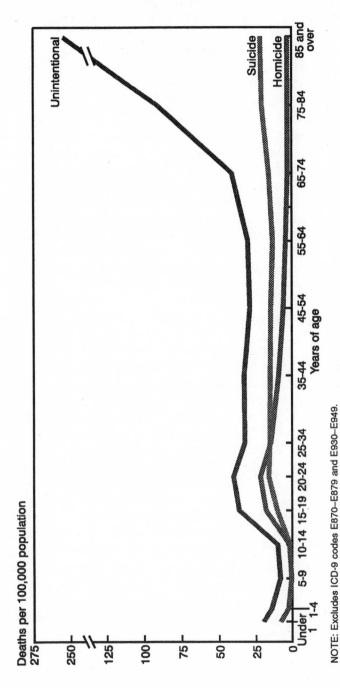

Figure 8.2. *Injury death rates by age and manner of death: United States, 1995. NOTE: Excludes ICD-9 codes E870-E879 and E930-E949. SOURCE: Centers for Disease Control and Prevention, National Center for Health Statistics, National Vital Statistics System.*

NOTE: Excludes ICD-9 codes E870–E879 and E930–E949.

SOURCE: Centers for Disease Control and Prevention, National Center for Health Statistics, National Vital Statistics System.

Homicide rates for infants were close to 3 times the rate for children ages 1-4 years, and about 10 times the rate for children 5-9 years of age.

Homicide rates were highest at ages 20-24 years. Age-specific rates then decline until ages 65-74 years when they hold constant.

From ages 10-14 years to 20-24 years, age-specific homicide rates exceed suicide rates; from ages 25 years and over, suicide exceeds homicide.

At ages 15-19 years and 20-24 years, homicide rates for males were 5-6 times the rates for females. For infants and for children ages 1-9 years, homicide rates for males and females were similar. At ages 35-74 years, the sex ratio averaged 2-3:1.

Intent was not determined for 2 percent of injury deaths in 1995. Age-specific death rates were constant at 1-2 per 100,000 for infants and ages 15 years and over, and lower among children 1-14 years of age. Other means of injury include legal intervention and injury resulting from war operations. In 1995 0.2 percent of all injury deaths were so classified.

Causes, Ages 0-14 Years

Motor vehicle traffic. Among children ages 1-4, 5-9, and 10-14 years, motor vehicle traffic injuries were the leading cause of all (not just injury) deaths, accounting for an average of 18 percent of all deaths and 37 percent of all injury deaths for these children. Death rates for motor vehicle traffic injuries were similar among infants and children 1-4 and 5-9 years, whereas for children ages 10-14 years, the death rate was about 30 percent higher than for the younger ages (4.5 per 100,000 population). Death rates for boys and girls were similar for infants and for children ages 1-4 years. At 5-9 and 10-14 years, death rates for boys were nearly 50 percent higher than for girls.

Among children 1-14 years of age, the majority of traffic victims (55-65 percent) were occupants of vehicles (as opposed to motorcyclist, pedestrians or pedal cyclists) and 94 percent of infant victims were occupants. For these childhood fatalities being struck by a vehicle as a pedestrian was more likely than being struck as a pedal cyclist.

Drowning. Drowning rates were higher for children ages 1-4 years than for younger and older children. At ages 1-4 years, 5-9 years, and 10-14 years, the risk of drowning was greater for boys than for girls. For example, at ages 10-14 years, the drowning rate for boys was 2.6 times that for girls (1.8 compared with 0.7 per 100,000). Among children

1-14 years of age, 97 percent of the drowning deaths were unintentional; among infants, 80 percent were unintentional.

Fires and burns. Death rates for fire and burns were higher for children 1-4 years of age than for older children 5-14 years or infants. The rate for boys aged 1-4 years was 1.4 times the rate for girls (3.6 compared with 2.6 per 100,000). At other ages, rates for boys and girls were similar. Ninety-one percent of fire and burn deaths among children under 15 years of age were unintentional and 8 percent were homicides.

Suffocation. Suffocation was the leading cause of injury death among infants, followed by motor vehicle traffic injuries. The suffocation rate among infants was 10 times the rates for children 1-4 years and 10-14 years. The rate for male infants was 1.3 times the rate for females (12.4 compared with 9.5 per 100,000 population). Seventy percent of the suffocations among infants were due to mechanical means (such as in a bed or cradle, by a plastic bag, or due to a lack of air in a closed space) rather than due to respiratory obstructions.

Firearms. Firearms were the second leading cause of death among children aged 10-14 years, accounting for 13 percent of all deaths and 24 percent of all injury deaths. The rate at ages 10-14 years was nearly 6 times the rate for children ages 1-9 years (3.4 compared with 0.6 per 100,000). Forty-eight percent of the firearm deaths among children 10-14 years of age were homicides, and 29 percent were suicides. The firearm death rate for boys ages 10-14 years was 3.8 times the rate for girls. The mortality sex ratios for firearm suicide and firearm homicide at ages 10-14 years were about 3:1 and 4:1, respectively. The ratio for unintentional firearm mortality was about 6:1. The five leading causes of injury death among children under 15 years of age, motor vehicle traffic injuries, fire and burns, drowning, suffocation, and firearms, accounted for 80 percent of injury deaths in this age group in 1995. Among infants, congenital anomalies were the leading cause of death followed by other diseases related specifically to infancy. Injury accounted for 4 percent of all deaths in infancy. For children ages 1-4 years, the death rate for congenital anomalies (4.4 per 100,000) was similar to the death rate for motor vehicle traffic injuries.

Malignant neoplasms were the second leading cause of death at ages 5-9 years after motor vehicle traffic-related injury deaths, and were the third leading cause at ages 10-14 years following motor vehicle traffic and firearm injuries.

Figure 8.3. Death rates for leading causes of injury among children under 15 years of age by age: United States, 1995. (Rate is based on fewer than 20 deaths.) SOURCE: Centers for Disease Control and Prevention, National Center for Health Statistics, National Vital Statistics System.

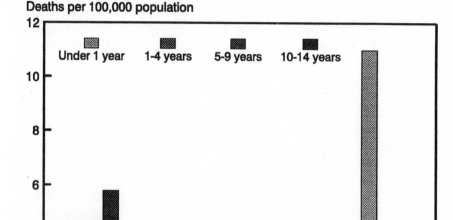

Deaths per 100,000 population

* Rate is based on fewer than 20 deaths.

SOURCE: Centers for Disease Control and Prevention, National Center for Health Statistics, National Vital Statistics System.

Causes, Ages 15-64 Years

Among teenagers 15-19 years of age, motor vehicle traffic injuries and firearm injuries were the first and second leading causes of all (not just injury) deaths. At ages 20-24 years motor vehicle traffic injuries and firearm injuries were the two leading causes of death. At ages 25-34 years, firearms and motor vehicle traffic deaths were second and third following deaths from Human Immunodeficiency Virus (HIV) infection.

At 35-44 years of age, the number of deaths from motor vehicle traffic injuries, firearm injuries, and from poisoning followed deaths from HIV, malignant neoplasms, and diseases of heart (each of which caused more than twice as many deaths as were caused by motor vehicles, firearms or poisoning).

By ages 45-54 years and 55-64 years, the number of deaths from diseases of heart and malignant neoplasms were 2-3 and 7-9 times the total number of injury deaths in those respective age groups.

Motor vehicle traffic. Motor vehicle traffic-related injuries were the cause of 31 percent of the injury deaths in people aged 15-64 years. Within this age group the death rates were highest for young persons ages 15-19 years and 20-24 years; by ages 35-64 years, the death rates were are about half what they were at 15-24 years of age (29 per 100,000). Death rates for males 15-64 years of age were 2-3 times the rates for females.

About 80 percent of motor vehicle traffic victims among persons 15-64 years of age were vehicle occupants. Occupant death rates for persons aged 15-24 years were about twice the rates for persons 25-64 years of age. Pedestrian death rates increase with age, from 1.7 per 100,000 at 15-19 years to 2.5 at 55-64 years. At 55-64 years of age, 17 percent of traffic deaths involved a pedestrian.

Firearms. Firearms were the cause of 29 percent of injury deaths among persons ages 15-64 years. The firearm death rate was highest for persons 20-24 years of age, at 29.9 per 100,000. At ages 15-64 years, 48 percent of firearm deaths were homicides, 46 percent were suicides, and 3 percent were unintentional.

At ages 15-19 years and 20-24 years, the firearm death rates for males were about 8 times the rates for females; for persons 25-64 years of age, the mortality sex ratio averaged 5:1.

Among persons 15-24 years of age firearm homicide rates exceeded firearm suicide rates by a factor of 2. For persons aged 45-64 years this reverses and the firearm suicide rates were 2-4 times the firearm homicide rates.

Poisoning. Poisoning was the third leading cause of injury death at ages 15-64 years, accounting for 14 percent of all injury deaths at these ages. The poisoning death rate peaked at 35-44 years of age. At this age the poisoning death rate was similar to the firearm death rate and only 6 percent lower than the motor vehicle traffic death rate. Across ages 15-64 years, 57 percent of poisoning deaths were unintentional, 30 percent were suicides, and 13 percent were of undetermined intent. At ages 35-44 years, 93 percent of the unintentional poisoning deaths were caused by drugs, medicinal substances, and biological agents.

For ages 15-64 years the death rate for poisoning among males was 2-3 times the rate among females, and the sex ratio was higher for unintentional poisoning deaths than for suicide by poisoning.

Motor vehicle traffic injuries, firearms, and poisoning were the three leading causes of injury deaths for persons 15-64 years, accounting for 74 percent of all injury deaths, and 13 percent of all deaths.

Figure 8.4. *Death rates for leading causes of injury among persons 15-64 years of age by age: United States, 1995. SOURCE: Centers for Disease Control and Prevention, National Center for Health Statistics, National Vital Statistics System.*

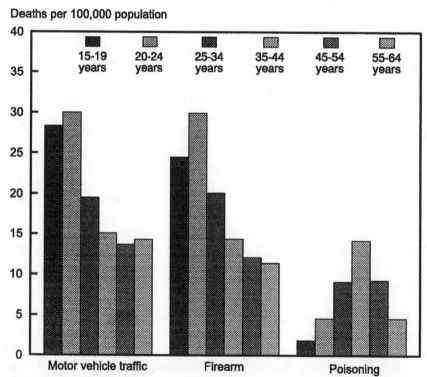

SOURCE: Centers for Disease Control and Prevention, National Center for Health Statistics, National Vital Statistics System.

Causes, Ages 65 Years and over

Among adults 65 years of age and over, two out of three injury deaths resulted from motor vehicle injuries, firearms, suffocation, and falls. For persons aged 65-74 years, motor vehicles and firearms were the two leading causes of injury deaths, accounting for one-half of injury mortality; at ages 75-84 years, motor vehicles and falls were the cause of close to one-half of all injury deaths, and for those 85 years of age and over, falls caused one-third of injury deaths.

Motor vehicle traffic. The motor vehicle traffic death rate for persons 65-74 years of age (17.3 per 100,000) was about 40 percent lower than the rates for persons aged 75-84 years and 85 years and over. The rate at ages 65-74 years was about 20 percent higher than the rate for persons 55-64 years of age. Motor vehicle traffic injuries were the cause of 22 percent of all injury deaths among persons 65 years and over.

Four of five motor vehicle traffic victims were occupants of vehicles and most of the others were struck as pedestrians. The risk for being killed as a pedestrian increases sharply after ages 65-74 years when the rate was 3.0 per 100,000; by ages 85 years and over, the rate was 7.1 per 100,000, 3-5 times the rates for persons 1-64 years.

For persons 65-84 years of age, motor vehicle traffic death rates for males were 1.6-1.8 times the rates for females. For persons 85 years and over the rate for males was 3.1 times the rate for females, (with similar differences by sex for occupants and pedestrians).

Falls. Falls accounted for 23 percent of injury deaths among persons 65 years and over, and for 34 percent of injury mortality among persons 85 years of age and over. The death rate due to falls increases dramatically for persons aged 85 years and over; the rate at those ages (94.6 per 100,000) was 3.6 times the rate for persons 75-84 years. At age 85 years and over the death rate for males was 1.5 times the rate for females (a smaller differential than for other causes of injury).

The death rate for falls is likely an underestimate of the true rate because the E-codes recommended and used to classify fall mortality exclude E887, "fracture, cause unspecified." In 1995 there were 3,503 deaths so classified; nearly 9 out of 10 were among persons 75 years of age and over. If all deaths coded to E887 were added to the specified E-codes for falls, the death rates for falls at ages 75-84 years and 85 years and over would have been 32 percent and 61 percent higher than their 1995 levels (26 and 95 per 100,000). An international comparison of mortality in the elderly provides insight on the failure of physicians to accurately record falls on the death certificate (1).

Firearms. Firearms were the cause of 14 percent of injury deaths among persons 65 years of age and over; nearly 9 out of 10 firearm deaths were suicides. The sex ratio for firearm suicides increases with age, from 11:1 at 65-74 years, to 19:1 at 75-84 years and 38:1 at 85 years and over (45.7 compared with 1.2 per 100,000).

Figure 8.5. *Death rates for leading causes of injury among adults 65 years of age and over by age: United States, 1995. SOURCE: Centers for Disease Control and Prevention, National Center for Health Statistics, National Vital Statistics System.*

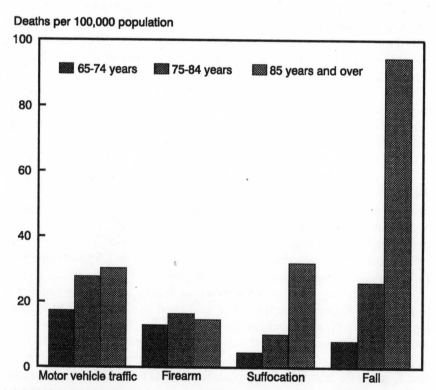

Deaths per 100,000 population

SOURCE: Centers for Disease Control and Prevention, National Center for Health Statistics, National Vital Statistics System.

Suffocation. Suffocation was the cause of 9 percent of injury deaths for persons 65 years of age and over, three-quarters of which were unintentional and most of the remainder were suicides (by hanging). Of the unintentional suffocations, 2 out of 3 were caused by non-food objects causing obstruction in the respiratory tract. The suffocation rate increases with age. The rate was highest for those aged 85 years and over, 7 times the rate for persons 65-74 years.

Reference

1. Langlois JA, Smith GS, Baker SP, Langley JD. International comparisons of injury mortality in the elderly: Issues and differences between New Zealand and the United States. Int J Epidemiol 24:136-43. 1995.

Trends, Leading Causes of Injury Death

From 1985 to 1995 the age-adjusted injury death rate declined 6 percent to 51.5 per 100,000 following a 16 percent decline in the preceding 5 years. During the 1985-95 period, however, there was considerable variation in the trends by cause of injury and by gender.

Motor vehicle traffic. The age-adjusted motor vehicle traffic death rate declined 15 percent from 1985 to 1993, with a larger decline for males than for females, 17 percent compared with 8 percent. From 1993 to 1995 the motor vehicle traffic death rate increased 2 percent with no change in the rate for males and a 4 percent increase in the rate for females. From 1985 to 1993 motor vehicle death rates decreased for persons ages 1-14 years, 15-24 years, 25-44 years, and 45-64 years. From 1993 to 1995 the rate for persons 45-64 years increased 5 percent and was relatively stable for other ages.

Firearms. Age-adjusted firearm death rates, on the other hand, increased 22 percent from 1985 to 1993, with larger increases for males than females (23 percent compared with 10 percent). The mortality sex ratio increased from 5:1 to 6:1. From 1993 to 1995 the firearm death rate declined 11 percent, 10 percent for males and 13 percent for females. From 1985 to 1993 age-specific firearm death rates increased for persons under 45 years of age, and most notably for persons 15-24 years. From 1993 to 1995 declines were observed in each age group.

Poisoning. From 1985 to 1991 age-adjusted death rates for poisoning remained fairly stable at about 5 per 100,000. From 1991 to 1995 the rate increased 18 percent from 4.9 to 5.8 per 100,000, with most of the increase taking place among males. The mortality sex ratio increased from 2:1 to nearly 3:1 during the 10 years. At ages 25-44 years (where the poisoning death rates were highest), death rates increased 44 percent from 1985 to 1995 while at ages 65 years and over, a 26 percent decrease was noted.

Suffocation. Age-adjusted death rates for suffocation were relatively unchanged for most of the 1985 to 1995 period, averaging 3 per 100,000. The mortality sex ratio averaged close to 3:1. Suffocation death rates were higher for infants and the elderly than for other ages. For those under 1 year of age, the rate increased 10 percent from 1985 to 1995 while among the elderly, the death rate declined 16 percent.

Falls. Mortality from falls declined 11 percent during this period, with a relatively unchanged mortality sex ratio of nearly 3:1. However, among the elderly where the rates are highest, the death rate increased slightly. For younger ages, fall mortality either declined or remained stable.

Drowning. Death rates for drowning declined 27 percent from 1985 to 1995. The mortality sex ratio averaged 4:1 throughout the 10 years. Age-specific declines were observed across all age groups.

Fire and burns. Age-adjusted death rates for fire and burns have also declined during this period, by 33 percent. The mortality sex ratio remained relatively stable, with rates for males close to twice the rates for females. Age-specific fire and burn death rates declined 27-42 percent across all age groups.

From 1985 to 1995 the age-adjusted unintentional injury death rate declined 12 percent to 30 per 100,000; the age-adjusted suicide rate declined slightly from 12 to 11 per 100,000. On the other hand, from 1985 to 1991 the age-adjusted homicide rate increased 32 percent to 11 per 100,000; from 1991 to 1995 the homicide rate decreased 15 percent to 9 per 100,000, with the largest annual decline (9 percent) taking place from 1994 to 1995.

NOTE: All injury excludes ICD-9 codes E870-E879 and E930-E949.

Figure 8.6. *Age-adjusted death rates for leading causes of injury: United States, 1985-95. SOURCE: Centers for Disease Control and Prevention, National Center for Health Statistics, National Vital Statistics System.*

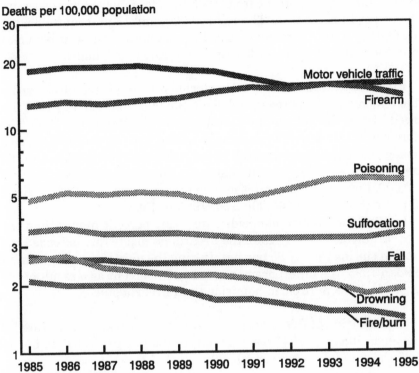

Deaths per 100,000 population

SOURCE: Centers for Disease Control and Prevention, National Center for Health Statistics, National Vital Statistics System.

Firearms and Motor Vehicles

In 1995, 18,003 persons aged 15-34 years died as a result of a firearm injury, accounting for 50 percent of all firearm deaths. From 1985 to 1993 the firearm injury death rate for persons 15-34 years of age increased 44 percent from 18.3 to 26.4 per 100,000 population; from 1993 to 1995 the rate declined 11 percent.

Firearm homicide. Changes in firearm homicide rates for persons aged 15-34 years have contributed more to the changes in total firearm mortality than have firearm suicide or unintentional firearm injury death rates. In this age group, the firearm homicide rate increased 83 percent from 1985 to 1993, followed by a 14 percent decline to 13.7 per 100,000 by 1995. Rates for males increased 89 percent and for females 47 percent from 1985 to 1993 followed by respective declines of 14 percent (to 23.5 per 100,000) and 18 percent (to 3.6 per 100,000) by 1995. Throughout most of this period, firearm homicide rates for males were about 6-7 times the rates for females.

Firearm suicide. The firearm suicide rate for persons 15-34 years of age increased 10 percent to 8.9 per 100,000 from 1985 to 1994 followed by a decline of about 6 percent to 8.4 per 100,000 in 1995. The increase is attributed to increases in the rate among males only, among whom the rate increased 13 percent from 1985 to 1994. In 1995 the firearm suicide rate for males declined 5 percent to 14.6 per 100,000. Firearm suicide rates for females, on the other hand, declined 13 percent to 2.1 per 100,000 from 1985 to 1995.

In 1985 the firearm homicide rate was 7 percent higher than the firearm suicide rate. By 1992 the firearm homicide rate exceeded the firearm suicide rate by 85 percent. During the most recent years, from 1993 to 1995, the difference narrowed to 63 percent as a result of the larger declines in firearm homicide than firearm suicide.

Unintentional firearm. The unintentional firearm death rate for the years 1985 to 1994 was constant at about 1 per 100,000, but in 1995 the rate fell to 0.8 per 100,000.

Motor vehicle traffic. In 1995, 18,428 persons 15-34 years of age died as a result of a motor vehicle traffic injury, accounting for 43 percent of all motor vehicle traffic deaths. From 1985 to 1993 the motor vehicle traffic death rate among young persons ages 15-34 years declined 18 percent to 23.7 per 100,000, with the largest proportional annual decline taking place from 1991 to 1992. From 1993 to 1995 the rate hovered around 24 per 100,000 thousand. From 1985 to 1993 the motor vehicle traffic death rate for males 15-34 years declined 21 percent and was stable through 1995. The rate for females fell 9 percent from 1985 to 1993 followed by a 5 percent increase by 1995.[1]

In 1995, 50 percent of all traffic fatalities among persons 15-34 years were alcohol-related, meaning that either the driver, occupant, or non-occupant (pedestrian or pedal cyclist) had a blood alcohol concentration of 0.01 grams per deciliter (g/dl) or greater.[2]

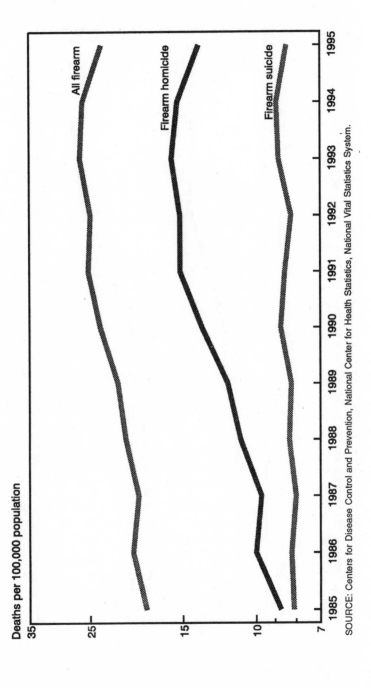

Figure 8.7. Firearm injury death rates by manner of death among persons 15-34 years of age: United States, 1985-95. SOURCE: Centers for Disease Control and Prevention, National Center for Health Statistics, National Vital Statistics System.

SOURCE: Centers for Disease Control and Prevention, National Center for Health Statistics, National Vital Statistics System.

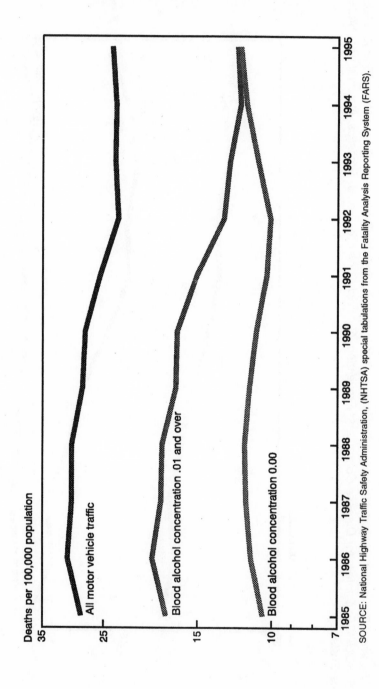

Figure 8.8. Motor vehicle traffic death rates by alcohol involvement among persons 15-34 years of age: United States, 1985-95. SOURCE: National Highway Traffic Safety Administration, (NHTSA) special tabulations from the Fatality Analysis Reporting System (FARS).

SOURCE: National Highway Traffic Safety Administration, (NHTSA) special tabulations from the Fatality Analysis Reporting System (FARS).

From 1985 to 1995 for persons ages 15-34 years, the alcohol-related traffic fatality rate declined 32 percent and the non-alcohol traffic fatality rate increased 13 percent for a net decline in the motor vehicle traffic crash death rate of 16 percent. Approximately 84 percent of the decline in the alcohol-related rate was a result of declines in the rates among persons who were considered intoxicated (persons with blood alcohol concentration of 0.10 g/dl or higher).

For drivers in all age groups involved in fatal crashes, intoxication rates decreased from 1985 to 1995. Intoxication rates were highest for motorcycle operators (20 percent) and lowest for drivers of large trucks (1 percent). For drivers ages 16-20 years involved in fatal crashes, the percent intoxicated dropped 47 percent to 13 percent. In 1995 the highest intoxication levels, 27-28 percent, were noted for drivers 21-34 years of age in fatal crashes. Nearly half of all pedestrians 25-34 years of age who died in traffic crashes were intoxicated compared with about 11 percent among pedestrians 65 years and over. NHTSA estimates that since 1975 minimum drinking age laws have reduced traffic fatalities involving drivers 18-20 years of age by 13 percent and have saved an estimated 15.7 thousand lives.

NHTSA estimates that alcohol-involved crashes resulted in $45 billion in economic costs in 1994, accounting for 30 percent of all crash costs. Seventy-eight percent of all alcohol-involved crash costs occur in crashes where a driver or pedestrian had a blood alcohol content of 0.10 g/dl or greater. The impact of alcohol involvement increases with injury severity. Alcohol-involved crashes accounted for 17 percent of property-damage-only crash costs, 29 percent of nonfatal injury crash costs, and 47 percent of fatal injury crash costs (1).

Reference

1. Blincoe LJ. Economic cost of motor vehicle crashes, 1994. NHTSA Technical Report. 1997.

Footnotes

1. These data are from the NCHS vital statistics system; however, the numbers of deaths for ages 15-34 based on FARS (Fatality Analysis Reporting System) in 1994 and 1995 were 18,068 and 18,393 respectively. Trends in the motor vehicle traffic death rates for the two systems are nearly identical; rates in any particular year differed by 2 percent or less.

2. Data on alcohol-related traffic crashes are from NHTSA, *Traffic Safety Facts, 1995* and from tabulations provided for the chartbook by NHTSA.

Geographic Variation

In 1994 motor vehicle injuries (traffic and non-traffic) were the leading cause of death for white males 15-24 years of age, and the second leading cause among black males ages 15-24 years. For the period 1988-92, the motor vehicle death rate for white males ages 15-24 years was about 1.4 times the rate for black males (51 compared with 36 per 100,000) Among white and black males 15-24 years of age, the motor vehicle death rates declined during this 4-year period, 28 and 14 percent.

Among teenage and young adult white males during the period 1988-92, motor vehicle injury death rates were highest in the east south central area of the United States. Other pockets of high death rates are seen in the Pacific area and the northern parts of the mountain States. Low motor vehicle death rates are seen in the New England and the Middle Atlantic areas. These patterns fit with the higher motor vehicle death rates noted in rural areas compared with urban areas.

Among teenage and young adult black males in the same age group, the motor vehicle death rate was higher in the southern half of the South Atlantic States (in the area from the Carolinas south to Florida) than in any other part of the country. In addition, pockets of high rates were also noted in the east south central and southern half of the mountain States. Areas of low rates are noted particularly in the northern half of the country.

Despite the higher death rates among white males compared with black males, the geographic patterns are relatively similar.

Geographic variation in injury mortality has been the subject of many analyses; motor vehicle death rates have been consistently found to be higher in more rural areas of the West and in the South (1, 2).

NOTE: Motor vehicle injuries are more broadly defined by ICD E-codes E810-E825 to be consistent with the *Mortality Atlas* and therefore include incidents that occurred in non-traffic areas (off public roads).

Figure 8.9. Geographic mortality patterns for motor vehicle injuries among white and black males 20 years of age: United States, 1988-92. SOURCE: Pickle LW, Mungiole M, Jones GK, White AA. Atlas of United States Mortality. Hyattsville, Maryland: National Center for Health Statistics. 1996.

White

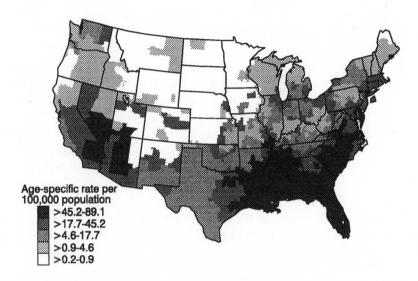

Age-specific rate per 100,000 population
- >45.2-89.1
- >17.7-45.2
- >4.6-17.7
- >0.9-4.6
- >0.2-0.9

Black

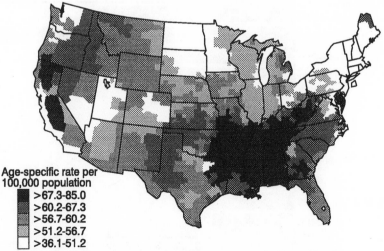

Age-specific rate per 100,000 population
- >67.3-85.0
- >60.2-67.3
- >56.7-60.2
- >51.2-56.7
- >36.1-51.2

SOURCE: Pickle LW, Mungiole M, Jones GK, White AA. Atlas of United States Mortality. Hyattsville, Maryland: National Center for Health Statistics. 1996.

References

1. Baker SP, Whitfield MA, O'Neil B. Geographic variation in mortality from motor vehicle crashes. N Engl J Med 316:1384-7. 1987.

2. Baker SP, O'Neil B, Ginsburg MJ, Li G. The injury fact book, second edition. 1992.

International Comparisons

In 1994 the motor vehicle traffic injury death rate among males 15-24 years of age was 41 per 100,000 population in the United States. Compared with a group of selected developed countries, only New Zealand (in 1992-93) had a higher death rate (63 per 100,000) than the United States. The rate in France was similar to the U.S. rate. Death rates in Australia, Canada, Denmark and Israel ranged from

Figure 8.10. *Motor vehicle traffic injury death rates among males 15-24 years of age for selected countries and selected years, 1992-95. SOURCE: Data provided by members of the International Collaborative Effort (ICE) on Injury Statistics.*

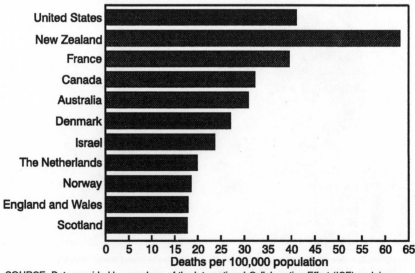

SOURCE: Data provided by members of the International Collaborative Effort (ICE) on Injury Statistics.

55-75 percent of the U.S. rate, and in Norway, Scotland, England and Wales, and The Netherlands, the death rates were about one-half the U.S. rate.

The firearm death rate among males 15-24 years of age in the United States was 54 per 100,000, from 4.5 to more than 60 times the rates in the comparison countries. Death rates in Canada, Israel, and Norway were similar (about 11-12 per 100,000), all averaging about a fifth of the U.S. rate. Death rates in Scotland, The Netherlands, and England and Wales were the lowest, averaging 1 per 100,000.

The firearm death rate among males 15-24 years in the U.S. was 32 percent higher than the motor vehicle traffic death rate. In none of the comparison countries did the firearm death rate exceed the motor vehicle death rate. In Norway the relative difference between the two rates was smaller than in the other countries, with 12.2 firearm deaths compared with 18.6 motor vehicle traffic fatalities per

Figure 8.11. Firearm injury death rates among males 15-24 years of age for selected countries and selected years, 1992-95. SOURCE: Data provided by members of the International Collaborative Effort (ICE) on Injury Statistics.

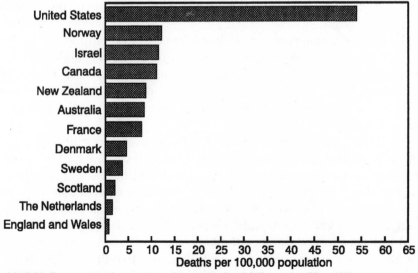

SOURCE: Data provided by members of the International Collaborative Effort (ICE) on Injury Statistics.

100,000 population. In Israel the motor vehicle death rate was twice the firearm death rate; in Canada and Australia, the ratios were 3-4:1; in New Zealand, Denmark, and Scotland the traffic death rates were 6-9 times the firearm death rates; and in The Netherlands and in England and Wales, the ratios were 13 and 24: 1.

The distribution of firearm deaths by intent differs by country. In the United States 63 percent of the firearm deaths among males ages 15-24 years were homicides, and 30 percent were suicides. In no other country, except for The Netherlands, were more than 25 percent of the firearm deaths homicides. Firearm suicide accounted for at least 70 percent of firearm deaths in Norway, Canada, New Zealand, Australia, France, and Sweden. NOTE: Countries were selected based on their representation in the International Collaborative Effort (ICE) on Injury Statistics.

Occupation

In 1995 occupational injuries in the United States cost $119 billion in lost wages and productivity, administrative expenses, health care, and other costs (1). From 1980 to 1992, 77,675 civilian workers died as a result of occupational injuries, at an average annual occupational injury death rate of 5.5 per 100,000 workers (2). The 1994 and 1995 occupational fatality rates were estimated to be 5 per 100,000 workers (3). In 1995, 6,210 fatal work injuries were reported by the Census of Fatal Occupational Injuries, 6 percent fewer than in 1994.

In 1994-95 transportation-related incidents accounted for an average of 41 percent of all occupational injury fatalities; highway traffic incidents were the leading cause of transportation incidents and accounted for 21 percent of all occupational injury fatalities. Highway traffic incidents were the leading cause of occupational injury death for male workers.

In 1994-95 assaults and violent acts accounted for 20 percent of all occupational injury fatalities, with homicide as the highest ranking component (16 percent of all fatalities) making it the second leading cause of workplace injury fatalities. Workplace homicides declined 5 percent from 1994 to 1995 (despite the fact that 12 percent of the occupational homicides in 1995 resulted from the bombing of the Federal building in Oklahoma). Robbery was indicated as the primary motive for workplace homicide; in 1995 about two-fifths of the homicide victims worked in retail establishments. An average of four out of five workplace homicides were committed with a firearm in 1994-

95. In 1995 homicide was the leading cause of death for female workers, accounting for 46 percent of their fatal work injuries.

These findings are due in part to the fact that females are not exposed, to the same extent as their male counterparts, to other high-risk working conditions such as work with heavy machinery and work at elevations (4).

Being "struck by an object" (mostly falling ones) was the largest component, 59 percent, of the category "contact with objects and equipment."

Figure 8.12. *Percent distribution of fatal occupational injuries, according to event: United States, 1994-95. SOURCE: Bureau of Labor Statistics, Census of Fatal Occupational Injuries.*

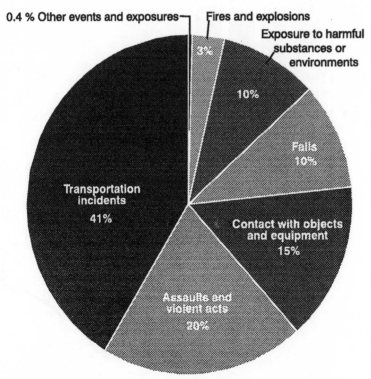

SOURCE: Bureau of Labor Statistics, Census of Fatal Occupational Injuries.

Figure 8.13. Fatal occupational injury death rates by occupation: United States, 1994-95. SOURCE: Bureau of Labor Statistics, Census of Fatal Occupational Injuries.

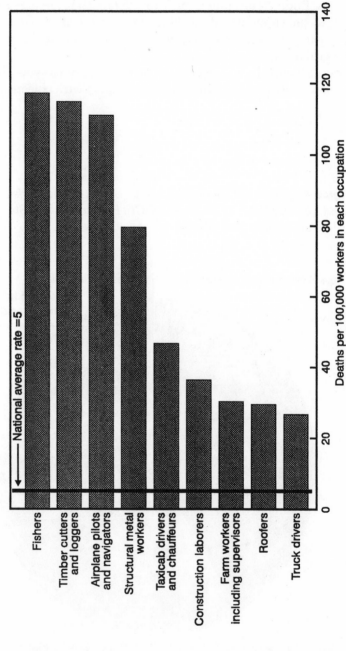

SOURCE: Bureau of Labor Statistics, Census of Fatal Occupational Injuries.

Falls to lower levels accounted for 9 of 10 falls, and contact with electric currents accounted for 56 percent of the "exposures to harmful substances or environments" fatal injuries.

Injury death rates for specific occupations measure the risk of incurring a fatal injury at work adjusting for the number of persons in the occupation. The average 1994-95 national rate of 5 per 100,000 workers is very low compared with rates in "high-risk" occupations (3). Occupations with large numbers of fatalities are not always those with the highest rate. The average annual number of deaths in 1994-95 was highest for truck drivers (756); their fatal injury risk, however, is much lower than for fishers, timber cutters, and airplane pilots (27 compared with 111-117 per 100,000 workers). Based on data from 1993, about three-fourths of fatalities among fishers resulted from falling from a boat or a capsizing boat; timber cutter deaths were often the result of falling trees or of transportation-related events (5).

The 1994-95 fatality rate for structural metal workers was 1.7 times the rate for taxicab drivers and 2-3 times the rates for construction laborers, farm workers, roofers, and truck drivers.

Structural metal workers were most likely to die as a result of a fall (5). Seventy percent of the fatalities in 1995 among taxicab drivers were homicides (6). The workplace homicide rate in 1993 was estimated to be highest for taxi drivers and chauffeurs, at 43 per 100,000 employed compared with the next highest rates of 11 per 100,000 for gas station attendants, sales clerks, and police (7). Despite different methods of data collection, the National Traumatic Occupational Fatalities Surveillance System is consistent in showing these occupations as high risk for homicide (4, 8).

Higher injury fatality rates in 1995 were noted for self-employed workers than for wage and salaried employees (11 compared with 4 per 100,000); for men than for women (8 compared with 1 per 100,000), and for older than for younger workers (9 per 100,000 for workers 55 years of age and over compared with 4 per 100,000 for workers aged 16-54 years) (3).

References

1. National Safety Council. Accident facts. Itasca, Illinois: National Safety Council. 1996.

2. NIOSH, personal communication based on data from the National Traumatic Occupation Fatality system. 1996.

3. BLS home page [WorldWide Website]. (Washington): Bureau of Labor Statistics; 1996 URL address: www.bls.gov/ oshcftab.htm.

4. Jenkins EL. Violence in the workplace. NIOSH CIB 57. 1996.

5. Toscano G, Windau J. The changing character of fatal work injuries. Fatal workplace injuries in 1993: A collection of data and analysis. BLS. Report 891. 1995.

6. 1995 News Release. CFOI report. August 8 1996.

7. Toscano G, Weber W. Violence in the workplace. Fatal workplace injuries in 1993: A collection of data and analysis. BLS. Report 891. 1995.

8. Jenkins EL. Workplace homicide: Industries and occupations at high risk. Occupational Medicine. State of the Art Reviews 11(2):219-25. 1996.

Section 8.2

Hospitalization

Extracted from NIH Publication No. 97-1232.
Health United States 1996-97 and Injury Chartbook.

Sex and Age

Hospital discharge rates from non-Federal short-stay hospitals for persons with a first-listed diagnosis of injury increase with age. In 1993-94 the average annual rates for children under 5 years of age and 5-14 years of age were 57 percent and 42 percent of the rate for young persons ages 15-24 years (90 discharges per 10,000 persons), and that rate is about one-half the rate for persons aged 65-74 years, and about a fifth of the rate for persons 75 years of age and over (412 per 10,000 persons).

Although injury discharge rates for males and females were similar (108 compared with 99 per 10,000 persons) for all ages combined, injury discharge rates vary considerably by age. At ages 15-24 years the discharge rates for males were twice those for females (119 compared with 60 per 10,000), while for the elderly 75 years of age and over, the rate for males was about 70 percent of the rate for females (322 compared with 463 per 10,000 persons).

Injury discharge rates for black males under 15 years, 15-44 years, and 45-64 years of age were 1.8-2.0 times the rates for white males. At ages 65 years and over, the rates for white and black males were similar. Among females, discharge rates for black children were 1.9 times the rates for white children and differences narrowed with age. For persons 65 years of age and over, injury discharge rates for white females were 1.4 times the rates for black females.

The average length of stay for injuries in short-stay general hospitals in 1993-94 was 6.1 days, similar to all non-injury causes (5.8 days). Length of stay for injury increases with age from about 4-5 days for children under 15 years of age to 7-8 days for persons aged 65 years and over. Average lengths of stay for males and females by age were similar.

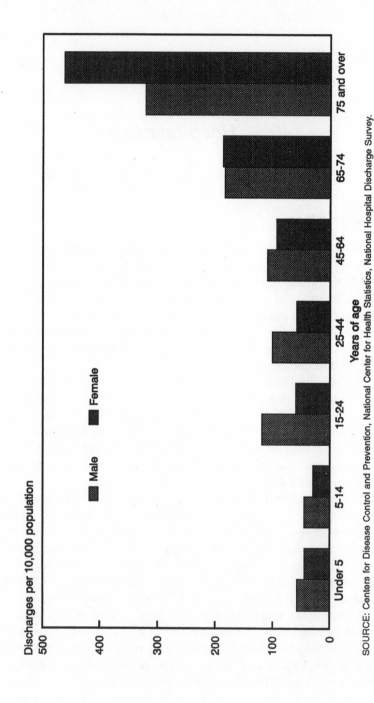

Figure 8.14. Hospital discharge rates for injury by age and sex: United States, 1993-94. SOURCE: Centers for Disease Control and Prevention, National Center for Health Statistics, National Hospital Discharge Survey.

SOURCE: Centers for Disease Control and Prevention, National Center for Health Statistics, National Hospital Discharge Survey.

In 1993-94, 9 percent of all discharges were for a first-listed diagnosis of injury. At ages 5-14 years and 15-24 years, 17 percent and 10 percent of all discharges were for an injury. For persons 25 years and over, 7-9 percent of discharges were for an injury. Differences by sex were greater for persons ages 15-24 years (31 percent among males compared with 4 percent among females) and for persons 25-44 years of age (17 percent for males compared with 5 percent for females) than for other ages. For both white and black males 15-44 years, 20 percent of all hospital discharges were for an injury compared with about 5 percent among females.

Hospital discharge data can include readmissions for the same injury and often include diagnoses not considered "true injuries"[1].

Reference

1.   Smith GS, Langlois JA, Buechner JS. Methodological issues in using hospital discharge data to determine the incidence of hospitalized injuries. Am J Epidemiol 134:1146-58. 1991.

First-Listed Diagnosis

In 1993-94 *fractures* accounted for 38 percent of all first-listed injury diagnoses among patients discharged from short-stay general hospitals. Poisoning and toxic effects (poisoning), open wound and injury to blood vessel (*open wounds and lacerations*), intracranial injuries, excluding those with skull fracture (*intracranial injuries*), and sprains and strains of joints and adjacent muscles (*sprains and strains*) were the next leading injury diagnoses accounting for an additional 25 percent of first-listed injury discharges.

Discharge rates for males for *open wounds and lacerations*, and for internal injury of thorax, abdomen and pelvis (*internal injuries*) were 3.1-3.4 times the respective rates for females.

Similarly, discharge rates among males for *intracranial injuries* and for *sprains and strains* were 1.8 and 1.5 times the respective rates among females. On the other hand, discharge rates among males for *fractures* and for *poisoning* were about 80 percent of the rates for females.

The average lengths of stay for fractures, intracranial and internal injuries were higher than for the other leading diagnoses of hospitalized injuries, about 6-7 days per person. For other leading injury diagnoses, the average length of stay was about 3-4 days. Average length of stay was similar for males and females for the leading injury of diagnoses.

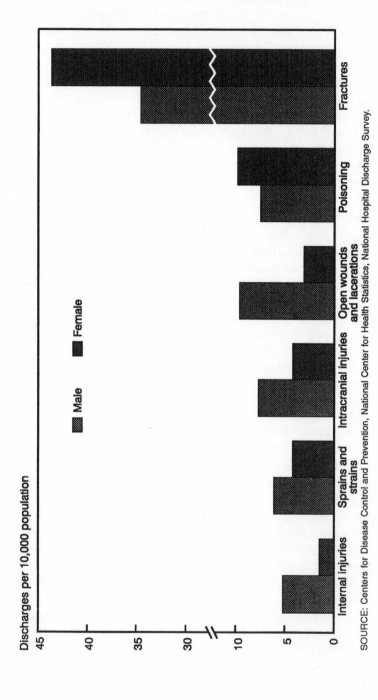

Figure 8.15. Hospital discharge rates for leading first-listed injury diagnoses by sex: United States, 1993-94. SOURCE: Centers for Disease Control and Prevention, National Center for Health Statistics, National Hospital Discharge Survey.

SOURCE: Centers for Disease Control and Prevention, National Center for Health Statistics, National Hospital Discharge Survey.

National hospitalization data cannot be used to study external causes of injury. In 1994 only 50 percent of discharges in which the first-listed diagnosis was an injury had an associated E-code.

Multiple injury diagnoses are not uncommon. In addition to the 1993-94 average annual 2.7 million discharges in which injury was the first-listed diagnosis, there were an average annual 3.3 million more discharges in which there was at least one secondary injury diagnosis on the patient's medical record. For both sexes fractures, and among males open wounds and lacerations were the most common second injury diagnoses.

NOTE: Complications of surgical and medical care, not elsewhere classified, accounted for about 23 percent of all first-listed and for 39 percent of all second-listed injury diagnoses. These diagnoses are not considered separately in the chartbook. They are included in the total count of first-listed diagnoses.

Fractures

Fractures were the leading cause of injury hospitalization, accounting for nearly two out of five discharges in each year, 1992, 1993 and 1994, in which the first-listed diagnosis was an injury. In 1992-94 the average annual discharge rate was 39.3 per 10,000 persons. The average length of stay for fractures was 7.4 days.

In 1992-94 among children under 5 years of age, fractures accounted for nearly a quarter of all injury hospitalizations at an average annual rate of 12.6 discharges per 10,000 persons. At ages 5-14 years, fractures accounted for 40 percent of injury hospitalizations at a rate of 16.5 per 10,000. At ages 15-24 years, 25-44 years, and 45-64 years, the fracture rates were higher than for younger persons averaging about 24-30 per 10,000. Fractures, however, accounted for a smaller proportion, about 30 percent, of injury hospitalizations than at the younger ages. By ages 65-74 years, the fracture rate rose to 67.3 per 10,000, and to 248.0 per 10,000 among persons aged 75 years and over. Three of five injury hospitalizations among the elderly 75 years of age and over were for fractures. The average length of stay for fractures increased with age from about 4 days for children under 15 years of age to 10 days for the elderly aged 75 years and over.

Among children 5-14 years of age, teenagers and adults ages 15-24 years and 25-44 years, fracture rates for males were 1.6, 2.7, and 2.2 times the respective rates for females. For younger children and for people aged 45-64 years, fracture discharge rates for males and

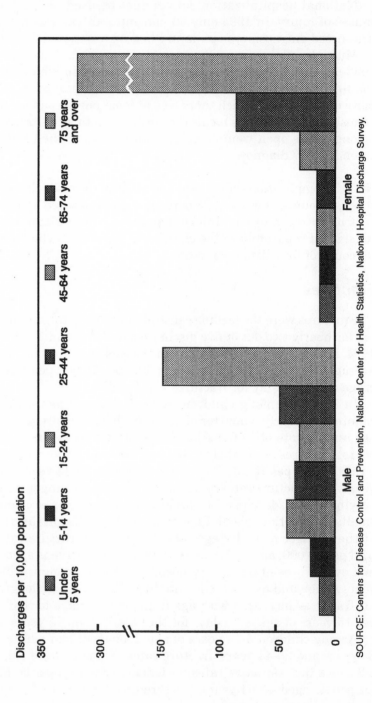

Figure 8.16. Hospital discharge rates for first-listed diagnosis of fracture by age and sex: United States, 1992-94. SOURCE: Centers for Disease Control and Prevention, National Center for Health Statistics, National Hospital Discharge Survey.

females were similar. For persons 65-74 years of age and ages 75 years and over, the fracture rates for males were about half the rates for females.

In 1992-94 29 percent of all fractures were to the hip (neck of femur). Among persons 75 years of age and over, three out of five fractures were to the hip; hip fracture rates at that age for females were twice the rates for males (186.1 compared with 90.2 per 10,000 population). The average length of stay was the same for elderly males and females, about 11 days. Among males 15-24 years and 25-44 years, fractures of the tibia and fibula, and ankle, as well as fractures of face bones were equally prevalent, accounting for 40 percent of all fractures in these age groups in 1992-94. Among females, fractures of the ankle were the most common fracture diagnosis, accounting for 19 percent of fractures among those 15-24 years of age and 30 percent of all fractures among females ages 25-44 years.

Other First-Listed Diagnoses

Poisonings, open wounds, intracranial injuries, and sprains and strains follow fractures as the leading causes of injury hospitalizations.

Poisoning. The average annual hospital discharge rate for 1992-94 for poisoning was highest among persons 15-24 years of age and lowest for children 5-14 years of age. Discharge rates for persons aged 45-64 years, 65-74 years, and 75 years and over were similar to the rate for children under 5 years of age (averaging 6-9 per 10,000).

Discharge rates for females 15-24 years and 45-64 years were 1.6 times the respective rates for males, and among young children ages 5-14 years, the rate for females was 2.5 times the rate for males. The average length of stay for a poisoning hospitalization was about 3 days for persons younger than 65 years of age, with slightly longer stays for persons aged 65 years and over.

The most common poisoning diagnosis among persons 5-14 years of age and 15-24 years of age was "poisoning by analgesics, antipyretics, and antirheumatics."

Open wounds and lacerations. Discharge rates for open wounds and lacerations were highest for persons 15-24 years of age, 12 per 10,000, and were similarly low for children under 15 years of age and for ages 45-74 years, at 4 per 10,000. Rates for males were higher than for females at ages 5-14- 65-74 years. At ages 15-24 years, the average annual 1992-94 rate for males was 4.5 times the rate for females,

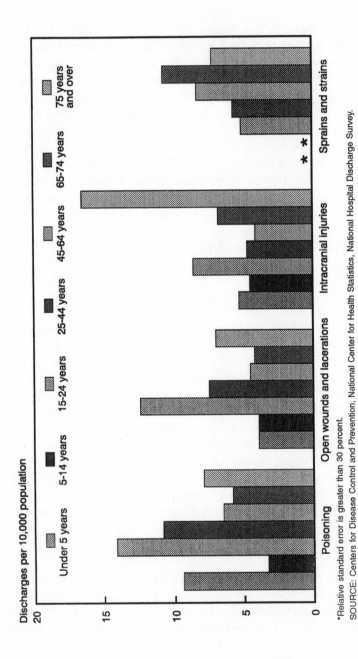

Figure 8.17. Hospital discharge rates for leading first-listed injury diagnoses by age: United States, 1992-94. (Relative standard error is greater than 30 percent.) SOURCE: Centers for Disease Control and Prevention, National Center for Health Statistics, National Hospital Discharge Survey.

*Relative standard error is greater than 30 percent.

SOURCE: Centers for Disease Control and Prevention, National Center for Health Statistics, National Hospital Discharge Survey.

20.2 compared with 4.5 per 10,000 persons. Average length of stay was about 4 days, with little variation by age or sex.

Intracranial Injury. Intracranial injury discharge rates were highest, 16.5 per 10,000, among the elderly 75 years of age and over. Rates for children under 15 years of age and for adults aged 25-64 years were similarly low, averaging 4-5 per 10,000 persons. At ages under 5 years to 45-64 years, discharge rates for males were 2-3 times the rates for females.

At 75 years of age and over, the most common diagnoses were brain (specifically, subarachnoid, subdural, and extradural) hemorrhage, following injury, and concussions. The average length of stay among the elderly for intracranial injuries was about 8 days.

At ages 5-14 years and 25-44 years, discharges after concussions was the cause of the largest source of gender differences.

Sprains and strains. Discharge rates for sprains and strains for persons 45-74 years of age and over were higher than rates for younger persons. The rates for males aged 25-44 and 45-64 years were about twice the rates for females at those ages.

At ages 45-64 years and 65-74 years, sprains and strains of the shoulder and upper arm region were responsible for most hospitalizations. At ages 25-44 years, in addition to the shoulder and upper arm area, knee and leg sprains and strains were more frequent among males and were the two regions of the body with large gender differences.

Section 8.3

Emergency Department

Extracted from NIH Publication No. 97-1232.
Health United States 1996-97 and Injury Chartbook.

Sex and Age

In 1993-94, 40.9 percent of all visits made to emergency departments were for injuries; the average annual number of injury-related visits made to emergency departments was 37.5 million. Forty-seven percent of all visits among males and 35 percent among females were injury-related. Injury visit rates for males 5-14 years of age, 15-24 years, and 25-44 years of age were, 1.2-1.8 times the non-injury visit rates for the respective groups. Among females 5-14 years of age, injury and non-injury visit rates were similar. For all other age groups among females injury visit rates were lower than non-injury visit rates.

For all ages, average annual injury visit rates for males were 1.3 times the rates for females (16.6 compared with 12.7 per 100 persons). Visit rates for injury were similarly high for children under 5 years of age and for persons 15-24 years of age and were similarly lower for people aged 45-64 years and 65-74 years compared with other age groups. At ages 5-14 years, 15-24 years, and 25-44 years, injury visit rates for males were 1.4 times the rates for females, and among those 75 years of age and over, the visit rate for females was 1.3 times the rate for males.

Emergency department visit rates for black males and females were higher than for white males and females, 23 and 17 per 100 persons compared with 16 and 12 per 100 persons. Rates for black males and females were higher than for white persons among children under 5 years of age and among persons aged 15-24 years, 25-44 years, and 45-64 years. Racial differences were larger for males ages 25-44 years and 45-64 years than for younger or older persons and were larger for females 25-44 years of age than for other groups. (Visit rates by ethnicity were not considered reliable.)

212

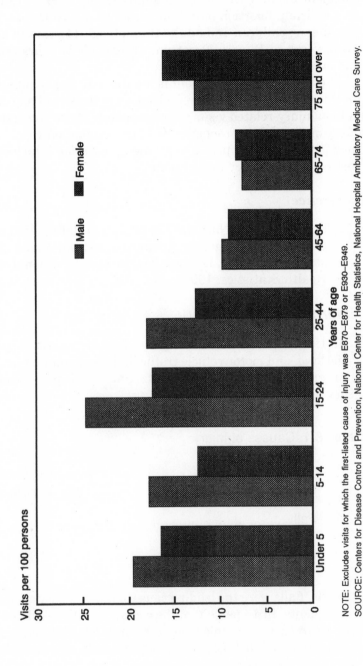

Figure 8.18. Emergency department visit rates for injury by age and sex: United States, 1993-94. NOTE: Excludes visits for which the first-listed cause of injury was E870-E879 or E930-E949. SOURCE: Centers for Disease Control and Prevention, National Center for Health Statistics, National Hospital Ambulatory Medical Care Survey.

NOTE: Excludes visits for which the first-listed cause of injury was E870–E879 or E930–E949.

SOURCE: Centers for Disease Control and Prevention, National Center for Health Statistics, National Hospital Ambulatory Medical Care Survey.

In 1993-94, 6.5 percent of the injury visits to the emergency department resulted in a hospital admission with no overall difference by sex. The proportion admitted varied by age from less than 5 percent among children and adults through age 44 years to 8 percent at 45-64 years to 18 and 29 percent at ages 65-74 years and 75 years and over.

The emergency department is not the only site of ambulatory care for injury. In 1994 physicians' offices were the site of an estimated 85 million injury-related visits [1]. Unfortunately, there is currently no way of estimating what proportion of injury-related office visits were for "new" injuries as opposed to follow-up care for injuries that were treated in emergency departments.

Reference

1. Schappert SM. National Hospital Ambulatory Medical Care Survey: 1994 summary. Advance data from vital and health statistics; no 273. Hyattsville, Maryland: National Center for Health Statistics. 1996.

External Cause of Injury

In 1993-94, three causes of injury—falls, being struck by or against something, and motor vehicle traffic injuries accounted for 18 percent of all emergency department visits, and for 43 percent of all emergency department visits due to injury.

Table 8.1. Causes of Injury.

Cause	Average annual visits in millions
Fall	8.0
Struck by, against	4.3
Motor vehicle traffic	3.8

Falls. Falls were the leading cause of injuries treated in emergency departments. In 15 percent of the cases, the fall was classified as one that occurred on the same level from slipping, tripping, or stumbling. In more than half (54 percent) of visits for falls, no detail existed about how the fall occurred.

Age-specific visit rates for falls are "Q-shaped" with rates nearly as high for the youngest as the oldest persons. In emergency department data, this age pattern was unique to falls. For persons aged 65-74 years and 75 years and over, rates for females are 1.6-1.7 times the rates for males. This is consistent with the higher fracture rates for elderly females. With advancing age, fall-related injuries, like all causes of injury, were more likely to result in hospitalization.

For example, among persons 75 years of age and over, one-third of visits caused by falls resulted in hospitalization, compared with less than 3 percent among persons under 25 years of age.

Impact. Being struck by or against a person or an object was the second leading cause of injuries treated in emergency departments. The shape of the age distribution curve is very different from that of falls. Rates were relatively high for persons 5-14 years of age and those aged 15-24 years and are lowest for persons 65 years of age and over.

Among persons younger than 45 years of age, visit rates were higher for males than for females. For ages 45-74 years, there were no differences by gender. At the oldest ages, rates for females exceeded those for males. It is not always possible to determine whether these incidents were "unintentional" or "assaultive" because if the intent was not specifically stated on the medical record, the coding default was unintentional. (This coding guideline was changed as of October 1996 to state that if the intent is not stated or unable to be determined, the intent code would be undetermined.)

Still, 12 percent of these visits for "struck" were for assaults. Unlike falls among the elderly, visits in this category are not likely to result in hospitalization.

Motor vehicle traffic. Motor vehicle traffic visit rates were highest for persons 15-24 years of age. Visit rates at each age group are similar for males and females. A comparison between the shapes of the age-specific death rate for motor vehicle traffic injuries and emergency department visit rates reveals that death rates were as high for those aged 65 years and over as they were for persons 15-24 years of age, while the visit rates were as low for the elderly as they are for young children under 15 years. This is likely the result of the severe consequences of motor vehicle traffic injuries among the elderly; once injured, they die before reaching the emergency department. Less than 10 percent of persons under the age of 75 years who were treated in emergency departments for a motor vehicle related injury were admitted to the hospital compared with 24 percent of persons 75 years and over.

Among teenagers and young adults 15-24 years of age, visit rates for falls, being struck, and motor vehicle traffic crashes were similar.

Other leading causes of injury visits include: being cut with a knife or other instrument (3.1 million average annual visits) overexertion (1.6 million average annual visits), insect or animal bites and stings (1.2 million average annual visits), and poisoning (1 million average annual visits).

Figure 8.19. *Emergency department visit rates for leading first-listed causes of injury by age: United States, 1993-94. (Relative standard error is greater than 30 percent. SOURCE: Centers for Disease Control and Prevention, National Center for Health Statistics, National Hospital Ambulatory Medical Care Survey.)*

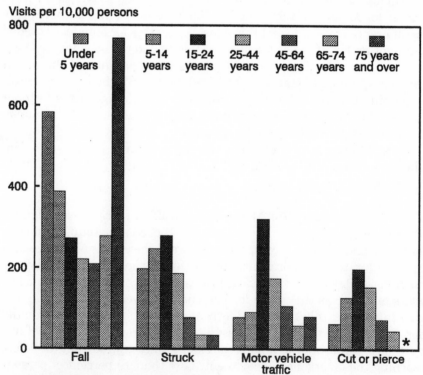

*Relative standard error is greater than 30 percent.

SOURCE: Centers for Disease Control and Prevention, National Center for Health Statistics, National Hospital Ambulatory Medical Care Survey.

Injury Diagnoses

Open wounds and lacerations, superficial injuries, sprains and strains, and fractures were the four leading principal injury diagnoses in emergency departments in 1993-94, accounting for 63 percent of all first-listed principal injury diagnoses.

Open wounds and lacerations. Open wounds and lacerations were the most common principal diagnosis among children under 5 years of age and 5-14 years, occurring at rates of 527 and 415 visits per 10,000 persons. The visit rate was as high as among persons aged 15-24 years (436 per 10,000). With increasing age, visit rates for open wounds and lacerations decline. For the youngest children through the adults ages 45-64 years, rates among males were two-three times the rates for females. Among those 75 years of age and over, rates by gender were similar.

Superficial injury. Superficial injury visit rates were higher for persons ages 15-24 years than for other ages (and were as high as the rates for open wounds and lacerations, and for sprains and strains.) Rates were lowest among persons ages 45-64 and 65-74 years, and were similarly high for children, for people 25-44 years of age, and for the elderly. Visit rates among males 25-44 years of age were higher than among females of those ages. At other ages, rates by gender were similar.

Strains and sprains. Visit rates for *sprains and strains* peaked at ages 15-24 years (435 per 10,000). There were no significant gender differences by age. Sprains and strains of the back were the most common site.

Fractures. Fractures were the leading type of injury visit to the emergency department among the persons aged 75 years and over. Rates among females ages 65-74 years and 75 years and over were 2 and 3 times the respective rates for males. In contrast, the fracture rate among males at ages 15-24 years was twice the fracture rate of females.

Among young children under 5 years of age, visit rates for poisoning were as high as for fractures, about 106 per 10,000. Visits for poisoning are highest in this age group. In addition, the visit rate for intracranial injuries in the 4 years and under age group was also as high as for fractures and poisoning. At ages 5-14 years, the intracranial injury visit rate for boys was 3 times that for girls.

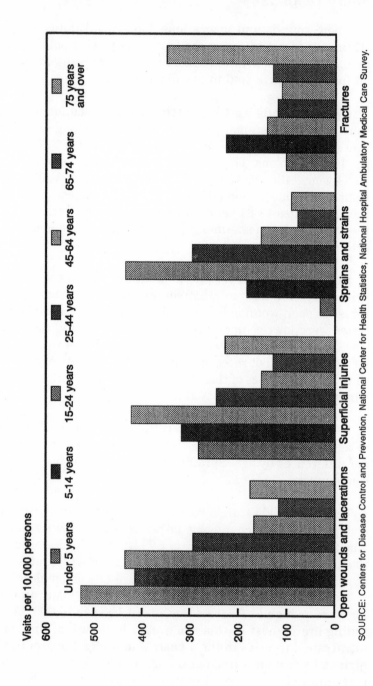

Figure 8.20. Emergency department visit rates for leading first-listed injury diagnoses by age: United States, 1993-94. SOURCE: Centers for Disease Control and Prevention, National Center for Health Statistics, National Hospital Ambulatory Medical Care Survey.

SOURCE: Centers for Disease Control and Prevention, National Center for Health Statistics, National Hospital Ambulatory Medical Care Survey.

Cause and Diagnosis

Of the average annual 8 million emergency department visits for falls in 1993-94, approximately one-fifth of each of the principal diagnoses were fracture, superficial injury, open wounds and lacerations, and sprains and strains. Sprains and strains, and superficial injuries were the principal diagnoses for three-fifths of the visits related to motor vehicle traffic injuries. In all, 18 percent of the visits had diagnoses not coded as injuries, half of these were categorized as "diseases of the musculoskeletal system and connective tissue disease."

An additional fifth were coded as "observation and evaluation for suspected conditions not found." For visits related to motor vehicle injuries, about one in four visits for children under 5 years of age were for observation for a suspected, but not found, condition (part of the non-injury codes).

In all, 86 percent of the principal diagnoses for falls were injuries (ICD-9-CM codes 800-999). The remaining 14 percent had first-listed ICD-9-CM codes that were not injuries. One-third of these were categorized as "diseases of the musculoskeletal system and connective tissue disease," and the remainder had diagnoses spread across the other disease categories.

Among young children who visited the emergency department for a fall-related injury, the most likely diagnosis was open wound and laceration while for persons 15-44 years, sprains and strains were more likely and among the elderly falls more often resulted in a fracture than in other types of injury.

Of the average annual 4.3 million emergency department visits for "being struck by or against an object or a person" superficial injuries, and open wounds and lacerations were the principal diagnoses for about three-fifths of the visits; 12 percent of the visits had a diagnosis of fracture. Nine percent of these visits had first-listed diagnoses that were not coded as injuries; 17 percent of these were categorized as "diseases of the musculoskeletal system and connective tissue disease." Regardless of age, most people were likely to have a diagnosis of open wound or superficial injury, although among the elderly 75 years and over, one-fifth had a fracture diagnosis.

NOTE: Because of the way in which the data are abstracted in the emergency department, there is no way to verify that the first-listed cause of injury corresponds to the first-listed diagnosis code.

Sports and Recreational Activities

Data from the Consumer Product Safety Commission (CPSC) can be used to estimate the number and rate of injuries associated with sports and recreation products that are treated in emergency rooms. In 1994 an estimated 4.4 million visits were made for all categories of sports and recreational activities. (CPSC data from the NEISS system.)

In 1994 the product groupings with the greatest number of associated injuries were basketball, bicycle and accessories, football, baseball and softball, and playground equipment. The CPSC estimated 2.4 million visits for these product groups. Basketball related injuries were higher among persons 15-24 years of age (955 injuries per 100,000 persons) than for younger or older persons. The rate of injuries associated with bicycles among children 5-14 years of age (908 per 100,000 persons) was similarly high. The rate for baseball and softball injuries was higher among children aged 5-14 years (411 per 100,000) than for younger or older persons, and was similar to the rates for football injuries among children 5-14 years of age and for injuries from playground equipment among young children under 5 years of age and children aged 5-14 years.

Estimates of sports and recreation injuries based on morbidity data from the NHAMCS-Emergency Department component are difficult to derive because there are many different external cause of injury codes that mention sports or recreational activities in the *International Classification of Diseases* (ICD), the system most often used to classify cause of injury in the United States. Some of the codes are only sports-related and some are partially sports-related. Further, there are few product codes in the ICD, making it more difficult to produce estimates. Using only the ICD-9-CM external cause codes that are specific to sports or recreational activities(and not the codes that are partially sports or recreation related), data from the NHAMCS-ED were used to make a conservative estimate of the number of sports and recreation-related visits made— approximately 1.6 million visits to emergency departments in 1994.

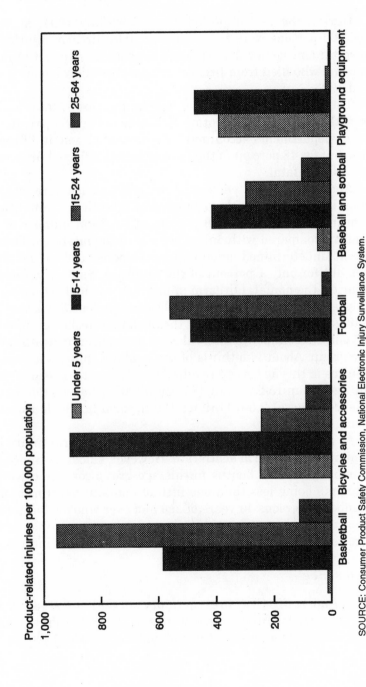

Figure 8.21. Selected sports and recreational product injury rates among persons under 65 years of age by age treated in hospital emergency departments: United States, 1994. SOURCE: Consumer Product Safety Commission, National Electronic Injury Surveillance System.

SOURCE: Consumer Product Safety Commission, National Electronic Injury Surveillance System.

Firearm Injuries

During the 2-year period June 1992-May 1994, an estimated 200,000 persons were treated for nonfatal firearm injuries in U. S. hospital emergency departments [1], about 2.6 times the number of persons who died from firearm injuries during calendar years 1992 and 1993.

The distribution of nonfatal firearm injuries by intent is different from the mortality distribution. Self-inflicted injuries treated in emergency departments accounted for 6 percent of nonfatal firearm injuries, but for 48 percent of the fatalities. Self-inflected firearm injuries are usually fatal.

Approximately 62 percent of nonfatal injuries were interpersonal assaults compared with 47 percent of fatalities. Unintentional firearm injuries comprised 18 percent of the total number of nonfatal injuries compared with only 4 percent of the fatalities. The category intent undetermined accounted for 14 percent of the nonfatal injuries but for only 1 percent of the fatalities. Similar to fatal firearm injuries, the nonfatal firearm injury rate was highest for persons 15-24 years of age and lowest for children under 15 years of age. For young people aged 15-24 years, the nonfatal rate, however, was 4 times (95 percent confidence interval 2.5-5.8) the firearm death rate in that age group. About two-thirds of the nonfatal injuries as well as fatal injuries in this age group resulted from assaults. The assault rate for the age group 15-24 years, (85 per 100,000) was 4.4 (95 percent confidence interval 2.6-6.1) times the firearm homicide rate for these young people.

At ages 45 years and over, the nonfatal firearm injury rate was similar to the firearm death rate. However, suicides comprised three-fourths of firearm deaths in this age group compared with suicide attempts being less than one-fifth of nonfatal firearm injuries. The number of persons 45 years of age and over who died as a result of a firearm suicide was five times the number who were treated for firearm related suicide attempts (95 percent confidence interval 4 to 10).

Reference

1. Annest JL. CDC firearm injury surveillance study. National Center for Injury Prevention and Control. Atlanta, Georgia: Centers for Disease Control and Prevention. 1996.

Section 8.4

Poisoning

Extracted from NIH Publication No. 97-1232.
Health United States 1996-97 and Injury Chartbook.

In 1993-94 the average annual emergency room visit rate for poisoning (106 per 10,000 children under 5 years of age) among young children and infants was similar to that for fractures, making poisoning tied for the third leading cause of injury visits to emergency departments. The average annual number of visits in which poisoning was the principal diagnosis in children younger than 5 years of age was about 210,000 (1).

In 1995 poison control centers managed over 1 million (1,070,497) potentially poisonous exposures among children under 6 years of age, accounting for 53 percent of all human poisoning exposures reported by the toxic exposure surveillance system (TESS). This effort by the poison control centers redirects exposures of limited toxicity from the emergency room to treatment within the home.

The child's home was the site of the exposure in 94 percent of cases reported to the poison control center. The frequency of exposures to substances in this age groups reflects not only the size of the market for the product, but its accessibility in the home.

Cosmetics and personal care products exposures caused the most calls to poison control centers for children under 6 years of age, accounting for 12 percent of all exposures among children in this age group. Cleaning substances accounted for 11 percent of the exposures, with 10 percent of the cases managed in a health care facility. Analgesics accounted for 8 percent of exposures, with nearly 17 percent of those cases managed in a health care facility. Plants, and cough and cold remedies each accounted for about 7 percent of childhood exposures; topical preparations for 5 percent, antimicrobial for 4 percent (64 percent of which were systemic antibiotics), and vitamins and gastrointestinal preparations for 3 percent of childhood exposures.

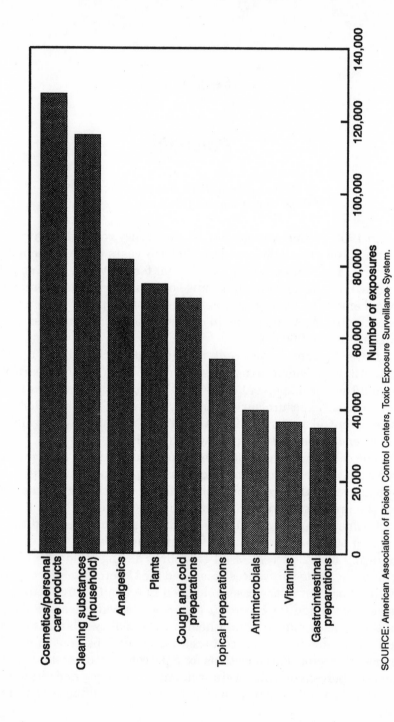

Figure 8.22. Leading exposures managed by poison control centers for children under 6 years of age: United States, 1995

SOURCE: American Association of Poison Control Centers, Toxic Exposure Surveillance System.

Reference

1. NHAMCS-ED. Public-use data tapes. 1993 and 1994.

Section 8.5

Injury

Extracted from NIH Publication No. 97-1232.
Health United States 1996-97 and Injury Chartbook.

In 1993-94 an estimated average annual 58 million episodes of injury, occurring at a rate of 23 episodes per 100 people, were reported in household interviews of the civilian non-institutionalized population of the United States. The rate was higher for persons under 45 years of age than for older persons. An injury episode was more likely to be reported by males ages 15-24 years and 25-44 years than by females of those ages. On the other hand, for persons 65 years of age and over, females were more likely than males to report an injury.

For infants and young children under 5 years of age and for people over age 65 years, the majority of injuries (53 percent and 56 percent) occurred in the home.

For the population aged 15-24 years and 45-64 years, 8-9 percent of all injury episodes involved a moving motor vehicle.

Among all currently employed persons ages 18-44 years, about a third of all reported injuries happened at work, 43 percent for males compared with 21 percent among females.

Injury episodes were more likely to be reported by persons who lived alone rather than by those who lived with others. At ages 15-24 years through 65-74 years, the rate of injury episodes for people who lived alone was 2 times the rate for those who lived with other people.

It is important to realize that the number of episodes of injury is equal to or less than the incidence of injury conditions because a person may

Figure 8.23. Episodes of injury by age and sex: United States, 1993-94. SOURCE: Centers for Disease Control and Prevention, National Center for Health Statistics, National Health Interview Survey.

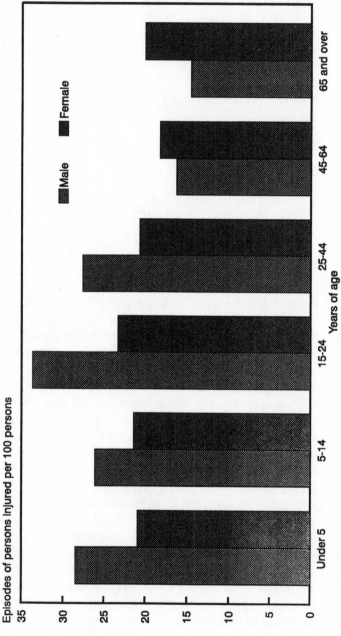

Episodes of persons injured per 100 persons

SOURCE: Centers for Disease Control and Prevention, National Center for Health Statistics, National Health Interview Survey.

incur more than one injury in a single episode. In 1994 there were an estimated 62 million reported injury conditions in the United States at a rate of 23.8 per 100 persons per year. Ninety-two percent of reported injuries were medically attended. The most often reported injury conditions were sprains and strains, contusions and superficial injuries, open wounds and lacerations, and fractures and dislocations, all accounting for about three-fourths of current injuries.

Chapter 9

Chronic Obstructive Pulmonary Disease

COPD—What Is It?

Chronic Obstructive Pulmonary Disease (COPD) is a term which refers to a large group of lung diseases which can interfere with normal breathing. It is estimated that 11 percent of the U.S. population has COPD and the incidence is increasing (2).

For a better understanding, it would be best to consider the two most important conditions that compose COPD: Chronic Bronchitis and Emphysema.

Chronic Bronchitis

Chronic bronchitis is a long-standing inflammation of the breathing tubes (airways) which are called bronchi. This inflammation causes increased production of mucous and other changes. The patient's symptoms are cough and expectoration of sputum (the spitting of mucus). The cough and expectoration must occur most days for at least 3 months per year, 2 years in a row. Other causes of these symptoms, such as tuberculosis or other lung diseases, must be excluded.

Chronic bronchitis can lead to more frequent and severe respiratory infections, narrowing and plugging of the breathing tubes (bronchi), difficult breathing and disability.

Emphysema

Emphysema is a chronic lung disease which affects the alveoli (air sacs) and/or the ends of the smallest bronchi (breathing tubes). The lung loses its elasticity (similar to an overused rubber band), and therefore these areas of the lungs become enlarged. These enlarged areas trap "stale" air and do not effectively exchange it with fresh air. This results in difficult breathing and may result in insufficient oxygen being delivered to the blood. In some cases, the patients also have difficulty getting rid of a waste gas called carbon dioxide. The predominant symptom in patients with emphysema is shortness of breath.

Bullous Disease

Bullous disease refers to spaces in the lungs greater than one centimeter in diameter when distended. Bullae can occur as one or many. In bullous disease, the lung structure between the bullae is normal; but in those with C.O.P.D. it may be grossly abnormal. In this condition usually there are no symptoms or signs. Only in advanced cases will there be symptoms of shortness of breath on exertion. Occasionally a bulla will rupture and produce a condition called pneumothorax (collapsed lung).

Note: While some patients with COPD have only chronic bronchitis or emphysema, most have some combination of both.

Causes of COPD

The causes of COPD are not fully understood. It is generally agreed that the most important cause of chronic bronchitis and emphysema is cigarette smoking. Causes such as air pollution and occupational exposures may play a role, especially when combined with cigarette smoking. Heredity also plays a contributing role in some patients' emphysema, and is especially important in a rare form due to alpha 1 anti-trypsin deficiency.

Symptoms (What the Patients Feel)

Patients with predominantly Chronic Bronchitis usually have cough and sputum for many years before they develop shortness of breath.

Patients with predominantly Emphysema usually have shortness of breath and develop cough and sputum during a respiratory infection or in the later stages of the illness.

Signs (What the Doctor Finds on Examination)

Chronic Bronchitis. Initially the patient looks normal, however as time passes the lips and skin may appear blue (cyanosis), there may be abnormal lung sounds, swelling of the feet and heart failure.

Emphysema. Initially the patients do not usually appear blue at rest but eventually appear underweight and visibly short of breath. The chest may increase in size from front to back (the so-called barrel chest) and lung sounds may be diminished.

Diseases Which May Complicate COPD

- **Cancer of the Lung.** It is well known that cancer and COPD are closely related. It has now been shown that patients with airflow obstruction have a higher incidence of cancer of the lung than those without obstruction.

- **Heart Disease**

- **Pneumonia**

- **Pneumothorax** (collapsed lung)

- **Sleep Disorders**

- **Pulmonary Embolism** (blood clot in the lungs)

Pulmonary Function Tests

Pulmonary function tests (PFT's) are various tests used to determine several characteristics and capabilities of your lungs. Your test results are compared to values considered healthy for your age, height, weight, gender, and race.

These tests will determine:

- The amount of air your lungs can hold. (Total Lung Capacity)

- How quickly you move the air in and out? (Forced Expiratory Volume)

- How well your lungs can transfer oxygen from the air into your blood? (Arterial Blood Gas, Pulse Oximetry)

- How well carbon dioxide can be removed from the blood? (Arterial Blood Gas)

- The response of your lungs to bronchodilators.

Your doctor will utilize this information to ascertain whether you do or do not have a lung problem. He or she will also use this information to help define your illness.

Some of the less complex tests are:

- **Spirometry:** While breathing through a tube connected to a recording machine the patient takes a deep breath in and blows it out as quickly and completely as possible. The results are recorded and analyzed. This test can be performed before and after the use of bronchodilators.

  This is probably the most useful and yet underused test in the management of obstructive pulmonary disease. Measuring the amount of air that can be forced out in one second (FEV_1) and the amount of air that can be completely and forcibly exhaled (FVC) and measuring the ratio of the FEV_1/FVC will give an excellent assessment of the amount of airway obstruction. This relatively inexpensive and reproducible test should be done during periodic physical examination, similar to an electrocardiogram and other routine tests.

- **Peak Flow:** This can be done by you conveniently and quickly anytime of the day. A portable, hand held device called a Peak Flow meter is used to take this measurement. It simply involves taking a deep breath and blowing into the Peak Flow meter as quickly and forcefully as possible. This test is especially useful in asthma, where it can be used to evaluate the changes in the severity of your asthma and your response to medication. An individual daily log of Peak Flows is useful to monitor asthma. Comparing any day's value to the patients' "personal best" will help determine the severity of your asthma at any particular time.

- **Arterial Blood Gas (ABGs):** An ABG is done from a sample drawn from one of your arteries. The blood is then analyzed by a special machine, which records the amount of carbon dioxide (waste gas) and oxygen in your blood. One of the uses of this test is to determine whether or not you need any extra oxygen.

- **Pulse Oximetry**: This test is performed by placing a special light clip on you finger, earlobe or forehead. The pulse oximeter uses light waves to indirectly measure the amount of oxygen in your blood. Done without the use of needles, the pulse oximetry can be performed at rest, while you are walking or even overnight while you sleep.

- **X-Ray Appearance in COPD**: In the early stages of the disease the x-ray of the chest may be completely normal. But in the moderate to severe cases a reasonably accurate diagnosis of COPD can be made with the plain chest x-ray and C.T. (Computerized Axial Tomography) scanning. The most common appearances in the chest x-rays are hyperinflation of the lung, depressed diaphragms, loss of blood vessel markings, reduced size of the heart, the presence of bullae and sometimes increased lung markings.

Treatment of COPD

There are a number of treatments which can help patients with COPD. The most important step, of course, is to stop smoking. An important self help maneuver must be emphasized at this time:

- **Pursed Lip Breathing.**

The various treatments can be separated into several categories:

Bronchodilators

(albuterol, pirbuterol, isoetherine, metaproteranol, terbutaline, salmeterol)

- **Beta-agonists:** This class of medication is most commonly used in an inhaled form. This can be either as a small canister that sprays a fine mist when pushed (known as an metered dose inhaler or MDI), or in a liquid form made into a mist to breathe by a machine at home. There are short and long-acting forms of both the inhaled and pill forms. NEVER USE THE LONG-ACTING FORMS (salmeterol) TO HELP ACUTE SYMPTOMS!! They take much, much longer to work than the short acting versions, and your symptoms may get worse before your medication takes effect. The advantage of the inhaled forms is that the medication is absorbed directly by the lung. This leads to fewer side effects from the medication. Correct use of your inhaler is very important. If you have difficulty using your inhaler correctly make sure to let your doctor know. Your doctor can prescribe either a different form of the medication, a different type of inhaler, or more instructions on the proper use of your inhaler. (See end of this section).

- **Theophylline:** Theophylline is a type of medication that can have multiple effects on your body's ability to breathe better. It can cause your airways to relax and open further, thereby making it easier to breathe. It can also improve the diaphragm's ability to contract. Also, theophylline can increase the clearance of mucus from your airways and help you clear excessive phlegm. However, theophylline can have side-effects that can limit its use. You may feel nervous, have tremors, or even feel nauseated. That is why your doctor may want to check the blood level from time to time to ensure that you are getting the correct dose. Theophylline can be given either in a pill form or as a continuous infusion when you are in the hospital.

- **Anticholinergics:** (Ipratropium bromide) This is a type of medication most commonly given by the inhaled route. There is also a liquid form available which can be used in a nebulizer. This medication can also help the small airways of the lung relax and open further, thereby making it easier to breathe. This type of medication works best when used on a regular basis and is not for acute symptoms.

Anti-inflammatories (Steroids)

(prednisone, methylprednisolone)

Since COPD may have an inflammatory component, your doctor may prescribe a steroid containing medication. The type of steroid contained in these preparations is not the type that builds muscle. Your body normally makes its own anti-inflammatory steroids, however, extra doses may benefit selected patients.

Steroids also can be given in several forms. The inhaled form delivers the medication right where you want it, straight to the lungs. If your breathing does not respond to the inhaled form your doctor may chose to place you on a pill form. An intravenous form is also available. Steroids have many side effects. This is why your doctor will try to get you off steroids as soon as possible. There is much less concern with side effects when using inhaled steroids, and this is the preferred form.

A Special Note on Inhaled Medications. Metered dose inhalers (MDIs) or hand held inhalers are a convenient, effective and safe way to deliver medications to the lungs. Because they are delivered locally and directly to the lungs, smaller doses of medication can be used. The beneficial effects of the medication can occur while the side effects are minimized. But, if the inhalers are not used correctly the medication will not get to the right place. At best, using perfect technique, only 10-20 percent of the medication gets to the right place. So, you see why it's important to use good technique.

Using Your Inhaler Correctly

- Begin by controlling your breathing. Use pursed lip breathing to help you slow down your rate of breathing and to help you coordinate the remainder of the steps.

- Remove the cap from the mouthpiece of the inhaler.

- Shake your inhaler for 5-10 seconds.

- Place the mouth piece in one of three acceptable positions.

- In your mouth with your tongue and teeth out of the way

- Resting on your lower lip with your mouth wide open or 1-1.5 inches in front of your wide open mouth.

- Begin to inhale as you press the inhaler. This is a very important step and will take practice to perfect.

- Inhale slowly for 5-6 seconds if you can manage. This helps the medication to get deeply into the lungs. Contrary to what most people think inhaling quickly makes most of the medication deposit on the back of your throat, not in your lungs.

- Slow is the way to go.

- At the end of the inhalation hold your breath for about 10 seconds.

- Exhale through pursed lips.

- If more than one puff is prescribed, wait a few minutes before taking your second puff and repeat the steps above.

- After your last puff, rinse your mouth and throat with mouthwash or water to help prevent dryness. This is essential if you are using inhaled steroids.

Rinse the mouthpiece thoroughly with warm water at least once a day. Let it air dry before assembling and storing it. If you are carrying your inhaler in your pocketbook, put it in a ziplock bag to keep it lint free.

Other Facts About Inhalers

- Do not use your inhaler more often than ordered or it may not be as effective when you really need it.

- Inhaled medicines obtained over the counter should not be used unless ordered by your doctor. Some of these medications can interact with your prescribed medicines in an adverse way.

- It is a good idea to mark the date you first started using a new inhaler so you can keep track of when it is getting empty. For example, if you use 2 puffs 4 times a day of your inhaler and it holds 200 inhalations, you will need to replace it in 25 days.

Spacer Devices

A spacer device is a tube that allows you to spray the medication into it before you inhale. It may also be useful in training first-time users of metered dose inhalers (MDI) and for people who are having trouble using their inhalers correctly. There are several commercially available spacer devices.

You may benefit from a spacer if you:

- have trouble pressing your inhaler as you breathe in.
- get yeast infections from inhaled steroids
- cough when you use the inhaler, or
- feel more comfortable using a spacer

The basic steps for using a spacer are:

- Control your breathing with pursed lip breathing
- Shake the inhaler and take off the caps of the mouthpieces of the inhaler and the spacer
- Place the inhaler into the spacer driver
- Place your lips around the mouthpiece of the spacer
- Depress the spray into the spacer
- Inhale slowly
- Hold your breath for 5-10 seconds

As you can see the steps are similar to using your inhaler without a spacer. A spacer eliminates the need to breathe in as you press the inhaler. *It is still important to inhale slowly and hold your breath.*

Oxygen

If your lung function is impaired severely there may come a time when your body cannot absorb enough oxygen from the air. That is when extra oxygen can be of benefit. Some patients only require extra oxygen while walking or exercising, some only at night. Others will benefit from around-the-clock use of extra oxygen.

The most common form of extra oxygen is delivered by nasal cannula. (A small tube carries oxygen from a tank to your nose.) You can have large tanks in your house for long-term use, or small lightweight and portable tanks for when you are on "the go". There are even machines that can concentrate the oxygen normally present in the air; these are stationary devices designed to be used in the home.

To decide if you will benefit from extra oxygen, your doctor should perform some special testing. Usually your doctor will want to measure the level of oxygen in your blood — a test called an arterial blood gas. Another instrument called the pulse oximeter can measure the oxygen of your blood without the discomfort of needles. This can be done at rest, while you walk, or even overnight while you sleep. Please Note: Long term oxygen therapy prolongs life in COPD patients who have low blood oxygen levels (Hypoxemia).

Lung Reduction Surgery

For certain types of COPD and in carefully selected patients a special type of lung surgery may offer improvement in lung function. This surgery removes damaged areas of the lung so that any remaining normal lung can function better.

In certain patients with COPD, parts of the lung enlarge greatly and form large 'balloons' (bullae) in the lung. This most commonly takes place in the upper lung area. The large 'balloons' contain part of the lung that does not work well and can 'crush' the rest of the remaining lung. By pressing on the rest of the lung, the lung cannot function as well as it could if it was allowed to expand normally. The surgery removes the large 'balloon' parts of the lung and allows the rest of the lung to expand again.

While early data suggest there is benefit in a select group of patients, it is still a major surgical procedure and should not be undertaken lightly. Prospective patients need to undergo very careful testing prior to consideration for this type of surgery. Your pulmonary physician along with a thoracic surgeon will be best able to decide if you will benefit from this surgical procedure.

Furthermore, this should not just be considered a single procedure. This surgery differs from other surgeries in that you will need to take part in an aggressive pre and post-operative rehabilitation program. The surgery is only part of the whole procedure, and this needs to be a carefully orchestrated complete package for it to have the maximal effect.

Transplant Surgery

While lung transplantation is currently being performed for some patients with late stage COPD, this is a highly invasive, complex procedure, which carries substantial risk. There are strict criteria for lung transplant recipients and there is a long waiting list. For these reasons, as well as the possible complications of any organ transplant surgery, this option is viable only in a very small, select group of patients.

Restrictive Lung Disease

Restrictive lung disease is caused by a group of conditions which decrease the capacity of your lungs and can cause difficulties in your breathing. Some of these include:

- **Lung conditions:** Examples include scarring from pneumonia, tuberculosis, sarcoidosis, and certain interstitial lung disease

- **Neurologic and muscular diseases:** These can interfere with the nerve supply and/or muscular strength of the chest wall and the lungs, affecting normal breathing. Examples: muscular dystrophy, multiple sclerosis and poliomyeletis

- **Structural abnormalities of the spine and chest wall deformities:** By physically altering the shape of the lung cage, these conditions can interfere with normal breathing. Example: kyphosis, scoliosis, and congenital or acquired deformities of the chest.

Asthma

Asthma is a breathing condition characterized by intermittent wheezing, shortness of breath, and widespread narrowing of the airways. It may abate either spontaneously or as a result of treatment. One characteristic feature of asthma is inflammation of the airways, resulting in swelling of the lining of the breathing passages. Another characteristic feature of asthma is airway hyper-responsiveness (which is an exaggerated airway narrowing). The inflammatory changes may be triggered or caused by extrinsic factors such as dust, pollen, animal dander, molds and other allergens. The airway hyperresponsiveness may be triggered by the above and in addition exercise, stress and cold dry air. There are a number of cases of asthma that are not brought on by any presently known external factors. This type of asthma is called intrinsic asthma and is also known as late life asthma.

Heredity, including allergies and certain occupational causes of asthma are also important and will be discussed at a later date.

Symptoms of Asthma

The severity of asthma may vary with season, climate, temperature and infection. There are usually symptom-free periods between attacks. The symptoms may eventually become more persistent.

- **Wheezing:** a very common symptom of asthma which is often present throughout the breathing cycle but most noticeably during expiration. This is often described as a high-pitched musical sound.

- **Breathlessness:** the most troublesome symptom of asthma. Patients describe a sensation of 'tightness' in the chest or an inability to catch their breath.

- **Cough:** a symptom in some patients with asthma. This can occasionally be the only symptom of asthma.

Diagnostic Tests

Physical exam, chest x-rays, and breathing are usually normal during symptom free periods. Routine lung function tests may be normal in between episodes of asthma. If asthma is suspected, your physician may order special testing. This testing, which is performed under careful supervision, requires inhaling a substance (methacholine or cold dry air) to help confirm the diagnosis of Asthma. An important pulmonary test which you can administer to yourself is called the Peak Flow.

Treatment of Asthma

The aims of asthma therapy are more than just the alleviation of symptoms, but the elimination of the cause of the condition itself.

There are effective therapies available now to control asthma. The step-wise approach to asthma treatment is as follows:

Step One-Avoidance. There are factors that are known to initiate (trigger) an attack of asthma.

(**Note:** These steps are for extrinsic asthma. They may not play a role in the so called intrinsic asthma for which there is no obvious cause.)

Among these factors are:

- Dust and especially dust mite
- Mold
- Animal Dander (e.g. hair)
- Pollen
- Cold, Dry Air
- Air Pollution, Cigarette Smoke
- Respiratory Infections
- Rarely, exercise can trigger the symptoms of asthma.

Things you can do to avoid/minimize your exposure to these factors are:

1. Thoroughly clean your home environment with special attention towards dust attracting items such as carpets, drapes, and bedding.

    - If possible, carpeting should be replaced with tile or linoleum.
    - Walls should be as bare as possible.
    - Drapery should be replaced with easier cleaning items such as vertical blinds.
    - Blankets and comforters should be washed frequently.

2. If you are allergic to a particular type of pet, and if complete avoidance is not possible, then you should at least not allow the pet into your bedroom or other rooms in which you spend a majority of your time. Shampoo pet frequently, especially cats.

3. Avoid contacts with people who have active respiratory infections.

4. Frequent handwashing decreases the transmission of infection

5. You may ask your doctor about yearly vaccination to prevent influenza (flu) and other infections.

Step Two—Medications

- **Bronchodilators:** (albuterol, pirbuterol, isoetherine, metaproteranol, terbutaline, salmeterol)

  This class of medication is most commonly used in an inhaled form. This can be either as a small canister that sprays a fine mist when pushed (known as an inhaler or MDI), or in a liquid form made into a mist to breathe by a machine at home. There are short and long-acting forms of both the inhaled and pill forms. NEVER USE THE LONG-ACTING FORMS (salmeterol) TO HELP ACUTE SYMPTOMS!! They take much, much longer to work than the short acting versions, and your symptoms may get worse before your medication takes effect. The advantage of the inhaled forms is that the medication is absorbed directly by the lung. This leads to fewer side effects from the medication. Correct use of your inhaler is very important. If you have difficulty using your inhaler correctly make sure to let your doctor know. Your doctor can prescribe either a different form of the medication, a different type of inhaler, or more instructions on the proper use of your inhaler.

- **Anti-Inflammatory Medications:** (prednisone, methylprednisolone) **Inhalers:** fluonisolide, triamcinolone, acetonide, beclomethasone, fluticasone

  Since asthma may have an inflammatory component, your doctor may prescribe a steroid containing medication. The type of steroid contained in these preparations is not the type that builds muscle. Your body normally make its own anti-inflammatory steroids, however, extra doses may be of benefit in selected patients.

  Steroids also can be given in several forms. Again, the inhaled form delivers the medication right where you want it, straight to the lungs. If your breathing does not respond to the inhaled form, your doctor may chose to place you on a pill form. An intravenous form is also available. Steroids may have many side effects. There is much less concern with side effects when using inhaled steroids, and this is the preferred form.

- **Theophylline:** Theophylline is a type of medication that can have multiple effects on your bodies ability to breathe better. It can cause your airways to relax and open further, thereby making it easier to breathe. It can also improve the diaphragm's ability to contract. Also, theophylline can increase the clearance of mucus from your airways and help you clear excessive phlegm. However, theophylline can have side effects that can limit its use. You may feel nervous, have tremors, or even feel nauseated. That is why your doctor may want to check the blood level from time to time to ensure that you are getting the correct dose.

The Next Step. There is impressive amount of research in asthma management, and in the near future we will undoubtedly see several novel and even more effective therapies. Keep an eye out, since we will post information as these new treatments become available. But, as always, the best source of information is your own doctor.

Chapter 10

Pneumonia and Influenza

Chapter Contents

Section 10.1

Facts about Lung Diseases

Extracted from NHLBI FY 1996 Fact Book,
Chapter 4, Disease Statistics.

- Lung diseases, excluding lung cancer, caused an estimated 228,000 deaths in 1995.

- Chronic obstructive pulmonary disease caused 99,000 deaths in 1995 and is the fourth leading cause of death.

- The four leading causes of infant mortality are lung diseases or have a lung disease component; rates declined between 1985 and 1995 for three of them:

  —Congenital anomalies (-26 percent).

  —Sudden infant death syndrome (-40 percent).

  —Respiratory distress syndrome (-62 percent).

  —Disorders relating to short gestation (+13 percent).

- Lung diseases account for 46 percent of all deaths under 1 year of age in 1994.

- Between 1985 and 1995, the total death rate for COPD increased by 13 percent in contrast with declines for other major causes except lung cancer; however, the age-specific trend in COPD is downwards for men under age 75 years and for women under age 45 years (not shown).

- Between 1984 and 1994, the percent increase in death rate for COPD and asthma was greater in women than in men.

- Asthma and emphysema are among the leading chronic conditions causing limitation of activity.

- Asthma is the fourth leading chronic condition causing bed disability days.

244

- Asthma and chronic bronchitis are present in at least 5 percent of the population in each age group from childhood to adulthood.

- Among 28 industrialized countries, the United States ranked twelfth for COPD mortality in men ages 35 to 74 years and seventh in women in that age group in 1993.

- Between 1984 and 1994, the prevalence of asthma increased for all age groups. Presently, 14.6 million Americans have the disease.

- The estimated economic cost of these lung diseases is expected to be $114.7 billion in 1997:
  - —$78 billion in direct health expenditures.
  - —$20 billion in indirect cost of morbidity.
  - —$16 billion in indirect cost of mortality.

See also charts and tables in Chapter 2, "Facts and Figures: Rates and Comparisons of Injury and Disease by Gender, Race and Age" and Chapter 5, "Diseases of the Heart: Facts About Major Cardiovascular Diseases."

Deaths From Lung Diseases, U.S., 1995

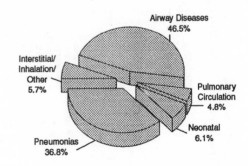

Figure 10.1.

245

Figure 10.2.

Death Rates for Chronic Obstructive Pulmonary Disease and Allied Conditions* by Gender, Ages 35-74 Years, Selected Countries, 1993†

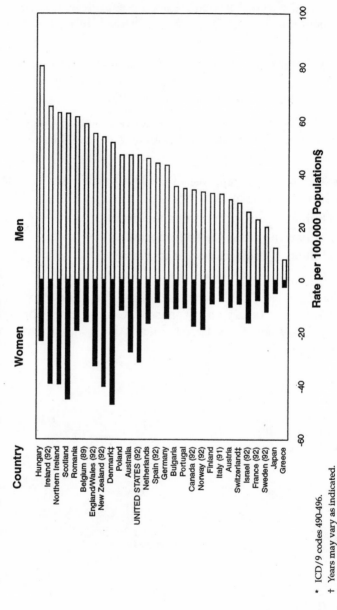

* ICD/9 codes 490-496.
† Years may vary as indicated.
‡ ICD/8 codes 490-493.
§ Rates are age adjusted to the European standard population.
Source: Published and unpublished data from WHO.

Figure 10.3.

Prevalence of Asthma by Age, U.S., 1984 and 1994

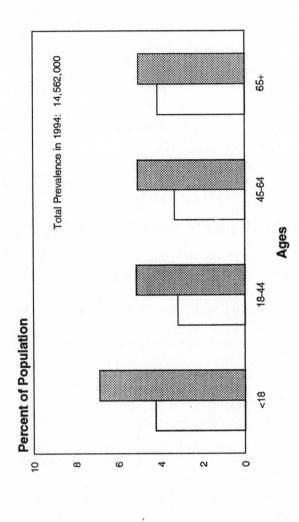

Percent of Population

Total Prevalence in 1994: 14,562,000

1984
1994

Ages

<18   18-44   45-64   65+

Source: NHIS, NCHS.

Section 10.2

Pneumonia

When You Can't Breathe, Nothing Else Matters

"Pneumonia" encompasses many different diseases that infect or inflame the lungs. Pneumonia is caused by a variety of agents such as bacteria, viruses, and mycoplasmas, among others. Pneumonia remains an important cause of morbidity and mortality in the United States; in 1994, there were an estimated 4.2 million cases of pneumonia, resulting in 64 million restricted-activity days and 40.0 million bed days.

- In 1993, pneumonia costs were estimated to be $7.8 billion in the U.S. This includes $1.7 billion in direct health care costs and $6.1 billion in lost earnings due to sickness or death.

- People considered at high risk for pneumonia include the elderly, the very young, and those with underlying health problems, such as chronic obstructive pulmonary disease (COPD), diabetes mellitus, and congestive heart failure. Patients with diseases that impair the immune system, such as AIDS, or patients with other chronic illnesses, such as asthma, or those undergoing cancer therapy or organ transplantation are particularly vulnerable.

- Pneumonia affects the lungs in two ways. Lobar pneumonia affects a lobe of the lungs, and bronchial pneumonia can affect patches throughout both lungs.

- The major types of pneumonia are bacterial pneumonia, viral pneumonia, and mycoplasma pneumonia. Other pneumonia include pneumocystis carinii pneumonia (PCP), which is caused by an organism long thought of as a parasite but now believed to be a fungus. Other less common pneumonia may be caused by the inhalation of food, liquid, gases or dust, and by fungi. Other diseases, such as tuberculosis, can cause pneumonia.

- Approximately 50 percent of pneumonia are believed to be caused by viruses and tend to result in less severe illness than do bacterial-caused pneumonia. The symptoms of viral pneumonia are similar to influenza symptoms, including fever, dry cough, headache, muscle pain, weakness, high fever, and increasing breathlessness.

- Viral pneumonia are less common in normal adults with a fully functioning immune system. However, most pneumonia in the very young are caused by viral infection, including respiratory syncytial virus (RSV).

- Pneumococcus is the most common cause of bacterial pneumonia. In healthy individuals, but especially when the body defenses are weakened, the bacteria can multiply and cause serious damage. Pneumococcus can cause serious infections of the lungs (pneumonia), the bloodstream (bacteremia), the covering of the brain (meningitis), and other parts of the body. Pneumococcal pneumonia accounts for 50 percent of all community-acquired pneumonia, and an estimated 40,000 deaths yearly.

- The onset of bacterial pneumonia can vary from gradual to sudden. In most severe cases, the patient may experience shaking/chills, chattering teeth, severe chest pains, sweats, cough that produces rust colored or greenish mucus, increased breathing and pulse rate, and bluish color lips or nails due to lack of oxygen.

Mycoplasmas are the smallest free living agents of disease in man, unclassified as to whether bacteria or viruses, but having characteristics of both. The agents generally cause a mild and widespread pneumonia. The most prominent symptom of mycoplasma pneumonia is a cough that tends to come in violent attacks, but produces only sparse whitish mucus. Mycoplasma are responsible for approximately 20 percent of all cases of pneumonia.

- Early treatment with antibiotics can cure bacterial pneumonia and speed recovery from mycoplasma pneumonia and a certain percentage of rickettsia cases. There are no effective treatments for most types of viral pneumonia, which usually heal on their own.

- Pneumococcal vaccination is effective in preventing invasion of pneumococcal infections. People in high risk groups are advised to receive the pneumonia vaccine.

- Pneumonia vaccine is covered by Medicare, as well as some state and private health insurance.

- The pneumonia vaccine is generally given once, although revaccination after 3-5 years should be considered for children with nephrotic syndrome, splenia, or sickle cell anemia who would be less than 11 years old at revaccination. Revaccination should also be considered for high-risk adults who received their first shot six years ago or more, and for those who are shown to have rapid decline in pneumococcal antibody levels.

More information about pneumonia, including the following materials, are available from the American Lung Association, 1-800-LUNG-USA (1-800-586-4872):

- Facts About Pneumonia: (Order #0029)
- Pneumonia News: (Order #1176)
- Pneumonia? Not Me: (Order #1326)

For more information on lung health, programs, and special events, call your local American Lung Association at 1-800-LUNG-USA.

Section 10.3

Colds and Flu: Time Only Sure Cure

FDA Consumer, October 1996 with revisions made March 1997.

It's not chicken soup. Believe it or not, a much more unorthodox therapy of warm-and-cold showers has recently been proposed—though not proven—for the prevention of the common cold. Shower therapy joins an ever-growing spectrum of suggested preventers and treatments for the common cold—among them, hand washing, vitamin C, interferon, seclusion, and various over-the-counter cough and cold medications.

"An efficient, practical and inexpensive prophylaxis [preventive measure] against one of the most frequent (and 'expensive') diseases has been identified at last," claims water therapy researcher Edward Ernst, M.D., in the April 1990 issue of *Physiotherapy*. Though some may doubt his shower theory, Ernst is right about one thing, the common cold is a frequent and expensive disease, striking some people as many as 12 times a year and leading to some 15 million days lost from work annually in the United States. Influenza, or flu, likewise, is a frequent and expensive disease, reaching epidemic levels in the United States each year.

Identify the Enemy

Flu is like the cold in many ways most basically, they're both respiratory infections caused by viruses. If a cold is misdiagnosed as flu, there's no problem. At worst, a cold can occasionally lead to secondary bacterial infections of the middle ear or sinuses, which can be treated with antibiotics. But if the flu is misdiagnosed as a bad cold, potentially life-threatening flu complications like pneumonia may be overlooked.

Some of the symptoms of a cold and flu are similar, but the two diseases can usually be distinguished (see Table 10.1). Typically, colds begin slowly; two to three days after infection with the virus. The first symptoms are usually a scratchy, sore throat, followed by sneezing and a runny nose. Temperature is usually normal or only slightly elevated. A mild cough can develop several days later.

Table 10.1. Is It a Cold or the Flu?

Symptoms	Cold	Flu
fever	rare	characteristic, high (102–104 F); lasts 3–4 days
headache	rare	prominent
general aches, pains	slight	usual; often severe
fatigue, weakness	quite mild	can last up to 2-3 weeks
extreme exhaustion	never	early and prominent
stuffy nose	common	sometimes
sneezing	usual	sometimes
sore throat	common	sometimes
chest discomfort, cough	mild to moderate; hacking cough	common; can become severe

Symptoms tend to be worse in infants and young children, who sometimes run temperatures of up to 102 degrees Fahrenheit (39 degrees Celsius). Cold symptoms usually last from two days to a week.

Signs of the flu include sudden onset with a headache, dry cough, and chills. The symptoms quickly become more severe than those of a cold. The flu sufferer often experiences a "knocked-off-your-feet" feeling, with muscle aches in the back and legs. Fever of up to 104 degrees Fahrenheit (40 degrees Celsius) is common. The fever typically begins to subside on the second or third day, and then respiratory symptoms like nasal congestion and sore throat appear. Fatigue and weakness may continue for days or even weeks.

"The lethargy, achiness and fever are side effects of the body doing its job of trying to fight off the infection," according to Dominick

Iacuzio, Ph.D., influenza program officer with the National Institutes of Health (NIH).

Influenza rarely causes stomach upset. What is popularly called "stomach flu" with symptoms like nausea, diarrhea and vomiting, is technically another malady: gastroenteritis.

Cold and flu-like symptoms can sometimes mimic more serious illnesses like strep throat, measles, and chickenpox. Allergies, too, can resemble colds with their runny noses, sneezing, and general miserable feeling.

If symptoms persist, become severe or localized in the throat, stomach or lungs, or if other symptoms such as vomiting and behavioral changes occur, consult your physician.

"With the typical symptoms, it's not necessary to contact your physician immediately," Iacuzio says.

The Treatment Arsenal

There is no proven cure for colds or flu but time. However, over-the-counter medications are available to relieve the symptoms. "OTC cough-cold products can make you more comfortable while you suffer," says Debbie Lumpkins, a scientist with the Food and Drug Administration's division of over-the-counter drug products. "They are intended to treat the symptoms of minor conditions, not to treat the underlying illness."

Don't bother taking antibiotics to treat your flu or cold; antibiotics do not kill viruses, and they should be used only for bacterial complications such as sinus or ear infections. Overuse of antibiotics has become a very serious problem, leading to a resistance in disease-causing bacteria that may render antibiotics ineffective for certain conditions.

Children and teenagers with symptoms of flu or chickenpox should not take aspirin or products containing aspirin or other salicylates. Use of these products in young flu and chickenpox sufferers has been associated with Reye syndrome, a rare condition that can be fatal. Because cold symptoms can be similar to those of the flu, it's best not to give aspirin to people under 20 with these types of symptoms.

The active ingredients FDA considers safe and effective for relieving certain symptoms of colds or flu fall into the following categories:

- **Nasal decongestants** open up the nasal passages. They can be applied topically, in the form of sprays or drops, or taken orally. But using sprays or drops longer than three days may cause nasal congestion to worsen.

- **Antitussives**, also known as cough suppressants, can quiet coughs due to minor throat irritations. They include drugs taken orally, as well as topical medications like throat lozenges and ointments to be rubbed on the chest or used in a vaporizer.

- **Expectorants**, taken orally, help loosen mucus and make coughs more productive.

Until recently, another category of over-the-counter drugs called "antihistamines" was approved only for use by sufferers of hay fever and some other allergies. In October, clemastine fumarate, the active ingredient in products such as Tavist-1 and Tavist-D, was approved to treat cold symptoms. The effectiveness of other OTC antihistamines for this use is still being studied.

Most nonprescription cough-cold remedies contain a combination of ingredients to attack multiple symptoms. These combination products often contain antipyretics to reduce fever and analgesics to relieve minor aches, pains and headaches.

Users of OTC medicines should carefully follow the labeling instructions and warnings. To help people understand the OTC labels, FDA is working with industry on new labeling that would use more consumer-friendly language and standardize the placement of important information from product to product.

The Cold War

OTC cough and cold medication sales totaled 3.2 billion dollars in 1995, according to a national industry survey. That's no surprise, considering Americans endure about one billion colds each year.

Children get the most colds—six or eight a year. By contrast, adults average two to four a year, with a greater frequency in the parents of children.

The high rate in children is blamed on their lack of a built-up resistance to infection and the close contacts with other kids in schools and day care. Women's closer contact with children may also explain the greater prevalence of colds in women than in men.

Adults over 60 usually suffer less than one cold a year, probably because they have built up a natural immunity.

Most colds strike Americans in the fall and winter. Contrary to what many people believe, the increased rate of colds during this time is actually not due to the cold weather. So why do more people feel "under the weather" during the winter months? Probably, say researchers at NIH's National Institute of Allergy and Infectious Diseases, because of the greater time spent indoors in cold weather, increasing the opportunity for viruses to spread among people. Also, the lower humidity during the colder months helps cold-causing viruses to thrive and may dry the lining of the nasal passages, making them more susceptible to infection.

Because the symptoms of the common cold are caused by more than 200 different viruses—most by the so-called "rhinoviruses" (from the Greek rhin, meaning "nose")—the development of a vaccine isn't feasible. To minimize the spread of colds, people should try to keep their defenses up and their exposure down.

First Line of Defense

Cold viruses can be transmitted in one of two ways: by touching respiratory secretions on a person's skin (when shaking hands, for example) or on environmental surfaces (like doorknobs or handrails) and then touching the eyes, nose or mouth, or by inhaling infectious particles in the air (like respiratory secretions from a cough or sneeze).

The best way to break the chain of infection? Hand washing is the key, according to Iacuzio, along with not touching the nose, eyes or mouth.

"Your mucus membranes are your first line of defense against infection," according to Iacuzio. "Interference with the constant passage of mucus raises the chances for entry of the virus." That's why drinking liquids and maintaining a humid environment with a vaporizer may lower susceptibility.

To minimize the spread, other helpful measures include avoiding close, prolonged exposure to people with colds, and always sneezing or coughing into a facial tissue and immediately throwing it away. Cleaning environmental surfaces with a virus-killing disinfectant is also recommended.

The Flu Fighters

Flu typically affects 20 to 50 percent of the U.S. population each winter. It's a highly contagious disease, spreading mostly by direct person-to-person contact. "With the flu, coughing, even more than sneezing, is the most effective method of transmission," Iacuzio says.

The flu virus can linger in the air for as long as three hours. In close quarters, conditions are ripe for the spread of the virus. That explains why the highest incidence of the flu is in 5- to 14-year-olds, who spend much of their time in school, in close contact with their classmates. The most serious complications occur in older adults, however.

Years ago, there were no practical tools to protect people from flu. In 1918 to 1919, a global flu epidemic, or pandemic, struck half the world's population and claimed the lives of 20 million. Still today, 10,000 to 20,000 Americans (almost all of them elderly, newborns, or chronically ill) die each year from flu complications, usually pneumonia.

The challenge for scientists trying to protect us from the disease is that influenza viruses can change themselves, or mutate, to become different viruses. Scientists have classified flu viruses as types A, B and C. Type A is the most common and leads to the most serious epidemics. Type B can cause epidemics, but usually produces a milder disease than type A. Type C viruses have never been associated with a large epidemic.

Vaccine a Powerful Weapon

The most important tool for fighting the ever-changing flu virus is immunization by a killed virus vaccine licensed by FDA. The vaccine is made from highly purified, egg-grown viruses that have been made noninfectious.

Vaccination is available to anyone who wants to reduce their chances of getting the flu. Studies have shown the vaccine's effectiveness rate to be 70 to 90 percent in healthy young adults. In the elderly and in people with certain chronic illnesses, the vaccine sometimes doesn't prevent illness altogether, but it does reduce its severity and the risk of complications.

The government's Advisory Committee on Immunization Practices strongly recommends vaccination for the following high-risk groups:

- people aged 65 or older

- residents of nursing homes and other facilities that provide care for chronically ill persons

- people over the age of six months, including pregnant women, who have certain underlying medical conditions that required hospitalization or regular doctors' visits during the preceding year. These conditions include:

    - asthma, anemia, metabolic disease such as diabetes, or heart, lung or kidney disease

    - impaired immune system due to HIV infection, treatment with drugs such as long-term steroids, or cancer treatment with radiation or chemotherapy

- children and teenagers (6 months to 18 years) who must take aspirin regularly and therefore may be at risk of developing Reye syndrome if they get the flu.

To reduce the risk of transmitting flu to high-risk persons, and to protect themselves from infection, the advisory committee recommends flu shots for people with regular close contact with high-risk groups. Such people include health-care workers, nursing home personnel, home-care providers, and children. Police, firefighters, and other community service providers may also find vaccination useful.

Because it takes the immune system about six to eight weeks to respond to vaccination, the best time to get the flu vaccine is mid-October to mid-November, before the December-to-March U.S. flu season hits.

The vaccine's most common side effect is soreness at the vaccination site for up to two days. Some people may experience post-shot fever, malaise, sore muscles, and other symptoms resembling the flu that can last for one to two days. Actually, the flu vaccine can't cause flu because it contains only inactivated viruses.

The vaccine should be repeated annually, since the immunity is believed to last only about a year, and because the vaccine's composition changes each year based on the flu strains scientists expect to be most common.

To decide which strains of influenza virus should be incorporated into the vaccine for the coming flu season, FDA's Vaccines and Related Biologicals Advisory Committee meets in late January each year to consider reports from national and international surveillance systems. A World Health Organization panel meets in Geneva in mid-February to make final recommendations for the next season's flu vaccine.

The strains are labeled by their type (A, B or C) and the place where the strain was isolated. In 1996, the predominant strains were A/Johannesberg, A/Texas, and B/Beijing. The anticipated strains for the 1996-1997 flu season are largely the same: A/Texas, A/Wuhan-like, and B/Beijing.

"In the not-too-distant future," says Iacuzio, "consumers may have alternatives to the flu shot, including different delivery methods like nasal drops or a spray." Major pharmaceutical companies, in cooperation with scientists representing NIH, FDA's Center for Biologics Evaluation and Research, and academia, are making significant strides, also, toward an even more protective vaccine.

Some people, but not many, should avoid the flu shot. People allergic to eggs and people with certain other allergies and medical problems like bronchitis or pneumonia should consult a doctor before getting a flu shot. And those with a high fever should not receive the vaccine until they feel better.

Pregnant women who have a high-risk condition should be immunized regardless of the stage of pregnancy; healthy pregnant women may also want to consult their health-care providers about being vaccinated.

In the rare cases when the vaccine is not advisable, two prescription drugs are available for prevention of type A influenza: Symmetrel (amantadine), approved by FDA in 1976, and Flumadine (rimantadine), approved by FDA in 1993. Either drug also can be used to reduce symptoms and shorten the illness if administered within 48 hours after symptoms appear.

When Cold or Flu Strikes

If, despite precautions, you do get a cold or flu, besides taking an OTC medication if needed and as directed, drink fluids and get plenty of bed rest. "Your body is trying to attack the virus," Iacuzio says. "Give in, and give your body a chance to fight off the infection. It takes energy to do that."

Many people are convinced that vitamin C can prevent colds or relieve symptoms. There is no conclusive evidence of this, but the vitamin may reduce the severity or duration of symptoms, according to the National Institute of Allergy and Infectious Diseases. But taking vitamin C in large amounts over long periods can be harmful, sometimes causing diarrhea and distorting common medical tests of the urine and blood.

Another proposed therapy, interferon-alpha nasal spray, can prevent infection and illness but causes unacceptable side effects like nosebleeds, according to the institute.

Many patients have their own, unproven theories about what works. "As long as it's not harmful, why not try it?" says Iacuzio. "But be skeptical of something that hasn't been clinically proven in a well-designed, placebo-controlled study." So what about chicken soup? It may soothe a sore throat, unstuff clogged passageways, and hydrate a thirsty body. At the very least, according to Iacuzio, "It's good TLC. Psychologically, that's important when you're sick."

—Tamar Nordenberg is a staff writer for FDA Consumer.

Chapter 11

Human Immunodeficiency Virus Infection and Other Sexually Transmitted Diseases

Chapter Contents

Section 11.1

Human Immunodeficiency Virus (HIV) and Acquired Immune Deficiency Syndrome (AIDS)

Public Health Service, U.S. Department of Health and Human Services, May 1997. NIH Publication NIAID Fact Sheet. NIH Office of Communications Web Site: (http://www.niaid.nih.gov/factsheets/hivinf.html).

AIDS—acquired immune deficiency syndrome—was first reported in the United States in 1981 and has since become a major worldwide epidemic. AIDS is caused by the human immunodeficiency virus (HIV). By killing or impairing cells of the immune system, HIV progressively destroys the body's ability to fight infections and certain cancers. Individuals diagnosed with AIDS are susceptible to life-threatening diseases called opportunistic infections, which are caused by microbes that usually do not cause illness in healthy people.

More than 500,000 cases of AIDS have been reported in the United States since 1981, and as many as 900,000 Americans may be infected with HIV. The epidemic is growing most rapidly among minority populations and is a leading killer of African-American males. According to the U.S. Centers for Disease Control and Prevention (CDC), the prevalence of AIDS is six times higher in African-Americans and three times higher among Hispanics than among whites.

Transmission

HIV is spread most commonly by sexual contact with an infected partner. The virus can enter the body through the lining of the vagina, vulva, penis, rectum or mouth during sex. HIV also is spread through contact with infected blood. Prior to the screening of blood for evidence of HIV infection and before the introduction in 1985 of heat-treating techniques to destroy HIV in blood products, HIV was transmitted through transfusions of contaminated blood or blood components. Today, the risk of acquiring HIV from such transfusions is extremely small.

HIV frequently is spread among injection drug users by the sharing of needles or syringes contaminated with minute quantities of blood of someone infected with the virus. However, transmission from patient to health-care worker or vice-versa via accidental sticks with contaminated needles or other medical instruments is rare.

Women can transmit HIV to their fetuses during pregnancy or birth. Approximately one-quarter to one-third of all untreated pregnant women infected with HIV will pass the infection to their babies. HIV also can be spread to babies through the breast milk of mothers infected with the virus. If the drug AZT is taken during pregnancy, the chance of transmitting HIV to the baby is reduced significantly.

Although researchers have detected HIV in the saliva of infected individuals, no evidence exists that the virus is spread by contact with saliva. Laboratory studies reveal that saliva has natural compounds that inhibit the infectiousness of HIV. Studies of people infected with HIV have found no evidence that the virus is spread to others through saliva such as by kissing. However, the risk of infection from so-called deep kissing, involving the exchange of large amounts of saliva, is unknown. Scientists also have found no evidence that HIV is spread through sweat, tears, urine or feces.

Studies of families of HIV-infected people have shown clearly that HIV is not spread through casual contact such as the sharing of food utensils, towels and bedding, swimming pools, telephones or toilet seats. HIV is not spread by biting insects such as mosquitoes or bedbugs.

HIV can infect anyone who practices risky behaviors such as:

- sharing drug needles or syringes;
- having unprotected sexual contact with an infected person or with someone whose HIV status is unknown.

Having another sexually transmitted disease such as syphilis, herpes, chlamydia or gonorrhea appears to make someone more susceptible to acquiring HIV infection during sex with an infected partner.

Early Symptoms

Many people do not develop any symptoms when they first become infected with HIV. Some people, however, have a flu-like illness within a month or two after exposure to the virus. They may have fever, headache, malaise and enlarged lymph nodes (organs of the immune system easily felt in the neck and groin). These symptoms usually disappear within a week to a month and are often mistaken for those of another viral infection.

More persistent or severe symptoms may not surface for a decade or more after HIV first enters the body in adults, and within two years in children born with HIV infection. This period of asymptomatic infection is highly variable. Some people may begin to have symptoms in as soon as a few months, whereas others may be symptom-free for more than 10 years. During the asymptomatic period, however, HIV is actively infecting and killing cells of the immune system. HIV's effect is seen most obviously in a decline in the blood levels of CD4+ T cells (also called T4 cells)—the immune system's key infection fighters. The virus initially disables or destroys these cells without causing symptoms.

As the immune system deteriorates, a variety of complications begins to surface. One of the first such symptoms experienced by many people infected with HIV is lymph nodes that remain enlarged for more than three months. Other symptoms often experienced months to years before the onset of AIDS include a lack of energy, weight loss, frequent fevers and sweats, persistent or frequent yeast infections (oral or vaginal), persistent skin rashes or flaky skin, pelvic inflammatory disease that does not respond to treatment or short-term memory loss. Some people develop frequent and severe herpes infections that cause mouth, genital or anal sores, or a painful nerve disease known as shingles. Children may have delayed development or failure to thrive.

AIDS

The term AIDS applies to the most advanced stages of HIV infection. Official criteria for the definition of AIDS are developed by the U.S. Centers for Disease Control and Prevention (CDC) in Atlanta, Ga., which is responsible for tracking the spread of AIDS in the United States.

In 1993, CDC revised its definition of AIDS to include all HIV-infected people who have fewer than 200 CD4+ T cells. (Healthy adults usually have CD4+ T-cell counts of 1,000 or more.) In addition, the definition includes 26 clinical conditions that affect people with advanced HIV disease. Most AIDS-defining conditions are opportunistic infections, which rarely cause harm in healthy individuals. In people with AIDS, however, these infections are often severe and sometimes fatal because the immune system is so ravaged by

HIV that the body cannot fight off certain bacteria, viruses and other microbes.

Opportunistic infections common in people with AIDS cause such symptoms as coughing, shortness of breath, seizures, dementia, severe and persistent diarrhea, fever, vision loss, severe headaches, wasting, extreme fatigue, nausea, vomiting, lack of coordination, coma, abdominal cramps, or difficult or painful swallowing.

Although children with AIDS are susceptible to the same opportunistic infections as adults with the disease, they also experience severe forms of the bacterial infections to which children are especially prone, such as conjunctivitis (pink eye), ear infections and tonsillitis.

People with AIDS are particularly prone to developing various cancers such as Kaposi's sarcoma or cancers of the immune system known as lymphomas. These cancers are usually more aggressive and difficult to treat in people with AIDS. Hallmarks of Kaposi's sarcoma in light-skinned people are round brown, reddish or purple spots that develop in the skin or in the mouth. In dark-skinned people, the spots are more pigmented.

During the course of HIV infection, most people experience a gradual decline in the number of CD4+ T cells, although some individuals may have abrupt and dramatic drops in their CD4+ T-cell counts. A person with CD4+ T cells above 200 may experience some of the early symptoms of HIV disease. Others may have no symptoms even though their CD4+ T-cell count is below 200.

Many people are so debilitated by the symptoms of AIDS that they are unable to hold steady employment or do household chores. Other people with AIDS may experience phases of intense life-threatening illness followed by phases of normal functioning.

A small number of people initially infected with HIV 10 or more years ago have not developed symptoms of AIDS. Scientists are trying to determine what factors may account for their lack of progression to AIDS, such as particular characteristics of their immune systems or whether they were infected with a less aggressive strain of the virus or if their genetic make-up may protect them from the effects of HIV.

Diagnosis

Because early HIV infection often causes no symptoms, it is primarily detected by testing a person's blood for the presence of antibodies (disease-fighting proteins) to HIV. HIV antibodies generally do not reach detectable levels until one to three months following infection and may take as long as six months to be generated in quantities large enough to show up in standard blood tests.

People exposed to HIV should be tested for HIV infection as soon as they are likely to develop antibodies to the virus. Such early testing will enable them to receive appropriate treatment at a time when they are most able to combat HIV and prevent the emergence of certain opportunistic infections (see Treatment below).

Early testing also alerts HIV-infected people to avoid high-risk behaviors that could spread HIV to others. HIV testing is done in most doctors' offices or health clinics and should be accompanied by counseling. Individuals can be tested anonymously at many sites if they have particular concerns about confidentiality.

Two different types of antibody tests, ELISA and Western Blot, are used to diagnose HIV infection. If a person is highly likely to be infected with HIV and yet both tests are negative, a doctor may test for the presence of HIV itself in the blood. The person also may be told to repeat antibody testing at a later date, when antibodies to HIV are more likely to have developed.

Babies born to mothers infected with HIV may or may not be infected with the virus, but all carry their mothers' antibodies to HIV for several months. If these babies lack symptoms, a definitive diagnosis of HIV infection using standard antibody tests cannot be made until after 15 months of age. By then, babies are unlikely to still carry their mothers' antibodies and will have produced their own, if they are infected. New technologies to detect HIV itself are being used to more accurately determine HIV infection in infants between ages 3 months and 15 months. A number of blood tests are being evaluated to determine if they can diagnose HIV infection in babies younger than three months.

Treatment

When AIDS first surfaced in the United States, no drugs were available to combat the underlying immune deficiency and few treatments existed for the opportunistic diseases that resulted. Over the past 10 years, however, therapies have been developed to fight both HIV infection and its associated infections and cancers.

The Food and Drug Administration has approved a number of drugs for the treatment of HIV infection. The first group of drugs used to treat HIV infection, called reverse transcriptase (RT) inhibitors, interrupt an early stage of virus replication. Included in this class of drugs are AZT (also known as zidovudine), ddC (zalcitabine), ddI (dideoxyinosine), d4T (stavudine), and 3TC (lamivudine). These drugs may slow the spread of HIV in the body and delay the onset of opportunistic infections. Importantly, they do not prevent transmission of HIV to other individuals.

Non-nucleoside reverse transcriptase inhibitors (NNRTIs) such as delvaridine (Rescriptor) and nevirapine (Viramune) are also available for use in combination with other antiretroviral drugs.

More recently, a second class of drugs has been approved for treating HIV infection. These drugs, called protease inhibitors, interrupt virus replication at a later step in its life cycle. They include ritonavir (Norvir), saquinavir (Invirase), indinavir (Crixivan), and nelfinavir (Viracept). Because HIV can become resistant to both classes of drugs, combination treatment using both is necessary to effectively suppress the virus.

Currently available antiretroviral drugs do not cure people of HIV infection or AIDS, however, and they all have side effects that can be severe. AZT may cause a depletion of red or white blood cells, especially when taken in the later stages of the disease. If the loss of blood cells is severe, treatment with AZT must be stopped. DdI can cause an inflammation of the pancreas and painful nerve damage.

The most common side effects associated with protease inhibitors include nausea, diarrhea and other gastrointestinal symptoms. In addition, protease inhibitors can interact with other drugs resulting in serious side effects.

A number of drugs are available to help treat opportunistic infections to which people with HIV are especially prone. These drugs include foscarnet and ganciclovir, used to treat cytomegalovirus eye infections, fluconazole to treat yeast and other fungal infections, and TMP/SMX or pentamidine to treat *Pneumocystis carinii* pneumonia (PCP).

In addition to antiretroviral therapy, adults with HIV whose CD4+ T-cell counts drop below 200 are given treatment to prevent the occurrence of PCP, which is one of the most common and deadly opportunistic infections associated with HIV. Children are given PCP preventive therapy when their CD4+ T-cell counts drop to levels considered below normal for their age group. Regardless of their CD4+ T-cell counts, HIV-infected children and adults who have survived an episode of PCP are given drugs for the rest of their lives to prevent a recurrence of the pneumonia.

HIV-infected individuals who develop Kaposi's sarcoma or other cancers are treated with radiation, chemotherapy or injections of alpha interferon, a genetically engineered naturally occurring protein.

Prevention

Since no vaccine for HIV is available, the only way to prevent infection by the virus is to avoid behaviors that put a person at risk of infection, such as sharing needles and having unprotected sex.

Because many people infected with HIV have no symptoms, there is no way of knowing with certainty whether a sexual partner is infected unless he or she has been repeatedly tested for the virus or has not engaged in any risky behavior. The Public Health Service recommends that people either abstain from sex or protect themselves by using latex condoms whenever having oral, anal or vaginal sex with someone they aren't certain is free of HIV or other sexually transmitted diseases. Only condoms made of latex should be used, and water-based lubricants should be used with latex condoms.

Although some laboratory evidence shows that spermicides can kill HIV organisms, scientists are still evaluating the usefulness of spermicides in preventing HIV infection.

The risk of HIV transmission from a pregnant woman to her fetus is significantly reduced if she takes AZT during pregnancy, labor and delivery, and her baby takes it for the first six weeks of life.

Research

NIAID-supported investigators are conducting an abundance of research on HIV infection, including the development and testing of HIV vaccines and new therapies for the disease and some of its associated conditions. More than a dozen HIV vaccines are being tested in people, and many drugs for HIV infection or AIDS-associated opportunistic infections are either in development or being tested. Researchers also are investigating exactly how HIV damages the immune system. This research is suggesting new and more effective targets for drugs and vaccines. NIAID-supported investigators also continue to document how the disease progresses in different people.

For information about studies of new HIV therapies, call the AIDS Clinical Trials Information Service:

1-800-TRIALS-A
1-800-243-7012 (TDD/Deaf Access)

For federally approved treatment guidelines on HIV/AIDS, call the HIV/AIDS Treatment Information Service:

1-800-HIV-0440
1-800-243-7012 (TDD/Deaf Access)

NIAID, a component of the National Institutes of Health, supports research on AIDS, tuberculosis and other infectious diseases as well as allergies and immunology.

Section 11.2

AIDS Deaths Decline in 1996

HIV/AIDS Trends Provide Evidence of Success in HIV Prevention and Treatment, Centers for Disease Control *Update*, March 1997.

AIDS Deaths Decline for First Time

For the first time in the epidemic, there has been a marked decrease in deaths among people with AIDS. The decline in deaths is likely due to both the slowing of the epidemic overall and to improved treatments over the past several years, which have lengthened the lifespan of people with AIDS. While it is too soon to determine the impact protease inhibitors will have on these trends, these drugs promise to further lengthen the lifespan of individuals living with HIV. Additionally, the estimated number of people diagnosed with AIDS each year (AIDS incidence) continued to slow, with an increase of only 2 percent in 1995, reflecting in part the ongoing success of prevention efforts.

As treatment advances continue to improve survival, we will face a number of key challenges:

* First, if the number of new HIV infections each year (HIV incidence) remains stable or increases, and deaths continue to decrease there will be an increasing number of people living with HIV and AIDS. Additional resources will likely be needed for services, treatment, and care.

267

- Second, to continue to provide the necessary data to plan, direct, and evaluate HIV prevention efforts, HIV/AIDS surveillance systems must adapt to changes in medical practices which increase survive following diagnosis of HIV or AIDS. If progression to AIDS is successfully delayed for an increasing number of individuals, AIDS case reports may no longer provide a reliable indication of trends in the epidemic and will under-represent the need for treatment services. Surveillance systems will therefore need to improve methods to monitor the number of individuals with HIV infection.

- And finally, as we continue to work to develop better treatment options, we must not lose sight of the fact that preventing HIV infection reduces the number of people who need to undergo complex costly treatment regimens. Prevention remains our best and most cost-effective approach for bringing the HIV/AIDS epidemic under control and saving lives.

The 1996 Data: Trends in Case Reports, Estimated AIDS Incidence and Deaths

AIDS Cases Reported Through December 1996

- 581,429 people with AIDS have been reported to data.

- Of these, 488,300 (84 percent) were men, 85,500 (15 percent) were women, and 7,629 (1 percent) were children.

- In 1996 blacks accounted for a larger proportion of AIDS cases (41 percent) than whites for the first time.

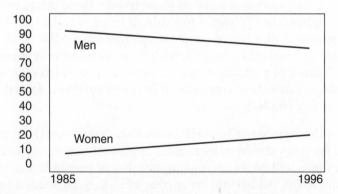

Figure 11.1. *Proportion of newly reported AIDS cases by gender.*

Women account for an increasing proportion of newly reported AIDS cases. The proportion of female adult and adolescent AIDS cases increased from 7 percent of the annual total in 1985 to 20 percent in 1996. In contrast, the proportion of male adult and adolescent AIDS cases decreased from 93 percent of the annual total in 1985 to 80 percent in 1996.

Trends in AIDS Incidence Through 1995

Between 1994 and 1995, the estimated number of people diagnosed with AIDS (AIDS incidence) increased 2 percent from 61,200 to 62,200 These estimates reflect a slowing in the growth of the epidemic, with an average of 15,200 people diagnosed each quarter between January 1994 and June 1996. Hopefully, with a combined strategy to prevent new infections and to provide early diagnosis and treatment for people who are infected, AIDS incidence will soon begin to decline.

During 1995:

- AIDS incidence rates per 100,000 people in the population were seven times higher among backs (99) than among whites (15) and three times higher among Hispanics (50) than among whites.

- AIDS incidence rues were much lower among women (10) than among men (48).

- AIDS incidence remained relatively constant among men who have sex with men (decline of 2 percent) and IDUs (increase of 2 percent), but continued to increase substantially among people infected heterosexually (17 percent increase).

Trends in Mortality

In 1995, the CDC AIDS surveillance system documented approximately 50,000 AIDS deaths. The year 1995 marked the smallest increase to date in AIDS deaths. During the first two quarters of 1996, the estimated number of AIDS deaths (22,000) was 13 percent less than the estimated number of AIDS deaths during the first two quarters of 1995 (24,900), marking the first decline in AIDS deaths since the beginning of the epidemic. Not surprisingly, trends in AIDS deaths closely parallel trends documented recently in AIDS incidence. AIDS deaths have not declined among women or among heterosexuals.

AIDS deaths declined in all four regions of the country (Northeast 15 percent, South 8 percent, Midwest 11 percent, West 16 percent). Deaths declined among men by 15 percent but increased among women by 3 percent. Deaths declined among MSM by 18 percent and 69 percent among IDUs but increased 3 percent among heterosexuals. Deaths declined among all racial/ethnic groups, but declines were greater among whites (21 percent) than among blacks (2 percent) and Hispanics (10 percent).

HIV infection remains the leading cause of death among 25-44 year olds, accounting for 19 percent of deaths in this age group.

Trends in Aids Prevalence:

- The number of people living with AIDS continues to increase. As of mid-1996, an estimated 223,000 people were living with AIDS.

- AIDS prevalence has increased 10 percent since mid-1995.

- The largest number of people living with AIDS by risk category are MSM (44 percent), followed by IDU (26 percent), and heterosexuals (12 percent).

- The greatest proportionate increase in AIDS prevalence from mid-1995 to mid-1996 occurred among those infected heterosexually (19 percent), while the greatest increase in the number of people living with AIDS occurred among MSM (5,100).

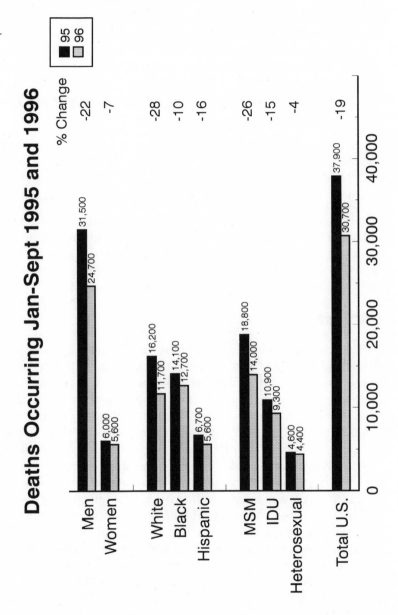

Figure 11.2. Estimated Number and Percent Change in AIDS-Deaths.

Section 11.3

New Ways to Prevent and Treat AIDS

NIH pub No. 97-1268. *FDA Consumer*, May 1997. This article originally appeared in the January-February 1997 *FDA Consumer*. The version below is from a reprint of the original article and contains revisions made in May 1997.

Preventing and treating AIDS is one of the Food and Drug Administration's top priorities. A new class of drugs, a home blood test collection kit, an oral diagnostic test, an HIV antigen test, an HIV-1 antigen test for blood supply, and an HIV viral load test are among the most recent in a long line of products FDA has approved to prevent, diagnose and treat infection with HIV, the virus that causes AIDS.

HIV Tests

The 1992 National Health Interview Survey by the Centers for Disease Control and Prevention found that only 20 percent of people at increased risk for HIV infection—such as intravenous drug users, male homosexuals, and prostitutes—agreed to be tested for HIV. More than twice that many people in the same risk group said they might use a home testing and counseling service if one were available. At the time, however, testing could only be done by a professional.

The situation changed when, on May 14, 1996, FDA approved Confide, the first HIV test system with a home-use blood collection kit. A second test kit was approved last July. It is hoped that home testing will make diagnosis easier and more accessible, especially in populations among whom the recent rise in cases of HIV is greatest, such as women, African Americans, and Hispanics. The tests are highly reliable and are designed to protect the user's anonymity.

FDA's approval on June 3, 1996, of OraSure Western blot, a laboratory test that does not require a blood sample, is also expected to increase participation in testing for HIV. Instead of pricking a finger—a procedure shunned by many individuals—OraSure uses a treated cotton pad to collect an oral specimen from between the gum and cheek.

The sample is tested for antibodies to HIV by a procedure that has been shown to be highly accurate. An earlier version of OraSure used a less reliable method to screen for HIV antibodies, and people who tested positive had to undergo a standard blood test to confirm the presence of the virus.

In March 1996, FDA approved the Coulter HIV-1 p24 Antigen Assay, the first blood screening test to detect antigens rather than antibodies. In screening routinely carried out since the mid-1980s, technicians check donated blood for HIV-1 antibodies by using enzyme-linked immunosorbent assay (ELISA) test kits. Since a small number of ELISA test results are nonspecific or falsely positive, the standard procedure uses a second, more specific test—the Western blot test—to validate the positive results from ELISA testing.

The Coulter test, which is used in addition to ELISA, screens blood for antigens—proteins found on the surface of the virus—that are detectable about one week earlier than HIV antibodies. The new test reduces the so-called "window" period, typically up to three months long, during which standard blood tests show no HIV antibodies, even though the donor may be infected.

The Amplicor HIV-1 Monitor Test, another new blood test approved last year, enables physicians to predict the risk of HIV disease progression by precisely measuring virus levels in blood. The test, which amplifies copies of genetic material from the virus by using polymerase chain reaction technology, is based on clinical studies showing that higher virus levels can be correlated with increased risk that the disease will progress to AIDS, and AIDS-related infection or death.

Condoms

Other than abstinence, latex-rubber condoms are the best protection against sexual transmission of HIV. Latex condoms should always be used for oral, anal and vaginal sex in any relationship that isn't mutually monogamous, and if there is any other chance that either partner may be infected. Condom manufacturers in the United States electronically test all condoms for holes and weak spots. In addition, FDA requires manufacturers to use a water test to examine samples from each batch of condoms for leakage. If the test detects a defect rate of more than 4 per 1,000, the entire lot is discarded.

The agency also encourages manufacturers to test samples of their products for breakage by using an air burst test in accordance with specifications of the International Standards Organization.

Under an FDA proposal, the labeling on latex condoms should state that "this product contains natural rubber latex." FDA has also requested manufacturers to state on the label that "[if] used properly, latex condoms will help reduce the risk of transmission of HIV infection (AIDS) and many other sexually-transmitted diseases."

Consumers should make sure the condom package is undamaged, and check each condom for damage as it is unrolled to be used. The condom should not be used if it is gummy or brittle, discolored, or has a hole. Condoms also should not be used after their expiration date or, if they don't have an expiration date, more than five years after the date of manufacture. Only water-based lubricants (for instance, glycerine or K-Y jelly) should be used with latex condoms, because oil-based lubricants such as petroleum jelly weaken natural rubber.

For people allergic to latex, FDA has approved several polyurethane condoms, which have been shown in laboratory tests to be comparable to latex condoms as a barrier to sperm and HIV virus. Each package of polyurethane condoms is labeled "For Latex Sensitive Condom Users." Natural membrane (lambskin) condoms, which are useful in preventing pregnancy, are not effective protection against HIV or other sexually transmitted diseases. Although sperm cannot pass through the lambskin material, small microorganisms, including HIV, can penetrate these condoms.

One product available for women—the polyurethane Reality Female Condom—provides limited protection against sexually transmitted diseases. FDA requires the labeling of Reality to indicate that "highly effective protection" against STDs is provided if the male partner uses a latex condom for men. Male and female condoms, however, should not be used at the same time because they won't stay in place.

Medical and Dental Equipment

To protect patients and health-care providers against exposure to potentially contaminated blood and other body liquids, FDA established quality standards for latex and synthetic rubber gloves used during surgery and patient examination. U.S. manufacturers of these products are requested to test samples from each lot to make sure they show no sign of leakage when filled for two minutes with 1,000 milliliters of water, and that they meet the standards of the American Society for Testing and Materials for stress resistance, tensile strength, materials, and dimensions. FDA also tests samples of domestic and imported surgical and patient examination gloves, using the same criteria.

FDA has joined CDC and the American Dental Association in urging dentists to autoclave—sterilize by steam under pressure—dental hand pieces and accessories between patients to remove possible contaminants. In addition, FDA requires that all such equipment must be designed to withstand autoclaving, and the labeling must include instructions for the sterilization process.

While most dentists are believed to comply with the recommendations for autoclaving, it's a good idea to ask what preventive measures the dentist follows before making an appointment.

Blood Transfusion

Each year, about 3.6 million Americans receive transfusions of blood products. FDA inspects the more than 3,000 donor centers where blood and blood components are collected and processed, and continuously updates requirements and standards designed to prevent disease transmission through transfusion.

Blood collection centers and manufacturers and distributors of blood products are responsible for maintaining five layers of overlapping safeguards.

First, potential donors must answer questions about their health and risk factors. Those whose blood may pose a health hazard are encouraged to exclude themselves. A trained and competent health professional then interviews potential donors about their medical histories.

Donors can be temporarily excluded from donating blood for such reasons as having a temperature, cold, cough, or sore throat on the day of the donation. Potential donors are permanently excluded from donating blood for reasons including evidence of HIV infection, male homosexual activity since 1977, and a history of intravenous drug abuse or viral hepatitis.

Second, blood establishments must keep current a list of deferred donors and check donor names against that list.

Third, after donation, the blood is tested for such blood-borne agents as HIV, hepatitis and syphilis.

The fourth layer of protection prevents general use of any blood products that have not been thoroughly tested.

The fifth layer of protection is FDA's requirement that blood establishments must investigate any breaches of safeguards and correct deficiencies. An error or accident can result from improper testing, incorrectly labeled components, improper interpretation of test results, improper use of equipment or failure to follow the manufacturers' directions for its use, or accepting units from donors who should have been deferred.

The system has helped reduce the risk of transfused HIV infection from 1 in 2,500 units of blood in 1985 to 1 in 440,000 to 640,000 units by the end of 1995. Since then, the Coulter test has shortened the typical window period when the HIV virus cannot be detected to less than three months. Health experts expect the use of this test to reduce the risk of transfused HIV infection even further.

Human Tissue Transplants

In December 1993, FDA issued an interim requirement that potential donors of all human tissues for transplantation—including tendons, bone, skin, and corneas—be tested for HIV-1, HIV-2, and hepatitis B and C viruses, and screened for symptoms of AIDS, hepatitis, and high-risk behaviors such as sex between males and intravenous drug abuse. Imported tissues must be accompanied by records showing that the tissues were similarly screened and tested. If such records are not available, the tissues must be shipped under quarantine.

The agency is preparing a final rule and a guideline to ensure uniformity in tissue testing and screening.

Drugs

In December 1995, a new class of drugs called protease inhibitors was added to the earlier approved class of nucleoside analogs, which included Retrovir (zidovudine, also known as AZT), Videx (didanosine, or ddI), Hivid (zalcitabine, or ddC), Zerit (stavudine, or d4t), and Epivir (lamivudine, or 3TC).

The protease inhibitors—Invirase (saquinavir), Norvir (ritonavir), and Crixivan (indinavir)—inhibit replication of HIV in a similar way as nucleoside analogs, but are active at different points in the replication process. Tested alone or in combination with the nucleoside analogs, the three protease inhibitors markedly reduced the viral load and increased the number of CD4 cells, which sharply declines in HIV infection and AIDS.

In June 1996, FDA approved Viramune (nevirapine), the first in a new class of drugs called non-nucleoside reverse transcriptase inhibitors. Viramune was approved for use in combination with nucleoside analogs to treat adults with HIV infection who have experienced clinical and/or immunological deterioration.

By the end of June, FDA also had approved 22 drugs for HIV- and AIDS-related conditions. Among them are NebuPent (aerosolized pentamidine isethionate) to prevent Pneumocystis carinii pneumonia, the most common life-threatening infection of people with AIDS, and Roferon-A (interferon alfa-2a) and Intron-A (interferon alfa-2b) for Kaposi's sarcoma, an aggressive cancer that affects primarily male homosexuals with AIDS.

Nutrition

Some patients with HIV have wasting syndrome, with symptoms that include major weight loss, chronic diarrhea or weakness, and constant or intermittent fever for at least 30 days. The syndrome is classified as an AIDS-defining illness. All people with HIV should carefully follow food safety practices, because their weakened immunity leaves them particularly vulnerable to food-borne illness. Diarrhea caused by such illness can lead to or worsen wasting syndrome.

To prevent food-borne illnesses, people with HIV should avoid nonpasteurized dairy products, wash hands and utensils with soap and hot water when preparing meals, and cook food thoroughly to kill harmful bacteria. Raw eggs and raw seafood such as oysters, clams, sushi, and sashimi should not be eaten. Additional information about food safety and HIV can be obtained from FDA.

Loss of appetite (anorexia) can be treated with two FDA-approved prescription medicines for HIV and AIDS patients. Marinol (dronabinol), a synthetic extract of marijuana, is indicated for anorexia associated with weight loss. Megace (megestrol acetate) can be used for anorexia, cachexia (emaciation), or any unexplained significant weight loss.

Unapproved Therapies

Recognizing the special needs of people with HIV infection and AIDS, FDA uses its discretion to allow them to import for their personal use unapproved but promising drugs for HIV and HIV-related life-threatening diseases. At the same time, the agency vigorously campaigns against AIDS health scams that have bilked their victims of as much as $10 billion a year.

As a result of FDA investigations, federal and state authorities have taken legal actions against individuals involved in hundreds of fraudulent cures for AIDS such as "energized" water, "ozone therapy," and hydrogen peroxide "treatment."

Because most of the scams are local enterprises, FDA initiated in 1989 an AIDS Health Fraud Task Force Network to monitor and counter the promotion of suspected fraudulent AIDS products. The task forces, so far established in 10 states, have built broadly based coalitions of federal, state and local authorities with the medical community and AIDS activists. They cooperate in explaining to individuals and organizations how to identify fraudulent health products and distribute general information about HIV infection.

For More Information

To learn more about food safety and HIV, write to FDA (HFE-88), 5600 Fishers Lane Rockville, MD 20857, and ask for the brochure "Eating Defensively—Food Safety Advice for Persons with AIDS." Be sure to include the publication number: (FDA) 92-2232.

More information about AIDS and HIV is also available from FDA's Office of AIDS and Special Health Issues on the World Wide Web. [http://www.fda.gov/oashi/aids/hiv.html]

—Mike Kubic

Mike Kubic is a member of FDA's public affairs staff.

Section 11.4

Sexually Transmitted Diseases (STDs)

NIH Publication No. 93–3057, April 1993.

Introduction

Sexually transmitted diseases, or STDs, are a major growing public health problem. The medical, social, and economic impact of STDs are far greater now than 20 years ago when syphilis and gonorrhea dominated a short list of major STDs. Today, physicians have a list of more than 30 infectious agents that can be sexually transmitted and which are epidemic among millions of people in the United States and abroad. More than 13 million people are affected by STDs every year.

STDs are associated with a wide range of disorders, including infertility, genital ulcers, and cervical cancer. STDs can result in miscarriage or premature birth, and the damage to newborns of infected mothers includes pneumonia, blindness, and mental retardation. Drugs can halt the progression of most STDs, particularly if the disease is diagnosed early. But left untreated, many of these diseases cause serious illness and death.

Early recognition of symptoms and treatment are crucial to stemming the damage caused by STDs. (Women with more than one sexual partner may need routine checkups for STDs even when they feel healthy because disease symptoms are often more difficult to detect in females than males.) But knowledge about what sexual behaviors place people at increased risk for STD infections may be one of the most effective means of controlling the epidemic of STDs.

During 1990, there were more than 130,000 new cases of syphilis, the largest increase since 1950. And the number of people with genital herpes continues to rise, with 500,000 new cases diagnosed in 1990. An estimated two million people are infected with gonorrhea and four million people are infected with chlamydia. Together, gonorrhea and chlamydia cause sterility in nearly 150,000 women a year in the United States.

AIDS, the deadliest of all STDs, was first described in 1981 in a report of an extremely rare type of pneumonia that had struck five otherwise healthy homosexual men in California. Two of the men died almost immediately after diagnosis. But by 1988, AIDS had become a tragic household word and a global epidemic. To date, the disease has killed more than 500,000 people worldwide, a death toll that includes children, drug users sharing contaminated needles, sexually active people of all persuasions, and persons who received AIDS-infected blood transfusions prior to rigorous blood-testing procedures instituted in 1985. In 1990, 45,000 new cases of AIDS were diagnosed. an 11 percent increase from 1989.

Why the Increase?

There are several reasons for the disturbing upswing in both incidence and variety of STDs. As the children of the baby boom era come of age, the United States has more adults and hence more sexually active people than ever before. At the same time, young people are becoming sexually active at an earlier age and with an increasing number of partners. For example, one study found that the proportion of 17-year-old women who had premarital intercourse rose from 25 percent in 1971 to 50 percent in 1980.

Widespread use of contraceptives, such as the pill, that do not protect against sexually transmitted infections also has contributed to the pandemic of STDs.

One piece of good news is that increased reporting of STDs is in part due to advances in microbiology that have enabled clinicians to diagnose infections and their associated complications more readily. Improved methods to culture the herpes simplex virus and to serologically diagnose the human immunodeficiency virus (HIV), the causative agent of AIDS, are two such advances. In addition, the emergence of AIDS has focused public attention on STDs in general, which may also have increased reporting and awareness of STDs. Physicians have come to understand that efforts to control AIDS must also focus on the control of all STDs.

AIDS

Facts about AIDS

Acquired immunodeficiency syndrome (AIDS) is a life-threatening illness that attacks the immune system. It is often transmitted by sexual contact and has alone claimed the lives of more than 500,000 young people worldwide. Treatment for this disease and all other STDs combined costs the nation billions of dollars annually.

AIDS is now a global pandemic, with more than one million cumulative cases documented or suspected in more than 165 countries. Researchers estimate that 10 million people worldwide may be infected with HIV. The most common route of infection is through sexual contact. However, HIV can be transmitted by exposure to infected blood from the sharing of needles or syringes among intravenous drug users, by transfusions of contaminated blood, or passing from a pregnant woman to her baby. In the United States, transmission of the virus among homosexual and bisexual men accounts for the largest number of AIDS cases, but the number of people who acquire the infection through heterosexual contact and intravenous drug use is increasing.

Controlling the AIDS Pandemic

HIV is intertwined with the same behaviors responsible for the transmission of other STDs. And as with all STDs, many people carry the infectious agent and can transmit it to others, but may have no symptoms. They may feel fine and have no outward signs of disease, but they pose a great danger to their prospective sexual partners. Unless people who are infected are tested, educated, and counseled, they are likely to spread AIDS and other STDs to more and more individuals.

Transmitting the AIDS Virus

To date, only three body fluids have been implicated in the transmission of the AIDS virus: semen, vaginal secretions, and blood. In contrast, there is no evidence that the virus has ever been transmitted by saliva, urine, sweat, or any other body fluids, even though the virus may be present in some of these secretions in small amounts. Casual contact—like shaking someone's hand, kissing someone on the cheek, sitting next to an infected person on the subway, or sharing the same office space—is not a factor in transmitting the AIDS virus. More than 96 percent of all people with AIDS have identifiable risk factors; sexual and drug-using behaviors are responsible for most AIDS cases.

Treatment for AIDS

Infection with other STDs can increase the likelihood of acquiring HIV infection. For example, herpes or syphilis can cause ulcerations or wounding of the skin around the genitals, creating a possible new entry route for the AIDS virus and increasing the likelihood of transmitting the disease during sexual contact with an infected person. Similarly, a person who already has AIDS and who has an open genital sore may be more likely to transmit the virus to someone else.

There is no magic bullet, no vaccine, and no cure for AIDS. This lethal disease attacks the immune system, leaving infected people susceptible to a variety of rare diseases, such as *Pneumocystis carinii* pneumonia, an unusual type of tuberculosis, or a cancer known as Kaposi sarcoma. Often the people who die of AIDS succumb, to one of these illnesses, known as an opportunistic infection, due to their weakened immune system. Currently, the U.S. government has approved one drug, AZT, also known as zidovudine, for treating early HIV infection and AIDS. AZT acts against the AIDS virus, and studies have shown that it can prolong the life of AIDS patients. Perhaps most important, AZT recently has been shown to slow the progression to illness, and possibly prolong the lives of people who are infected with the AIDS virus but who are not yet sick. AZT has several toxic side effects, including low red and white blood cell counts. Moreover, the drug can only slow the AIDS infection, not stop it. But the drug's promise of prolonging life may encourage more people who are at risk to be tested. People who carry the AIDS virus no longer have to wait until they get sick to do something about the disease.

AIDS Prevention

Many other drugs are now in clinical trials; some are similar to AZT but may be less toxic. Other experimental drugs appear to attack the AIDS virus in ways quite different from AZT. As scientists learn more about the structure of the AIDS virus and the way that it infects cells of the immune system, more and more drugs are being developed to destroy the virus or stop its reproduction.

Our only way of preventing this devastating disease is through education and prevention. Since the message in preventing sexual transmission of AIDS is identical to the message for preventing all the other STDS—use condoms and spermicide, understand the health risks associated with multiple sex partners and with particular sexual activity such as anal intercourse, get frequent checkups and appropriate treatment when needed—a concerted effort to control all STDs will have the effect of controlling the AIDS pandemic.

Gonorrhea

Gonorrhea is one of the most commonly reported diseases in the country, with 700,000 cases reported annually to the Centers for Disease Control. The infectious agent that causes gonorrhea, *Neisseria bacterium gonorrhoeae*, is usually found in white blood cells called polymorphonudear leukocytes. The bacterium infects membranes including the urethra of men and women, the uterine and cervical canals, the fallopian tubes, the portion of the scrotum known as the epididymis, the anal canal, the throat, and the conjunctiva of the eyes.

Symptoms

Although gonorrhea can cause pus-like discharges from the urethra and cervix, infections of the throat, anal canal, and cervix often have no visible symptoms. Moreover, early symptoms of gonorrhea are usually mild, and some people may have no symptoms at all. This is one reason why the disease is so readily transmitted from one person to another. If symptoms of infection do occur, they usually appear within two to 10 days after sexual contact with an infected partner. In women, early symptoms of gonorrhea include painful or burning sensation when urinating and a yellowish vaginal discharge. More advanced symptoms include abdominal pain, bleeding between menstrual periods, vomiting, and fever. Men may have a discharge from the penis and a burning sensation during urination that may be severe. Symptoms of rectal infection include a discharge, anal itching, and painful bowel movements. If the infection is not treated, it can spread to the bloodstream, and from there to the joints, heart valves, and the brain.

Special Concerns of Women

Women should be particularly alert to the complications of gonorrhea. Research shows that 90 percent of women will become infected with gonorrhea after a single episode of sexual intercourse with an infected partner, compared to one-third of men who have intercourse with an infected woman. The infection is also more severe in women, causing such complications as pelvic inflammatory disease, infertility, perihepatitis, and premature delivery of a baby.

About one million American women each year develop acute pelvic inflammatory disease (PID), a serious infection of the female pelvic organs. Gonorrhea causes a significant number of these cases. PID can cause scarring of the fallopian tubes, resulting in infertility in 20 percent of infected women. In other women, the scarring may block the passage of fertilized eggs into the uterus. If this happens, the egg may implant itself in the middle of the fallopian tube, resulting in an ectopic, or tubal, pregnancy—a life-threatening condition to the mother if not detected early.

A pregnant woman who has gonorrhea may also infect her infant as the baby passes through the cervical canal during delivery. Most states require that the eyes of all newborns be treated with medication to prevent gonococcal infection, which can lead to blindness if left untreated.

Diagnosis and Treatment

Gonorrhea is relatively easy to diagnose since the bacterium can be identified from infected secretions using a technique known as a gram stain. The gram-stain technique is highly accurate for men, predicting the infection in more than 90 percent of infected individuals. But this method is less accurate for women, predicting the disease in only 50 percent of infected individuals. For this reason, it is recommended that women have a culture taken of cervical secretions during a routine pelvic examination as a test for infection. Results of the test are known within two days.

Although the majority of gonorrhea strains are still sensitive to penicillin, ampicillin, or amoxicillin, some strains have developed resistance to penicillin. Fortunately, other antibiotics, like spectinomycin or ceftriaxone, can treat these resistant strains of infection. Because gonorrhea often occurs in tandem with other STDs, particularly chlamydia, a physician may prescribe a combination of antibiotics, such as ampicillin, or ceftriaxone, followed by tetracycline, to treat both diseases. Pregnant women should be treated with erythromycin rather than tetracycline.

Seven days after the end of medication, the physician should retest the patient to confirm that the infection has been eliminated. All sex partners of the patient should also be tested for gonorrhea. The partners should receive treatment if they are positive for gonorrhea by culture or gram stain, even if they have no symptoms of the disease.

Gonorrhea Prevention

Because gonorrhea is so readily transmissible, all men and women who have had sexual contact with more than one partner should be tested regularly for the disease. Using condoms during intercourse is highly effective in preventing the spread of this and other STDs. Diaphragms used with spermicidal foams, creams, and jellies that contain nonoxynol 9, also reduce the risk of infection.

Chlamydia: The Silent STD

Chlamydia trachomatis is known as the silent STD because its early symptoms are so mild. A disease that has been studied intensively only for the past five to ten years, chlamydial infection has rapidly become one of the most common STDs in the United States, with three to five million people diagnosed with the infection each year.

Chlamydiae are unique bacteria that resemble viruses, surviving and reproducing only within certain cells of the body. Also like viruses, the bacteria can lie dormant in infected individuals for long periods without symptoms, while in others the infectious agent causes severe complications including PID, infertility, and eye infection or pneumonia in the newborn.

Similarity to Gonorrhea

Symptoms of chlamydial infections are similar to those for gonorrhea. In addition, the same group of people—sexually active teenagers, particularly those in the inner city where these diseases are common—are at highest risk for developing gonorrhea and chlamydia. Moreover, in studies of patients at STD clinics in Baltimore and Washington, D.C., 20 percent of men with infections of the urethra caused by gonorrhea also had chlamydial infections; 40 percent of women treated for gonorrhea also had chlamydial infection of the cervix.

Chlamydia may cause PID in nearly half a million women; 150,000 each year become infertile as a result of PID. And also like gonorrhea, chlamydia infection can be passed to newborns during birth. Many physicians recommend that pregnant women be tested for both chlamydia and gonorrhea.

Symptoms of Chlamydial Infection

Early symptoms of chlamydial infections, if they appear at all, usually occur one to two weeks after infection. Fifty percent of infected women and 25 percent of infected men have no early symptoms of the disease and are not diagnosed until complications occur.

Chlamydiae cause inflammation of the urethra not associated with gonorrhea in about 40 percent of infected men. Common symptoms of the inflammation include discharge of mucus or pus from the penis and pain upon urination. The infection may also cause epididymitis, an inflammation of part of the male reproductive system located near the testes. Pain and swelling of the scrotal area accompanies this inflammation, and 10 to 30 percent of men with the condition may become permanently sterile.

Women with chlamydial infection also experience pain upon urination. There may be a vaginal discharge and abdominal pain; the cervix may be red with a mucus discharge from the cervical opening. In some women, the infection spreads to the uterus, the endometrium, and the fallopian tubes, causing pain and inflammation in the inner lining of the uterus and the fallopian tubes.

Diagnosis

Chlamydial infections are hard to diagnose for several reasons. Because early symptoms are mild or nonexistent, the disease is often overlooked. In addition, the infection can so closely resemble gonorrhea that physicians may mistake the symptoms. Moreover, diagnostic tests that rely on growing the bacterium in culture require a tissue culture facility, which may not be widely available to all physicians. More recently, however, a 30-minute test that can be performed in a doctor's office has been developed to detect the chlamydial organism.

Physicians recommend that all people with more than one sex partner, or who have sexual contact with someone who has multiple partners, should be tested annually for chlamydia, especially women under 35. In addition, physicians believe that men with inflammation of the urethra and women with inflammation of the cervix who have secretions containing white cells but who do not have gonorrhea should begin treatment for chlamydia even before tests confirm the problem.

Treatment and Prevention of Chlamydia

Chlamydial infections are highly sensitive to tetracycline and erythromycin. Penicillin, however, is ineffective against chlamydial bacteria. A follow-up visit to the physician is essential to make sure that the bacteria have been eradicated. As with many other STDs, use of condoms, diaphragms, or spermicide reduces the transmission of chlamydia. All sex partners of people infected with chlamydia should also be treated.

Herpes

Genital herpes is caused by the herpes simplex virus. Each year, about half a million new cases of genital herpes occur in the United States. The herpes simplex virus has two forms, HSV-I and HSV-II. HSV-I is commonly associated with oral herpes or fever blisters, which do not pose a serious health problem for most people. HSV-II is the form of herpes that most often infects the genitals, causing blisters, and that is spread through sexual contact. Because oral herpes can be transmitted to the genital area through oral-genital sex, genital herpes may sometimes be caused by HSV-I as well.

Genital herpes is usually spread through sexual contact with someone who has an outbreak of genital sores. But in some cases, herpes infection may be transmitted by a person who has no noticeable symptoms. The first or primary episode of genital herpes usually occurs within two to 10 days after exposure to infection and lasts for about three weeks.

Symptoms

Early symptoms of a primary episode include a burning sensation while urinating, pain in the legs or genital area, a vaginal discharge, or a feeling of pressure in the abdominal area. There may also be fever, headache, or swollen glands. Within a few days, red bumps develop into blisters and painful, open sores on the penis, on the vulva or in the vagina, around the anus, buttocks, or thighs, or in the cervix of women and the urinary tract of men. Over a period of days, the sores become crusted and heal without leaving any visible scars.

During this early part of the infection, the herpes virus travels up the sensory nerves to the ganglia at the end of the spinal cord. Even after the visible lesions have disappeared, the virus remains within the nerve cells in an inactive state. In some people, the virus reactivates from time to time. When this happens, the virus travels back down the nerve pathways to the skin, where it multiplies at or near the site of the original sores, often causing new sores to develop. Other times, the virus reactivates without any new symptoms, and the infected person may be unaware he or she is contagious during this period.

Symptoms during recurring episodes usually are milder than those of the first episode and typically last about a week. A recurring outbreak usually is preceded by a tingling sensation in the genital area or pain in the buttocks that radiates down the back of the leg. These are called prodromal symptoms and are caused by migration of the virus down the nerve pathway.

The frequency and severity of recurrences vary greatly. Many people may have only one or two recurrences in a lifetime, while others may have six to 10 episodes a year. Moreover, the pattern of recurrences changes over time in each individual. Some people report that recurrences are triggered by illness, stress, or menstruation, but most recurrences are not predictable. What is predictable is that individuals with herpes are most contagious during a recurrent outbreak.

Protecting the Newborn

Genital herpes poses a serious health threat for babies born to women who have a primary episode or an active recurrence of the virus during delivery. The virus can cause blindness, brain damage, and death of the newborn. Because of the risk of infecting the infant during a recurrence, physicians recommend that if there are signs that the mother has an active herpes infection at the time of labor, the child should be delivered by caesarean section to prevent transmission of the infection.

Diagnosis and Treatment of Herpes

Genital herpes is usually diagnosed based upon observation of genital sores visible to the naked eye. There are also laboratory tests. One rapid test relies on scraping a genital sore and staining the sample with a monoclonal antibody. Under an immunofluorescent microscope, the active herpes infection is clearly visible in cells.

The infected area should be kept clean and dry to prevent secondary infections. Patients should avoid touching the sore and should wash their hands immediately if there is any hand contact. During an active outbreak of herpes, patients should avoid sexual contact until the sores are completely healed.

An oral drug, acyclovir, has been proven effective in shortening the healing time and in reducing the seventy of a herpes outbreak. Acyclovir, however, is not a cure; it suppresses viral replication, helping to keep the virus inactive and prevent recurrences. People who have frequent recurring episodes can take acyclovir daily for a period of months to a year to prevent recurrences.

Syphilis

Syphilis is one of the oldest known STDs. A chronic illness that affects the entire body, syphilis is caused by *Treponema pallidum*, a spirochete (corkscrew-shaped bacterium). Syphilis has been called the great imitator because it can mimic the symptoms of so many diseases.

Until recently, the number of cases of syphilis had remained stable at about 70,000 cases a year, but 1988 saw a 33 percent increase, occurring almost entirely among heterosexuals. (Because of the AIDS epidemic and active educational campaigns for safer sex practices among homosexuals, syphilis, once a prominent disease among gay men, has declined rapidly in this population.) Among heterosexuals, the resurgence of syphilis has been linked to the exchange of sex for drugs, especially at crack houses where individuals trade sex for crack cocaine. The incidence of congenital syphilis (infection in a newborn) has increased dramatically as well.

Syphilis is acquired by direct contact with the sores of a person who is infected, although the bacterium can also be transmitted through contact with the mucous membranes of the genital area, mouth, or anus. A pregnant woman with syphilis can transmit the disease to her unborn child, who may be born with serious mental and physical impairments.

Symptoms

The first symptom of syphilis is usually a painless, open sore called a chancre. Appearing within 10 days to three months after sexual contact with an infected individual, the painless chancre may go unnoticed. Usually found on the part of the body that is exposed to the bacterium, such as the penis, vulva, or vagina, a chancre also can develop on the cervix, tongue, lips, or fingertips—any part of the body that comes into direct contact with the open sore on an infected person.

The chancre usually disappears within a few weeks without any treatment. But the disease is likely to progress through two more increasingly serious stages if not diagnosed and treated properly. The second, highly infectious stage is marked by a skin rash that appears from two to 12 weeks after the chancre vanishes. The rash may cover the whole body or appear in just a few areas, such as the palms of the hands or the soles of the feet. Because these minute sores contain active bacteria, any physical contact—sexual or nonsexual—with broken skin of the infected person can spread the disease. The rash may be accompanied by flu-like symptoms such as mild fever, fatigue, headache, and sore throat, as well as patchy hair loss, swollen lymph nodes throughout the body, and other disorders. The rash usually heals within several weeks or months, but signs of second-stage syphilis may recur for as long as two to three years after the initial infection.

About 15 to 40 percent of people infected with syphilis who go untreated reach the third stage. This stage, called the late or tertiary stage, although not contagious can be life-threatening. The bacteria can invade the heart, eyes, brain, nervous system, bones, and joints. Nearly every part of the body is susceptible to attack during this stage, which can last for years and even decades. Mental illness, blindness, heart disease, and death can occur among infected individuals who do not receive treatment.

Diagnosis and Treatment of Syphilis

To diagnose syphilis, the physician must identify the bacteria in a small amount of tissue taken directly from the chancre. If no sores are present to examine, a blood test that searches for characteristic antibodies is performed instead. Although blood tests are a good indicator of infection, they sometimes give false negative results during the first six weeks of syphilis infection. This is because it takes that long for antibodies against the disease to develop. Occasionally a false positive occurs; this is most common among the elderly and those with autoimmune diseases.

Syphilis is effectively treated with penicillin. Nevertheless, it is crucial to take a repeat blood test two months after treatment to make sure the infectious agent has been completely destroyed. If the syphilis bacterium has penetrated into the central nervous system, additional, higher doses of penicillin may be needed. Spectinomycin is an alternative effective drug for the treatment of syphilis for people allergic to penicillin.

Human Papillomavirus

The human papillomavirus (HPV) is more commonly by the condition it causes—genital warts. These warts, known as venereal warts or condyloma acuminatum, frequently are seen in people who have multiple sex partners. HPV affects up to 40 million people in the United States. One million new patients are diagnosed each year with genital warts.

About two-thirds of people who have sexual contact with an infected individual will go on to develop this common STD. But like so many other STDs, HPV infection often occurs without any symptoms. In many cases, small growths develop within three weeks to three months after exposure. If left untreated, the warts may develop into a fleshy, cauliflower-like structure. Women typically develop warts on the vulva, inside the vagina, or around the anus, but warts may also occur in the early stages as flat, virtually invisible lesions inside the cervix.

HPV infection may be detected on a Pap smear, which is a microscopic examination of cells taken from the cervix in order to detect cervical cancer. Because some types of HPV, specifically HPV-16 and HPV-18, may induce cancerous changes of the skin and cervix, it is strongly recommended that all women have annual Pap smears. This is especially important for women with multiple sex partners.

In men, genital warts usually appear at the tip or on the shaft of the penis, on the scrotum, or around the anus.

It is important for a person who may have warts to see a physician so that other types of similar-looking infections or conditions can either be ruled out or treated. Genital warts are usually diagnosed by visual examination. For women, the physician may perform a colposcopy, a painless examination in which a lighted magnifying instrument is used to view the internal reproductive organs of a woman, so that the flat cervical warts can be detected.

Questions and Answers

I had always heard that syphilis could only be transmitted through sexual contact. But is it true that in the secondary state of syphilis, if a person has sores on his hand, you could catch the disease by shaking his hand?

Yes. If a person has second-stage syphilis and has sores on his hand, someone else could get the disease if he or she has a break in skin or other type of lesion and that skin wound came into direct contact with the syphilis sores of the infected person. Fortunately, secondary syphilis today is rather rare because it is detected and treated effectively in its earlier stages.

What is perihepatitis, and how are hepatitis A and B transmitted sexually?

Perihepatitis is an inflammation of the surface lining of the liver. The inflammation can be part of a disorder called Fitz-Hugh-Curtis Syndrome, in which a woman first develops salpingitis (inflammation of the fallopian tubes) and lower abdominal pain, and then experiences severe pain in the upper right quadrant of the body, around the liver. Normally, the infection is caused by either chlamydia or gonorrhea, spreading from the fallopian tube up through the lymph nodes to involve the liver. (The disease is rare in men.)

Hepatitis A and B can both be transmitted through sexual contact. Hepatitis B was initially found to be sexually transmitted primarily among homosexual men, in a manner identical to AIDS. Anal intercourse is a high-risk behavior for the spread of both AIDS and hepatitis. The hepatitis B virus has been found in semen and, upon contact with mucous membranes such as the cervix or anal canal, can infect another person. Hepatitis A is more infectious, and can also be spread through contaminated food and water as well as by intimate sexual contact.

What are the chances that someone who is an asymptomatic carrier of the AIDS virus will develop the disease?

Persons who become infected with HIV, the virus that causes AIDS, may develop an acute flu-like infection that lasts perhaps two weeks, and then subsides. Subsequently, they feel totally normal, although they are still carrying the virus and are infectious to others through sexual activity and exchange of blood. These are the people we call asymptomatic. We have been monitoring a group of homosexual men in San Francisco who we know became infected with HIV in 1980. Eight years later, about 45 percent of these men had developed AIDS, while the others were still asymptomatic or had mild symptoms. Based on this and other studies, the mean incubation time for AIDS—the time it takes for 50 percent of an asymptomatic, infected group to develop the disease—appears to be 10 years. But what about the other 50 percent, will they ever develop AIDS? We haven't been following the disease long enough to know what will happen. But many researchers predict that more than 80 percent of infected individuals will eventually develop AIDS.

How do you define someone who is "infected" with AIDS if they show no symptoms?

We say that someone is infected if they are carrying the AIDS virus, as indicated by the presence of antibodies to the virus. If someone is infected, that means we can take that person's white blood cells, culture them, and grow the virus. There is a test, called the polymerase chain reaction, which amplifies the DNA of the AIDS virus in a latent form, meaning the virus is inactive inside the cells. All the people we have studied who tested positive for antibodies to the AIDS virus have this latent form of the virus. This means that if the lymphocytes become activated for some reason, the virus starts to replicate within these cells. It also means that if these infected lymphocytes are transmitted to another person through sexual contact, blood transfusion, or shared needles, HIV will also be transmitted. Anyone who tests positive for antibodies to HIV can infect their sexual partner, or partners with whom they share needles for intravenous drugs.

How well is blood used for transfusions being screened for the AIDS virus?

Federal law now requires that all donated blood be screened for HIV prior to transfusion. So, virtually all of the blood that is transfused today is free of the AIDS virus. Why do I use the qualifier "virtually" all? Because occasionally a person may be infected with AIDS, but may not have antibodies present, and so their blood might not be rejected by the antibody test. About one out of 100,000 units of blood may carry the virus. For a typical blood transfusion, the odds of receiving contaminated blood range from about one out of 100,000 to one out of 500,000. The odds are quite high that a person won't get infected through transfusion, but no one is 100 percent safe.

What role does nutrition play in the immune system? Can good nutrition increase the time it takes for infection with the AIDS virus to become an active disease?

Nutrition plays a key role in good health. Individuals who are malnourished certainly have weakened immune systems and are more susceptible to certain infectious agents. Moreover, when malnourished people do get sick, it seems that the disease, such as AIDS, progresses more rapidly through the body. But we are talking about extreme cases. For borderline cases, where someone might be slightly underweight or overweight, nutrition may not play as significant a role. We do recommend that HIV-infected people maintain an optimal nutrition state so as to avoid complications as long as possible.

How is the yeast infection candidiasis transmitted, and how common is this infection?

This condition is caused by a yeast organism called *Candida albicans*. There has been little research done on transmission of this infection. We know that a yeast infection can cause vaginitis in women, but whether transmission is from male to female or female to male has not been well studied. Yeast vaginitis is common in women who have multiple sex partners, so there is circumstantial evidence for sexual transmission. The infection is also common in pregnant women because their immune system is slightly weakened, and the yeast seems to thrive in this setting. Diabetic women also have a high incidence of yeast infection. No one has counted the number of cases, but in most STD clinics, about 10 percent of the women have a yeast infection, or vaginal candidiasis. Another 25 percent have a type of vaginitis known as *trichomonal vaginitis*. That disorder is caused by a protozoan agent called *Trichomonas vaginalis*, known as "Trich" for short. This infection has been better documented than yeast infection and is known to be sexually transmitted from male to female and vice-versa.

— Thomas Quinn, M.D., Senior Investigator,
Laboratory of Immunoregulation,
National Institute of Allergy and Infectious Diseases,
National Institutes of Health

Dr. Thomas Quinn, a specialist in the study of infectious diseases, is a professor of medicine in the division of infectious diseases at The Johns Hopkins University and a guest lecturer to the University of Maryland and Oxford University. Dr. Quinn has conducted investigations of several sexually transmitted diseases and has led international studies of the epidemiology of AIDS in Africa. He attended medical school at Northwestern University in Chicago and interned at Albany Medical Center in New York, specializing in internal medicine. He first came to the National Institutes of Health in 1977 as a research associate at NIAID, leaving two years later to become a senior fellow in medicine at the University of Washington in Seattle. Dr. Quinn rejoined NIAID in 1981.

Section 11.5

Using Condoms to Prevent HIV Infection and Other Sexually Transmitted Diseases (STDs)

NIH Publication No. HIV/NAIEP/10-93/035. DHHS and CDC Pamphlet.

Latex condoms are highly effective in preventing the transmission of HIV and other sexually transmitted diseases. They can greatly reduce a person's risk of acquiring or transmitting sexually transmitted diseases (STDs), including HIV infection. HIV is the virus that causes AIDS.

But for condoms to provide maximum protection, they must be used consistently and correctly.

Consistent use means using a condom from start to finish every time you have sex.

Correct use means to:

- Use a new latex condom for each act of intercourse—whether vaginal, anal, or oral.

- Be careful when opening the condom. Do not use teeth, fingernails, or other sharp objects to open the condom wrapper because you might tear the condom inside.

- Put the condom on after the penis is erect and before sexual contact.

- Hold the tip of the condom and unroll the condom all the way down the erect penis—the rolled rim should be on the outside. Leave space at the tip for semen, but make sure that no air is trapped in the condom's tip.

- If additional lubrication is needed, lubricate the outside of the condom if it is not prelubricated. **Use only water-based lubricants.** You can purchase lubricant at any pharmacy. Your pharmacist can tell you which lubricants are water-based. Oil-based lubricants, such as petroleum jelly, cold cream, hand lotion, cooking oil, or baby oil, weaken the condom.

- Withdraw from your partner while the penis is still erect. Hold the condom firmly to keep it from slipping off.

- Throw the used condom away in the trash. **Never re-use a condom**.

- If the condom breaks during sex, withdraw from your partner and put on a new condom.

Always keep condoms handy, but store them in a cool, dry place that is out of direct sunlight. Do not use a condom after its expiration date or if it has been damaged in any way.

Latex condoms are available in different sizes, colors, and textures. Find the one that is right for *you*.

Novelty products are not effective in preventing STDs.

Not having sex is the best way to avoid getting HIV infections or other STDs. However, if you do have sex, remember, condoms are highly effective, if used correctly from start to finish each time you have intercourse.

For more information on condoms or preventing HIV infection, contact:

CDC National AIDS Hotline **1-800-342-AIDS**
Spanish Service **1-800-344-7432**
TTY Service for the Deaf **1-800-243-7889**

Chapter 12

Diabetes

Chapter Contents

Section 12.1

Diabetes Overview

NIH Publication No. 96-3873.

Almost every one of us knows someone who has diabetes. An estimated 16 million people in the United States have diabetes mellitus—a serious, lifelong condition. About half of these people do not know they have diabetes and are not under care for the disorder. Each year, about 650,000 people are diagnosed with diabetes.

Although diabetes occurs most often in older adults, it is one of the most common chronic disorders in children in the United States. About 127,000 children and teenagers age 19 and younger have diabetes.

What Is Diabetes?

Diabetes is a disorder of metabolism—the way our bodies use digested food for growth and energy. Most of the food we eat is broken down by the digestive juices into a simple sugar called glucose. Glucose is the main source of fuel for the body.

After digestion, the glucose passes into our bloodstream where it is available for body cells to use for growth and energy. For the glucose to get into the cells, insulin must be present. Insulin is a hormone produced by the pancreas, a large gland behind the stomach.

When we eat, the pancreas is supposed to automatically produce the right amount of insulin to move the glucose from our blood into our cells. In people with diabetes, however, the pancreas either produces little or no insulin, or the body cells do not respond to the insulin that is produced. As a result, glucose builds up in the blood, overflows into the urine, and passes out of the body. Thus, the body loses its main source of fuel even though the blood contains large amounts of glucose.

What Are the Different Types of Diabetes?

The three main types of diabetes are:

- Insulin-dependent diabetes mellitus (IDDM) or Type I diabetes
- Noninsulin-dependent diabetes mellitus (NIDDM) or Type II diabetes
- Gestational diabetes.

Insulin-dependent Diabetes

Insulin-dependent diabetes is considered an autoimmune disease. An autoimmune disease results when the body's system for fighting infection (the immune system) turns against a part of the body. In diabetes, the immune system attacks the insulin-producing beta cells in the pancreas and destroys them. The pancreas then produces little or no insulin.

Someone with IDDM needs daily injections of insulin to live. At present, scientists do not know exactly what causes the body's immune system to attack the beta cells, but they believe that both genetic factors and viruses are involved. IDDM accounts for about 5 to 10 percent of diagnosed diabetes in the United States.

IDDM develops most often in children and young adults, but the disorder can appear at any age. Symptoms of IDDM usually develop over a short period, although beta cell destruction can begin months, even years, earlier.

Symptoms include increased thirst and urination, constant hunger, weight loss, blurred vision, and extreme tiredness. If not diagnosed and treated with insulin, a person can lapse into a life-threatening coma.

Noninsulin-Dependent Diabetes

The most common form of diabetes is noninsulin-dependent diabetes. About 90 to 95 percent of people with diabetes have NIDDM. This form of diabetes usually develops in adults over the age of 40 and is most common among adults over age 55. About 80 percent of people with NIDDM are overweight.

In NIDDM, the pancreas usually produces insulin, but for some reason, the body cannot use the insulin effectively. The end result is the same as for IDDM—an unhealthy buildup of glucose in the blood and an inability of the body to make efficient use of its main source of fuel.

The symptoms of NIDDM develop gradually and are not as noticeable as in IDDM. Symptoms include feeling tired or ill, frequent urination (especially at night), unusual thirst, weight loss, blurred vision, frequent infections, and slow healing of sores.

Gestational Diabetes

Gestational diabetes develops or is discovered during pregnancy. This type usually disappears when the pregnancy is over, but women who have had gestational diabetes have a greater risk of developing NIDDM later in their lives.

What Is the Scope and Impact of Diabetes?

Diabetes is widely recognized as one of the leading causes of death and disability in the United States. According to death certificate data, diabetes contributed to the deaths of more than 169,000 persons in 1992.

Diabetes is associated with long-term complications that affect almost every major part of the body. It contributes to blindness, heart disease, strokes, kidney failure, amputations, and nerve damage. Uncontrolled diabetes can complicate pregnancy, and birth defects are more common in babies born to women with diabetes.

Diabetes cost the United States $92 billion in 1992. Indirect costs, including disability payments, time lost from work, and premature death, totaled $47 billion; medical costs for diabetes care, including hospitalizations, medical care, and treatment supplies, totaled $45 billion.

Who Gets Diabetes?

Diabetes is not contagious. People cannot "catch" it from each other. However, certain factors can increase one's risk of developing diabetes. People who have family members with diabetes (especially NIDDM), who are overweight, or who are African American, Hispanic, or Native American are all at greater risk of developing diabetes.

IDDM occurs equally among males and females, but is more common in whites than in nonwhites. Data from the World Health Organization's Multinational Project for Childhood Diabetes indicate that IDDM is rare in most Asian, African, and Native American populations. On the other hand, some northern European countries, including Finland and Sweden, have high rates of IDDM. The reasons for these differences are not known.

NIDDM is more common in older people, especially older women who are overweight, and occurs more often among African Americans, Hispanics, and Native Americans. Compared with non-Hispanic whites, diabetes rates are about 60 percent higher in African Americans and 110 to 120 percent higher in Mexican Americans and Puerto Ricans. Native Americans have the highest rates of diabetes in the world. Among Pima Indians living in the United States, for example, half of all adults have NIDDM. The prevalence of diabetes is likely to increase because older people, Hispanics, and other minority groups make up the fastest growing segments of the U.S. population.

How Is Diabetes Managed?

Before the discovery of insulin in 1921, all people with IDDM died within a few years after the appearance of the disease. Although insulin is not considered a cure for diabetes, its discovery was the first major breakthrough in diabetes treatment.

Today, daily injections of insulin are the basic therapy for IDDM. Insulin injections must be balanced with meals and daily activities, and glucose levels must be closely monitored through frequent blood sugar testing.

Diet, exercise, and blood testing for glucose are also the basis for management of NIDDM. In addition, some people with NIDDM take oral drugs or insulin to lower their blood glucose levels.

People with diabetes must take responsibility for their day-to-day care. Much of the daily care involves trying to keep blood sugar levels from going too low or too high. When blood sugar levels drop too low—a condition known as hypoglycemia—a person can become nervous, shaky, and confused. Judgment can be impaired. Eventually, the person could pass out. The treatment for low blood sugar is to eat or drink something with sugar in it.

On the other hand, a person can become very ill if blood sugar levels rise too high, a condition known as hyperglycemia. Hypoglycemia and hyperglycemia, which can occur in people with IDDM or NIDDM, are both potentially life-threatening emergencies.

People with diabetes should be treated by a doctor who monitors their diabetes control and checks for complications. Doctors who specialize in diabetes are called endocrinologists or diabetologists. In addition, people with diabetes often see ophthalmologists for eye examinations, podiatrists for routine foot care, dietitians for help in planning meals, and diabetes educators for instruction in day-to-day care.

The goal of diabetes management is to keep blood glucose levels as close to the normal (nondiabetic) range as safely possible. A recent Government study, sponsored by the National Institute of Diabetes and Digestive and Kidney Diseases (NIDDK), proved that keeping blood sugar levels as close to normal as safely possible reduces the risk of developing major complications of diabetes.

The 10-year study, called the Diabetes Control and Complications Trial (DCCT), was completed in 1993 and included 1,441 people with IDDM. The study compared the effect of two treatment approaches—intensive management and standard management—on the development and progression of eye, kidney, and nerve complications of diabetes. Researchers found that study participants who maintained lower levels of blood glucose through intensive management had significantly lower rates of these complications.

Researchers believe that DCCT findings have important implications for the treatment of NIDDM, as well as IDDM.

What Is the Status of Diabetes Research?

NIDDK supports basic and clinical research in its own laboratories and in research centers and hospitals throughout the United States. It also gathers and analyzes statistics about diabetes. Other institutes at the National Institutes of Health also carry out research on diabetes-related eye diseases, heart and vascular complications, pregnancy, and dental problems.

Other government agencies that sponsor diabetes programs are the Centers for Disease Control and Prevention, the Indian Health Service, the Health Resources and Services Administration, the Bureau of Veterans Affairs, and the Department of Defense.

Many organizations outside of the Government support diabetes research and education activities. These organizations include the American Diabetes Association, the Juvenile Diabetes Foundation International, and the American Association of Diabetes Educators.

In recent years, advances in diabetes research have led to better ways to manage diabetes and treat its complications. Major advances include:

- New forms of purified insulin, such as human insulin produced through genetic engineering

- Better ways for doctors to monitor blood glucose levels and for people with diabetes to test their own blood glucose levels at home

- Development of external and implantable insulin pumps that deliver appropriate amounts of insulin, replacing daily injections

- Laser treatment for diabetic eye disease, reducing the risk of blindness

- Successful transplantation of kidneys in people whose own kidneys fail because of diabetes

- Better ways of managing diabetic pregnancies, improving chances of successful outcomes

- New drugs to treat NIDDM and better ways to manage this form of diabetes through weight control

- Evidence that intensive management of blood glucose reduces and may prevent development of microvascular complications of diabetes

- Demonstration that antihypertensive drugs called ACE-inhibitors prevent or delay kidney failure in people with diabetes.

What Will the Future Bring?

In the future, it may be possible to administer insulin through nasal sprays or in the form of a pill or patch. Devices that can "read" blood glucose levels without having to prick a finger to get a blood sample are also being developed.

Researchers continue to search for the cause or causes of diabetes and ways to prevent and cure the disorder. Scientists are looking for genes that may be involved in NIDDM and IDDM. Some genetic markers for IDDM have been identified, and it is now possible to screen relatives of people with IDDM to see if they are at risk for diabetes.

The new Diabetes Prevention Trial-Type I, sponsored by NIDDK, identifies relatives at risk for developing IDDM and treats them with low doses of insulin or with oral insulin-like agents in the hope of preventing IDDM. Similar research is carried out at other medical centers throughout the world.

Transplantation of the pancreas or insulin-producing beta cells offers the best hope of cure for people with IDDM. Some pancreas transplants have been successful. However, people who have transplants must take powerful drugs to prevent rejection of the transplanted organ. These drugs are costly and may eventually cause serious health problems.

Scientists are working to develop less harmful drugs and better methods of transplanting pancreatic tissue to prevent rejection by the body. Using techniques of bioengineering, researchers are also trying to create artificial islet cells that secrete insulin in response to increased sugar levels in the blood.

For NIDDM, the focus is on ways to prevent diabetes. Preventive approaches include identifying people at high risk for the disorder and encouraging them to lose weight, exercise more, and follow a healthy diet. The Diabetes Prevention Program, another new NIDDK project, will focus on preventing the disorder in high-risk populations.

Points to Remember

1. What Is Diabetes?

   - A disorder of metabolism—the way the body digests food for energy and growth.

2. What Are the Different Types of Diabetes?

   - Insulin-dependent diabetes (IDDM)
   - Noninsulin-dependent diabetes (NIDDM)
   - Gestational diabetes.

3. What Is the Scope and Impact of Diabetes?

   - Affects 16 million people
   - A leading cause of death and disability
   - Costs $92 billion per year.

4. Who Gets Diabetes?

   - People of any age
   - More common in older people, African Americans, Hispanics, and Native Americans.

Where Is More Information Available?

For more information about IDDM, NIDDM, and gestational diabetes, as well as diabetes research, statistics, and education, contact:

National Diabetes Information Clearinghouse
1 Information Way
Bethesda, MD 20892-3560
(301) 654-3327.

The following organizations also distribute materials and support programs for people with diabetes and their families and friends:

American Association of Diabetes Educators
444 North Michigan Avenue, Suite 1240
Chicago, IL 60611
(800) 832-6874
(312) 644-2233

American Diabetes Association
ADA National Service Center
1660 Duke Street
Alexandria, VA 22314
(800) 232-3472
(703) 549-1500

Juvenile Diabetes Foundation International
120 Wall Street
19th Floor
New York, NY 10005
(800) 223-1138
(212) 785-9500.

National Diabetes Information Clearinghouse
1 Information Way
Bethesda, MD 20892-3560
ndic@aerie.com

Section 12.2

Diabetes Statistics

NIH Publication No. 96-3926.

Prevalence of Diabetes in the United States

Total (diagnosed and undiagnosed): 16 million (1995 estimate)

- Diagnosed: 8 million

- Undiagnosed: 8 million

- Insulin-dependent diabetes (IDDM): Estimates range up to 800,000. (No national registry for diabetes exists. These estimates are extrapolated from several regional registries.)

- Noninsulin-dependent diabetes (NIDDM): About 7 to 7.5 million diagnosed cases (1993 estimate)

Cost

Studies of the cost of illness are based on many factors, and estimates may vary, depending on what an individual study includes in its analysis. The NIH, CDC, ADA, JDFI and other members of the diabetes community estimate the annual cost of diabetes to the country based on two major studies:

1. $91.1 billion for direct costs, including items such as inpatient and outpatient care for all diagnoses in diabetes patients; drugs, medical supplies[1] and nursing home care.[2]

2. $46.6 billion for indirect costs, such as loss of wages and productivity, and premature mortality.[2]

$137.7 billion is the total of both direct and indirect costs, derived by combining the above estimates.

Deaths

In 1993 about 400,000 deaths from all causes were estimated to have occurred in people with diabetes. This figure represents 5 percent of all persons known to have diabetes and 18 percent of all deaths in the United States in persons age 25 years and older. Based on death certificate data, diabetes contributed to the deaths of more than 169,000 persons in 1992. It is well known that death certificate data under-represent diabetes deaths. Diabetes was the seventh leading cause of death listed on U.S. death certificates in 1993, according to the National Center for Health Statistics. It is the sixth leading cause of death by disease.

Incidence

- Total new cases diagnosed every day: About 1,700 (1990-92 averaged)
- Total new cases diagnosed each year: 625,000 (1990-92 averaged)
- NIDDM: About 595,000 new cases per year
- IDDM: About 30,000 new cases per year

Prevalence

Number of people diagnosed with diabetes (1993 estimates)

- Women: 4.2 million
- Men: 3.6 million
- Children age 19 years or younger: About 100,000
- Adults age 65 years or older: 3.2 million

Percent of adults with diabetes by race and ethnicity (diagnosed and undiagnosed)

- African Americans: 9.6 percent
- Mexican Americans: 9.6 percent
- Cuban Americans: 9.1 percent
- Puerto Rican Americans: 10.9 percent
- White Americans: 6.2 percent
- American Indians: Ranges from 5 to 50 percent
- Japanese Americans: Among second-generation Japanese Americans 45 to 74 years of age residing in King County, WA, 20 percent of the men and 16 percent of the women had diabetes.

Treatment for Diabetes

Treatment emphasizes control of blood glucose through blood glucose monitoring, regular physical activity, meal planning, and attention to relevant medical and psychosocial factors. In many patients, oral medications and/or insulin injections are also required for appropriate glucose control. Treatment of diabetes is an ongoing process that is planned and regularly reassessed by the health care team, the person with diabetes, and his/her family. Patient and family education are important parts of the process.

- IDDM: By definition, people with IDDM require insulin injections.

- NIDDM: About 40 percent use insulin, 49 percent use oral agents, 10 percent use combination of insulin and oral medications.

Long-Term Complications

Heart disease

- Cardiovascular disease is two to four times more common in people with diabetes.

- Cardiovascular disease is present in 75 percent of diabetes-related deaths.

- Middle-aged people with diabetes have death rates twice as high and heart disease death rates about two to four times as high as middle-aged people without diabetes.

Stroke

- The risk of stroke is 2.5 times higher in people with diabetes.

High blood pressure

- Affects 60 to 65 percent of people with diabetes.

Blindness

- Diabetes is the leading cause of new cases of blindness among adults 20 to 74 years of age.

- From 12,000 to 24,000 new cases of blindness per year are caused by diabetic retinopathy.

Kidney disease (treatment by dialysis or transplantation)

- Diabetes is the leading cause of end-stage renal disease, accounting for 36 percent of new cases.

- 19,790 new cases occurred in 1992 in people with diabetes.

- 56,059 people with diabetes were undergoing dialysis or transplantation treatment in 1992.

Nerve disease

- About 60 to 70 percent of people with diabetes have mild to severe forms of diabetic nerve damage (with such manifestations as impaired sensation in the feet or hands, delayed stomach emptying, carpal tunnel syndrome, peripheral neuropathy).

- Severe forms of diabetic nerve disease are a major contributing cause of lower extremity amputations.

Amputations

- More than half of the lower limb amputations in the United States occur among people with diabetes; from 1989 to 1992, the average number of amputations performed each year among people with diabetes was 54,000.

Dental disease

- Studies show that periodontal disease, which can lead to tooth loss, occurs with greater frequency and severity in people with diabetes. In one study, 30 percent of IDDM patients age 19 years or older had periodontal disease.

- The rate of tooth loss is 15 times higher in Pima Indians with NIDDM, compared to those without diabetes, and the incidence of periodontal disease is 2.6 times higher.

Pregnancy

- The rate of major congenital malformations in babies born to women with preexisting diabetes varies from 0 to 5 percent in women who receive preconception care to 10 percent in women who do not receive preconception care.

- Three to 5 percent of pregnancies in women with diabetes result in death of the newborn; this compares to a rate of 1.5 percent in women who do not have diabetes.

Gestational Diabetes

Gestational diabetes is a type of diabetes that develops in some pregnant women; the condition disappears when the pregnancy is over. A history of gestational diabetes, however, is a risk factor for eventual development of NIDDM.

- Occurs in 2 to 5 percent of pregnancies, with higher rates in African Americans, Hispanics/Latino Americans, and American Indians (rates in American Indians range from 1 to 14 percent).

Impaired Glucose Tolerance (IGT)

IGT refers to a condition in which blood sugar levels are higher than normal but not high enough to be classified as diabetes (between 140 and 199 mg/dL in a 2-hour oral glucose tolerance test). IGT is a major risk factor for NIDDM.

- Present in about 11 percent of adults.

- About 40 to 45 percent of persons age 65 years or older have either NIDDM or IGT.

For More Information

The National Diabetes Information Clearinghouse (NDIC) is a service of the National Institute of Diabetes and Digestive and Kidney Diseases, part of the National Institutes of Health, under the U.S. Public Health Service. The clearinghouse, authorized by Congress in 1978, provides information about diabetes to people with diabetes and their families, health care professionals, and the public. NDIC answers inquiries; develops, reviews, and distributes publications; and works closely with professional and patient organizations and government agencies to coordinate resources about diabetes.

National Diabetes Information Clearinghouse
1 Information Way
Bethesda, MD 20892-3560

References

1. Rubin, R.J., Altman, W.M., and Mendelson, D.N. "Health Care Expenditures for People with Diabetes Mellitus, 1992*" *Journal of Clinical Endocrinology and Metabolism.* 78: 809A-809F, 1994. (Also known as the Lewin-VHI Study, 1993)

2. American Diabetes Association, "Direct and Indirect Costs of Diabetes in the United States in 1992," American Diabetes Association, 1993.

The Following Organizations Collaborated in Compiling This Section:

American Association of Diabetes Educators

American Diabetes Association

Centers for Disease Control and Prevention

Department of Veterans Affairs

Health Resource Services Administration

Indian Health Service

Juvenile Diabetes Foundation International

National Institute of Diabetes and Digestive and Kidney Diseases of the National Institutes of Health

Chapter 13

Stress, Depression, and Suicide

Chapter Contents

Section 13.1

Handling Stress

DHHS Publication No. (ADM) 91-502. Printed 1977 Revised 1983 Reprinted 1985. 1987. 1991. U.S. Department of Health and Human Services; Public Health Service; Alcohol, Drug Abuse, and Mental Health Administration; National Institute of Mental Health Office of Scientific Information.

You *need* stress in your life! Does that surprise you? Perhaps so, but it is quite true. Without stress, life would be dull and unexciting. Stress adds flavor, challenge, and opportunity to life. Too much stress, however, can seriously affect your physical and mental well-being. A major challenge in this stress-filled world of today is to make the stress in your life work for you instead of against you.

Stress is with us all the time. It comes from mental or emotional activity and physical activity. It is unique and personal to each of us. So personal, in fact, that what may be relaxing to one person may be stressful to another. For example, if you are an executive who likes to keep busy all the time, "taking it easy" at the beach on a beautiful day may feel extremely frustrating, nonproductive, and upsetting. You may be emotionally distressed from "doing nothing." Too much emotional stress can cause physical illness such as high blood pressure, ulcers, or even heart disease; physical stress from work or exercise is not likely to cause such ailments. The truth is that physical exercise can help you to relax and to handle your mental or emotional stress.

Hans Selye, M.D., a recognized expert in the field, has defined stress as a "non-specific response of the body to a demand." The important issue is learning how our bodies respond to these demands. When stress becomes prolonged or particularly frustrating, it can become harmful—causing distress or "bad stress." Recognizing the early signs of distress and then doing something about them can make an important difference in the quality of your life, and may actually influence your survival.

Reacting to Stress

To use stress in a positive way and prevent it from becoming distress, you should become aware of your own reactions to stressful events. The body responds to stress by going through three stages: (1) alarm, (2) resistance, and (3) exhaustion.

Let's take the example of a typical commuter in rush-hour traffic. If a car suddenly pulls out in front of him, his initial alarm reaction may include fear of an accident, anger at the driver who committed the action, and general frustration. His body may respond in the alarm stage by releasing hormones into the bloodstream which cause his face to flush, perspiration to form, his stomach to have a sinking feeling, and his arms and legs to tighten. The next stage is resistance, in which the body repairs damage caused by the stress. If the stress of driving continues with repeated close calls or traffic jams, however, his body will not have time to make repairs. He may become so conditioned to expect potential problems when he drives that he tightens up at the beginning of each commuting day. Eventually, he may even develop a physical problem that is related to stress, such as migraine headaches, high blood pressure, backaches, or insomnia. While it is impossible to live completely free of stress and distress, it is possible to prevent some distress as well as to minimize its impact when it can't be avoided.

Helping Yourself

When stress does occur, it is important to recognize and deal with it. Here are some suggestions for ways to handle stress. As you begin to understand more about how stress affects you as an individual, you will come up with your own ideas of helping to ease the tensions.

- **Try physical activity.** When you are nervous, angry, or upset, release the pressure through exercise or physical activity. Running, walking, playing tennis, or working in your garden are just some of the activities you might try. Physical exercise will relieve that "up tight" feeling, relax you, and turn the frowns into smiles. Remember, your body and your mind work together.

- **Share your stress.** It helps to talk to someone about your concerns and worries. Perhaps a friend, family member, teacher, or counselor can help you see your problem in a different light. If you feel your problem is serious, you might seek professional help from a psychologist, psychiatrist, social worker, or mental health counselor. Knowing when to ask for help may avoid more serious problems later.

- **Know your limits**. If a problem is beyond your control and cannot be changed at the moment, don't fight the situation. Learn to accept what is—for now—until such time when you can change it.

- **Take care of yourself.** You are special. Get enough rest and eat well. If you are irritable and tense from lack of sleep or if you are not eating correctly, you will have less ability to deal with stressful situations. If stress repeatedly keeps you from sleeping, you should ask your doctor for help.

- **Make time for fun.** Schedule time for both work and recreation. Play can be just as important to your well being as work; you need a break from your daily routine to just relax and have fun

- **Be a participant.** One way to keep from getting bored, sad, and lonely is to go where it's all happening. Sitting alone can make you feel frustrated. Instead of feeling sorry for yourself, get involved and become a participant. Offer your services in neighborhood or volunteer organizations. Help yourself by helping other people. Get involved in the world and the people around you, and you'll find they will be attracted to you. You will be on your way to making new friends and enjoying new activities.

- **Check off your tasks.** Trying to take care of everything at once can seem overwhelming, and, as a result, you may not accomplish anything. Instead, make a list of what tasks you have to do, then do one at a time, checking them off as they're completed. Give priority to the most important ones and do those first.

- **Must you always be right?** Do other people upset you—particularly when they don't do things your way? Try cooperation instead of confrontation; it's better than fighting and always being "right." A little give and take on both sides will reduce the strain and make you both feel more comfortable.

- **It's OK to cry**. A good cry can be a healthy way to bring relief to your anxiety, and it might even prevent a headache or other physical consequence. Take some deep breaths; they also release tension.

- **Create a quiet scene.** You can't always run away, but you can "dream the impossible dream." A quiet country scene painted mentally, or on canvas, can take you out of the turmoil of a stressful situation. Change the scene by reading a good book or playing beautiful music to create a sense of peace and tranquility.

- **Avoid self-medication.** Although you can use prescription or over-the-counter medications to relieve stress temporarily, they do not remove the conditions that caused the stress in the first place. Medications, in fact, may be habit-forming and also may reduce your efficiency, thus creating more stress than they take away. They should be taken only on the advice of your doctor.

The Art of Relaxation

The best strategy for avoiding stress is to learn how to relax. Unfortunately, many people try to relax at the same pace that they lead the rest of their lives. For a while, tune out your worries about time, productivity, and "doing right." You will find satisfaction in just being, without striving. Find activities that give you pleasure and that are good for your mental and physical well-being. Forget about always winning. Focus on relaxation, enjoyment, and health. If the stress in your life seems insurmountable, you may find it beneficial to see a mental health counselor. Be good to yourself.

—Louis E. Konolow. M.D.

Section 13.2

Plain Talk about Depression

NIH Publication No.94-3561 Printed 1994,
AHCPR Doc. No.95-5018 July 11, 1995

During any 1 year period, 17.6 million American adults or 10 percent of the population suffer from a depressive illness. The cost in human suffering cannot be estimated. Depressive illnesses often interfere with normal functioning and cause pain and suffering not only to those who have a disorder, but also to those who care about them. Serious depression can destroy family life as well as the life of the ill person.

Possibly the saddest fact about depression is that much of this suffering is unnecessary. Most people with a depressive illness do not seek treatment, although the great majority—even those with the severest disorders—can be helped. Thanks to years of fruitful research, the medications and psychosocial therapies that ease the pain of depression are at hand.

Unfortunately, many people do not recognize that they have a treatable illness. Read this section to see if you are one of the many undiagnosed depressed people in this country or if you know someone who is. The information briefly presented here may help you take the steps that may save your own or someone else's life.

What Is a Depressive Disorder?

A depressive disorder is a "whole-body" illness, involving your body, mood, and thoughts. It affects the way you eat and sleep, the way you feel about yourself, and the way you think about things. A depressive disorder is *not* the same as a passing blue mood. It is *not* a sign of personal weakness or a condition that can be willed or wished away.

People with a depressive illness cannot merely "pull themselves together" and get better. Without treatment, symptoms can last for weeks, months, or years. Appropriate treatment, however, can help most people who suffer from depression.

Types of Depression

Depressive disorders come in different forms, just as do other illnesses, such as heart disease. This section briefly describes three of the most prevalent types of depressive disorders. However, within these types there are variations in the numbers of symptoms, their severity, and persistence.

Major depression is manifested by a combination of symptoms (see symptom list) that interfere with the ability to work, sleep, eat, and enjoy once pleasurable activities. These disabling episodes of depression can occur once, twice, or several times in a lifetime.

A less severe type of depression, *dysthymia* involves long-term, chronic symptoms that do not disable, but keep you from functioning at "full steam" or from feeling good. Sometimes people with dysthymia also experience major depressive episodes.

Another type is *bipolar disorder* formerly called manic-depressive illness. Not nearly as prevalent as other forms of depressive disorders, bipolar disorder involves cycles of depression and elation or mania. Sometimes the mood switches are dramatic and rapid, but most often they are gradual. When in the depressed cycle, you can have any or all of the symptoms of a depressive disorder. When in the manic cycle, any or all symptoms listed under mania may be experienced. Mania often affects thinking, judgment, and social behavior in ways that cause serious problems and embarrassment. For example, unwise business or financial decisions may be made when an individual is in a manic phase. Bipolar disorder is often a chronic recurring condition.

Depression More Debilitating than Chronic Illness

A recent study sponsored by AHCPR has revealed that for many people depression—even mild depression—is more physically and socially debilitating than chronic medical conditions such as Type I and II diabetes, heart attack and hypertension. In fact, even though the depression may have improved considerably over time, two years after first consulting a doctor, depressed people still tended to be worse off than those with chronic illnesses.

The study, conducted by researchers at RAND Corporation in Santa Monica and the University of California, Los Angeles, looked at people with depression or chronic medical conditions two years after their initial visit to a physician. After two years, people with mild depression were significantly more limited in physical and role functioning, reported greater bodily pain, and had worse general health perceptions than did patients with hypertension, for example, even though the hypertensives' physical functioning had significantly deteriorated over the course of time. "Depressed people are often less able to perform their social roles as parents or workers," explains researcher Ron D. Hays, Ph.D., "and experience more physical pain and generally perceive their health as worse than persons with chronic medical conditions."

Symptoms of Depression and Mania

Not everyone who is depressed or manic experiences every symptom. Some people experience a few symptoms, some many. Also, severity of symptoms varies with individuals.

Depression

- Persistent sad, anxious, or "empty" mood
- Feelings of hopelessness, pessimism
- Feelings of guilt, worthlessness, helplessness
- Loss of interest or pleasure in hobbies and activities that were once enjoyed, including sex
- Insomnia, early-morning awakening, or oversleeping
- Appetite and/or weight loss or overeating and weight gain
- Decreased energy, fatigue, being "slowed down"
- Thoughts of death or suicide; suicide attempts
- Restlessness, irritability
- Difficulty concentrating, remembering, making decisions
- Persistent physical symptoms that do not respond to treatment, such as headaches, digestive disorders, and chronic pain.

Mania

- Inappropriate elation
- Inappropriate irritability
- Severe insomnia
- Grandiose notions
- Increased talking

- Disconnected and racing thoughts
- Increased sexual desire
- Markedly increased energy
- Poor judgment
- Inappropriate social behavior.

Causes of Depression

Some types of depression run in families, indicating that a biological vulnerability can be inherited. This seems to be the case with bipolar. Studies of families, in which members of each generation develop bipolar disorder, found that those with the illness have a somewhat different genetic makeup than those who do not get ill. However, the reverse is not true: Not everybody with the genetic makeup that causes vulnerability to bipolar disorder has the illness. Apparently additional factors, possibly a stressful environment, are involved in its onset.

Major depression also seems to occur, generation after generation, in some families. However, it can also occur in people who have no family history of depression. Whether inherited or not, major depressive disorder is often associated with having too little or too much of certain neurochemicals.

Psychological makeup also plays a role in vulnerability to depression. People who have low self-esteem, who consistently view themselves and the world with pessimism, or who are readily overwhelmed by stress are prone to depression.

A serious loss, chronic illness, difficult relationship, financial problem, or any unwelcome change in life patterns can also trigger a depressive episode. Very often, a combination of genetic, psychological, and environmental factors is involved in the onset of a depressive disorder.

Diagnostic Evaluation and Treatment

The first step to getting appropriate treatment is a complete physical and psychological evaluation to determine whether you have a depressive illness, and if so what type you have. Certain medications as well as some medical conditions can cause symptoms of depression and the examining physician should rule out these possibilities through examination, interview, and lab tests.

A good diagnostic evaluation also will include a complete history of your symptoms, i.e., when they started, how long they have lasted, how severe they are, whether you've had them before and, if so, whether you were treated and what treatment you received. Your doctor should ask you about alcohol and drug use, and if you have thoughts about death or suicide. Further, a history should include questions about whether other family members have had a depressive illness and if treated, what treatments they may have received and which were effective.

Last, a diagnostic evaluation will include a mental status examination to determine if your speech or thought patterns or memory have been affected, as often happens in the case of a depressive or manic-depressive illness.

Treatment choice will depend on the outcome of the evaluation. There are a variety of antidepressant medications and psychotherapies that can be used to treat depressive disorders. Some people do well with psychotherapy, some with antidepressants. Some do best with combined treatment: medication to gain relatively quick symptom relief and psychotherapy to learn more effective ways to deal with life's problems. Depending on your diagnosis and severity of symptoms, you may be prescribed medication and/or treated with one of the several forms of psychotherapy that have proven effective for depression.

At times, electroconvulsive therapy (ECT) is useful, particularly for individuals whose depression is severe or life-threatening or who cannot take antidepressant medication. ECT often is effective in cases where antidepressant medications do not provide sufficient relief of symptoms. In recent years, ECT has been much improved. The treatment is given in the hospital under sedation so that people receiving ECT do not feel pain.

Antidepressant Medications

Three groups of antidepressant medications are most often used to treat depressive disorders: tricyclics, monoamine oxidase inhibitors (MAOIs), and lithium. Lithium is the treatment of choice for bipolar disorder and some forms of recurring, major depression. Sometimes your doctor will try a variety of antidepressants before finding the medication or combination of medications most effective for you. Sometimes the dosage must be increased to be effective. Also, new types of antidepressants are being developed all the time, and one of these may be the best for you.

There are now two new classes of antidepressants which are neither tricyclics nor MAOIs, and which generally lack the side effects associated with these two traditional classes of drugs. The first of these is fluoxetine, a serotonin re-uptake inhibitor; the other is bupropion, believed to act on the dopaminergic system.

Patients often are tempted to stop medication too soon. *It is important to keep taking medication until your doctor says to stop, even if you feel better beforehand.* Some medications must be stopped gradually to give your body time to adjust. For individuals with bipolar disorder or chronic major depression, medication may have to become part of everyday life to avoid disabling symptoms.

Antidepressant drugs are not habit-forming, so you need not be concerned about that. However, as is the case with any type of medication prescribed for more than a few days, antidepressants have to be carefully monitored to see if you are getting the correct dosage. Your doctor will want to check the dosage and its effectiveness regularly.

If you are taking MAO inhibitors, you will have to avoid certain foods, such as cheeses, wines, and pickles. Be sure you get a complete list of foods you should not eat from your doctor and always carry it with you. Other forms of antidepressants require no food restrictions.

Never mix medications of any kind—prescribed, over-the-counter, or borrowed—*without consulting your doctor.* Be sure to tell your dentist or any other medical specialist who prescribes a drug that you are taking antidepressants. Some of the most benign drugs when taken alone can cause severe and dangerous side effects if taken with others. Some drugs, like alcohol, reduce the effectiveness of antidepressants and should be avoided. This includes wine, beer, and hard liquor.

Anti-anxiety drugs or sedatives are *not* antidepressants. They are sometimes prescribed along with antidepressants; however, they should not be taken alone for a depressive disorder. Sleeping pills and stimulants, such as amphetamines, are also inappropriate.

Be sure to call your doctor if you have a question about any drug or if you have having a problem you believe is drug related.

Side Effects

Antidepressants may cause mild and, usually, temporary side effects in some people. Typically these are annoying, but not serious. However, unusual side effects or those that interfere with functioning should be reported to your doctor. The most common side effects usually associated with tricyclic antidepressants and ways to deal with them, are:

- Dry mouth—drink lots of water; chew sugarless gum; clean teeth daily.

- Constipation—eat bran cereals, prunes, fruit, and vegetables.

- Bladder problems—emptying your bladder may be troublesome, and your urine stream may not be as strong as usual; call your doctor if there is any pain.

- Sexual problems—sexual functioning may change, if worrisome, discuss with your doctor.

- Blurred vision—this will pass soon; do not get new glasses.

- Dizziness—rise from bed or chair slowly.

- Drowsiness—this will pass soon; do not drive or operate heavy equipment if feeling drowsy or sedated.

The newer antidepressants have different types of side effects:

- Headache—this will usually go away.

- Nausea—even when it occurs, it is transient after each dose.

- Nervousness and insomnia—these may occur during the first few weeks; dosage reductions or time will usually resolve them.

- Agitation—if this happens for the first time after the drug is taken and is more than transient, consult your doctor.

Psychotherapies

There are many forms of psychotherapy effectively used to help depressed individuals, including some short term (10-20 weeks) therapies. "Talking" therapies help patients gain insight into and resolve their problems through verbal "give-and-take" with the therapist. "Behavioral" therapists help patients learn how to obtain more satisfaction and rewards through their own actions and how to unlearn the behavioral patterns that contribute to their depression.

Two of the short term psychotherapies that research has shown helpful for some forms of depression are Interpersonal and Cognitive/ Behavioral therapies. Interpersonal therapists focus on the patient's disturbed personal relationships that both cause and exacerbate the depression. Cognitive/Behavioral therapists help patients change the negative styles of thinking and behaving often associated with depression.

Psychodynamic therapies, sometimes used to treat depression, focus on resolving the patient's internal psychological conflicts that are typically thought to be rooted in childhood.

In general, the severe depressive illnesses, particularly those that are recurrent, will require medication (or ECT under special conditions) along with psychotherapy for the best outcome.

Helping Yourself

Depressive disorders make you feel exhausted, worthless, helpless, and hopeless. Such negative thoughts and feelings make some people feel like giving up. It is important to realize that these negative views are part of the depression and typically do not accurately reflect your situation. Negative thinking fades as treatment begins to take effect. In the meantime:

- Do not set yourself difficult goals or take on a great deal of responsibility.

- Break large tasks into small ones, set some priorities, and do what you can as you can.

- Do not expect too much from yourself too soon as this will only increase feelings of failure.

- Try to be with other people; it is usually better than being alone.

- Participate in activities that may make you feel better.

- You might try mild exercise, going to a movie, a ball game, or participating in religious or social activities.

- Don't overdo it or get upset if your mood is not greatly improved right away. Feeling better takes time. Do not make major life decisions, such as changing jobs, getting married or divorced, without consulting others who know you well and who have a more objective view of your situation. In any case, it is advisable to postpone important decisions until your depression has lifted.

- Do not expect to snap out of your depression. People rarely do. Help yourself as much as you can, and do not blame yourself for not being up to par.

- *Remember*, do not accept your negative thinking. It is part of the depression and will disappear as your depression responds to treatment.

Family and Friends Can Help

Since depression can make you feel exhausted and helpless, you will want and probably need help from others. However, people who have never had a depressive disorder may not fully understand its effect. They won't mean to hurt you, but they may say and do things that do. It may help to share this section with those you most care about so they can better understand and help you.

Helping the Depressed Person

The most important thing anyone can do for the depressed person is to help him or her get appropriate diagnosis and treatment. This may involve encouraging the individual to stay with treatment until symptoms begin to abate (several weeks), or to seek different treatment if no improvement occurs. On occasion, it may require making an appointment and accompanying the depressed person to the doctor. It may also mean monitoring whether the depressed person is taking medication.

The second most important thing is to offer emotional support. This involves understanding, patience, affection, and encouragement. Engage the depressed person in conversation and listen carefully. Do not disparage feelings expressed, but point out realities and offer hope. Do not ignore remarks about suicide. Always report them to the depressed person's therapist.

Invite the depressed person for walks, outings, to the movies, and other activities. Be gently insistent if your invitation is refused. Encourage participation in some activities that once gave pleasure, such as hobbies, sports, religious or cultural activities, but do not push the depressed person to undertake too much too soon. The depressed person needs diversion and company, but too many demands can increase feelings of failure.

Do not accuse the depressed person of faking illness or of laziness, or expect him or her "to snap out of it." Eventually, with treatment, most depressed people do get better. Keep that in mind, and keep reassuring the depressed person that, with time and help, he or she will feel better.

Where to Get Help

A complete physical and psychological diagnostic evaluation will help you decide the type of treatment that might be best for you. Listed above are the types of people and places that will make a referral to, or provide, diagnostic and treatment services.

Check the Yellow Pages under "mental health," "health," "social services," "suicide prevention," "hospitals," or "physicians" for phone numbers and addresses.

- Family doctors
- Mental health specialists, such as psychiatrists, psychologists, social workers, or mental health counselors
- Health maintenance organizations
- Community mental health centers
- Hospital psychiatry departments and outpatient clinics
- University—or medical school—affiliated programs
- State hospital outpatient clinics
- Family service/social agencies
- Private clinics and facilities
- Employee assistance programs
- Local medical and/or psychiatric societies

—Marilyn Sargent,
Office of Scientific Information,
National Institute of Mental Health

Further Information

Write To:

D/ART Public Inquiries
National Institute of Mental Health
Room 7C-02
5600 Fishers Lane
Rockville, MD 20857
1-800-421-4211

National Alliance for the Mentally Ill
2101 Wilson Boulevard, Suite 302
Arlington, VA 22201
(703) 524-7600; 1-800-950-NAMI

National Depressive and Manic Depressive Association
730 N. Franklin, Suite 501
Chicago, IL 60601
(312) 642-0049; 1-800-826-3632

National Foundation for Depressive Illness, Inc.
P.O. Box 2257
New York NY 10016
(212) 2684260; 1-800-248-4344

National Mental Health Association
1021 Prince Street
Alexandria, VA 22314-2971
(703) 684-7722; 1-800-969-6642

Section 13.3

Suicide Facts

NIH Publication Suicide Facts, June 1996.
Suicide in the Elderly, July 1991.

Completed Suicides, U.S. 1993

Suicide is the 9th leading cause of death in the United States, accounting for 1.4 percent of total deaths.

The 1993 age-adjusted rate was 11.3/100,000, or 0.0113 percent.

- Only 1.4 percent of total deaths were from suicide. By contrast, 33 percent were from diseases of the heart, 23 percent were from malignant neoplasms, and 6.6 percent from cerebrovascular disease, the three leading causes

Suicide by firearms is the most common method for both men and women, accounting for 61 percent of all suicides

More men than women die by suicide.

- The gender ratio is over 4:1.
- Over 72 percent of all suicides are committed by white men.
- Nearly 80 percent of all firearm suicides are committed by white men.

The highest suicide rates are for persons over 65; however, it is not a leading cause of death in this age group.

- The 1993 suicide rate for white men over 85 was 73.6/100,000.

Suicide is the third leading cause of death among young people 15 to 24 years of age, following unintentional injuries and homicide. In this age group:

- suicide rates are lower than for any other group except children less than 14 years of age;
- the rate was 13.5/100,000 in 1993, up from 13.0/100,000 in 1992;
- the total number of deaths in 1993 was 4,849. compared with 31,102 for all ages;
- The gender ratio was 5.5:1 (men:women).

Among young people 15 to 19 years of age the suicide rate was 10.9/ 100,000 in 1993.

- The total number of deaths was 1,884, compared with 31,102 for all ages.
- Rates among both young women and young men in this age group have increased since 1979; rates for young men have increased at a greater rate than rates for young women.
- The gender ratio was over 4.6:1 (men:women).

Among young people 20 to 24 years of age the suicide rate was 15.8/ 100,000 in 1993, up from 14.9/100,000 in 1992.

- The total number of deaths was 2,965, compared with 31,102 for all ages.
- Rates increased in 1993 for both young men and young women.
- The 1993 gender ratio was 6.1:1 (men:women).

Research Findings

Suicide is a complex behavior. The risk factors for suicide frequently occur in combination

- Scientific research has shown that almost all people who kill themselves have a diagnosable *mental* or *substance abuse* disorder; the majority have more than one disorder.

- Basic research has shown that alterations in neurotransmitters/ neuromodulators such as serotonin can increase risk for suicide. These altered levels have been found in patients with depression, violent suicide attempts and impulsive disorders, and also in postmortem brains of suicide victims.

- Adverse life events in combination with other strong risk factors such as mental or substance abuse disorders and impulsivity, may lead to suicide. However, suicide and suicidal behavior are not normal responses to the stresses experienced by most people. Many people experience one or more risk factors and are not suicidal.

More Research Findings

Familial factors in highly dysfunctional families can be associated with suicide, including:

- family history of mental or substance abuse disorder;
- family history of suicide;
- family violence, including emotional, physical, or sexual abuse.

Other risk factors include:

- prior suicide attempt
- firearm in the home
- incarceration
- exposure to the suicidal behavior of others, including family members, peers, and/or via the media in news or fiction stories.

Attempted Suicides

No national data on attempted suicide are available; reliable scientific research, however, has found that:

- There are an estimated 8-25 attempted suicides to one completion; the ratio is higher in women and youth and lower in men and the elderly.

- More women than men report a history of attempted suicide, with a gender ratio of about 2:1.

- The strongest risk factors for attempted suicide in adults are depression, alcohol abuse, cocaine use, and separation or divorce.

- The strongest risk factors for attempted suicide in youth are depression, alcohol or other drug use disorder, and aggressive or disruptive behaviors.

The majority of suicide attempts are expressions of extreme distress that need to be addressed, and not just a harmless bid for attention.

Prevention

Because suicide is a highly complex behavior, preventive interventions must also be complex and intensive if they are to have lasting effects over time.

Based on reliable findings from scientific research, recognition and appropriate treatment of mental and substance abuse disorders is the most promising way to prevent suicide and suicidal behavior in all age groups.

Because most elderly suicides have visited their primary care physician in the month prior to their suicides, recognition and treatment of depression in the medical setting is a promising way to prevent elderly suicide.

Limiting young people's access to firearms and other forms of responsible firearms ownership, especially in conjunction with the prevention of mental and addictive disorders, also may be beneficial avenues for prevention of firearm suicides.

Most school-based, information-only, prevention programs focused solely on suicide have *not* been evaluated to see if they work.

- New research suggests that such programs may actually increase distress in the young people who are most vulnerable.

School and community prevention programs designed to address sui-cide and suicidal behavior as part of a broader focus on mental health, coping skills in response to stress, substance abuse, aggressive behav-iors, etc., are most likely to be successful in the long run.

All suicide prevention programs need to be scientifically evaluated to demonstrate whether or not they work.

Suicide in the Elderly

Suicide is the eighth leading cause of death in the United States; over 30,400 people take their own lives each year. One person com-mits suicide every 17.3 minutes, over 83 per day. Perhaps as many as five million Americans have attempted to kill themselves. When suicide is discussed as a public health problem, emphasis is often placed upon the incidence among youth and young adults, a group accounting for 15.2 percent of the population and 16.2 percent of the suicides. However, less attention is paid to the startling fact that the highest rates of suicide actually are among the elderly, those over the age of 65. While representing only 12.4 percent of the population, older people take their own lives at a rate of 21 percent, a rate higher than found among members of any other age group in our nation.

Over the course of the century, the suicide rates for the elderly have fluctuated widely. While the long-term trend has been downward, the past decade has shown an increase, though not yet to the levels en-countered in the decade between 1930-1940. As our nation as a whole ages, the elderly have become the fastest growing segment of the popu-lation. When the large group of "baby boomers" reach old age, the absolute number of elderly suicides will likely rise sharply. Experts believe that to avoid a virtual epidemic of late life suicide, each of us must be better able to identify and help the people at risk.

A Profile of the Older Person at Risk

At all ages, men are more likely than women to commit suicide. Among the elderly, however, the difference becomes even more pro-nounced. In the general population, suicide rates for males are about four times that of females; among the "old-old" (age 75 and over), men have rates up to 13 times higher than women. Across the age spectrum, whites are at nearly 10 times the risk of non-whites. However, distinctions by race are substantially diminished with increased age.

Sex, race, marital status and socio-economic status are not the only factors implicated in suicide. Indeed, the decision to take one's own life is based on a complex constellation of factors. Among the elderly, three of these other risk factors, often working together include loss, physical illness and depressive disorder.

Loss: The elderly frequently encounter multiple losses in biological as well as psycho-social arenas. Greying hair and wrinkled skin are experienced by some as a loss of vitality; retirement may mean a loss of income, power and culturally sanctioned roles. Physical relocation, whether cross-country, to a neighboring community or to a nursing facility, may radically alter social patterns and networks. Friends and family die. The loss of a spouse can be an especially devastating event, increasing the risk for suicide by coupling loss and grief with isolation and loneliness. As a whole, the fear of becoming institutionalized or otherwise dependent on others, with the associated loss of physical integrity and autonomy, are common themes among elders who have contemplated, attempted or completed suicide.

Physical ill health: Numerous studies have found that deteriorating health is common among the suicidal elderly. The illnesses most closely linked are cancer, ulcers, brain disorders such as stroke or seizure, musculoskeletal disorders (such as arthritis), and bladder and prostate problems. For some terminally ill patients, suicide results from a reasoned choice of death over protracted illness. However, studies have shown that such circumstances are rare. The vast majority of patients with terminal illness do not choose to commit suicide, and those who are suicidal almost invariably have an associated severe clinical depression.

Depressive illness: Among the factors making the elderly vulnerable to suicide, mental illness is one of the most salient. Research has consistently shown that from 66-90 percent of persons taking their lives suffered from a diagnosable psychiatric illness at the time of death, most often a syndrome known as "clinical depression" or "major depression." Studies have found that up to 87 percent of elderly persons attempting or completing suicides were suffering from a form of this illness. Ironically, many effective treatments are available to treat depressive illness. Had their illness been detected and treated vigorously, suicide may well have been avoided.

Although substance abuse is less frequent among the elderly than among the young, it remains a major contributor to suicidal behavior.

Older persons who commit suicide frequently have abused alcohol, or prescription sedatives and painkillers.

Suicide Signals

Because clinical depression is so common in suicidal elderly, its early recognition can help to identify the majority of those at risk. Typical symptoms include thoughts of suicide, feelings of sadness, guilt and hopelessness, loss of interest in usually pleasurable activities, loss of appetite and energy, and sleep difficulty. In its most severe forms, the syndrome is easily recognized and should be treated by trained professionals. However, older people are often reluctant to see psychiatrists or other mental health personnel, whether as the result of fear or financial concerns. Instead, most suicidal elderly emphasize physical complaints to the exclusion of mood change, frequently visiting their family doctors for treatment of aches and pains actually symptomatic of the underlying depressive illness. Thus, exaggerated physical complaints may also be a signal of suicide risk. In fact, as many as three quarters of geriatric suicides have visited their personal physician within a month prior to the suicide or attempt.

People who make even vague comments about suicide or a desire to be dead should always be taken seriously. This is especially true for the elderly, who appear to make fewer attempts but use more lethal means to end their lives.

Studies have shown that over half of geriatric suicide victims have indicated their intent to others, but that such comments usually were not heeded. When statements about suicide are accompanied by changes in behavior, such as giving away possessions or changing a will, the risk of suicide is greatly increased.

How to Help

Once identified as being at risk, the suicidal person should be evaluated professionally. In the most dire cases, when the individual is at or near the point of harming himself, emergency rooms and hotlines are available to intervene quickly. Where time permits evaluation and treatment are also available through local mental health centers and in the private offices of mental health professionals. However, because the elderly tend not to self-refer to either mental health professionals or suicide prevention/crisis intervention services, family members, friends and services personnel who come in contact with older persons should be particularly vigilant.

A suicidal person may resist helping interventions; hopelessness is a part of the suicidal state. Moreover, depressive illness may cloud judgment. Complicating the situation still further are the facts that treatment may be perceived by the elderly as stigmatizing or financially prohibitive. Ironically, many of the conditions that may cause older people to feel suicidal can be treated by qualified professionals. With professional help that provides hope that both physical and psychological pain will lessen, the suicidal person usually will choose life.

−Barry D. Lebowitz, Ph.D., Chief
Mental Disorders of the Aging Research Branch.

Section 13.4

Posttraumatic Stress Disorder

It's been called shell shock, battle fatigue, accident neurosis and post rape syndrome. It has often been misunderstood or misdiagnosed, even though the disorder has very specific symptoms that form a definite psychological syndrome.

The disorder is post-traumatic stress disorder (PTSD) and it affects hundreds of thousands of people who have survived earthquakes; accidental disasters such as airplane crashes; or manmade disasters such as inner-city violence, domestic abuse, rape, war and the Holocaust.

Psychiatrists estimate that up to 10 percent of the population have been affected by clinically diagnosable PTSD. Still more show some symptoms of the disorder. While it was once thought to be mostly a disorder of war veterans who had been involved in heavy combat, researchers now know that PTSD afflicts both female and male civilians, and that it strikes more females than males.

In some cases the symptoms of PTSD disappear with time, while in others they persist for many years. It often occurs with—or leads to—other psychiatric illnesses, such as depression.

Not all people who experience trauma require treatment; some recover with the help of family, friends, pastor or rabbi. But many do need professional help to successfully recover from the psychological damage that can result from experiencing, witnessing or participating in an overwhelmingly traumatic event.

Although the understanding of post-traumatic stress disorder is based primarily on studies of trauma in adults, PTSD can occur in children as well. It is known that traumatic occurrences—birth trauma, child or domestic abuse, loss of parents, the disaster of war—often have a profound impact on the lives of children. Further research is needed, however, to establish the special characteristics of the disorder in children that distinguish it from its counterpart in adults. It is not clear, for example, how the development and resolution of the condition are affected by the type of trauma, the age at which it occurs and the type of treatment used.

Symptoms

Post-traumatic stress disorder usually appears within three months of the trauma, but sometimes the disorder surfaces months or even years later. Psychiatrists categorize PTSD's symptoms in four categories: intrusive symptoms, avoidant symptoms, symptoms of hyperarousal and associative features.

Intrusive Symptoms

Often people suffering from PTSD have an episode where the traumatic event "intrudes" into their current life. This can happen in sudden, vivid memories that are accompanied by very painful emotions and take over the victim's attention. This "re-experience" of the trauma is a flashback—a recollection that is so strong that the individual thinks he or she is actually experiencing the trauma again or seeing it unfold before his or her eyes. In traumatized children, this reliving of the trauma occurs in the form of action, through repetitive play.

When a person has a severe flashback, he or she is in a dissociative state, which sometimes can be mistaken for sleepwalking.

When that happens, the person acts as if he or she were actually experiencing the traumatic event again. But he or she isn't fully conscious of what he or she is doing. For example, a war veteran may begin prowling around his neighborhood as if patrolling hostile territory.

At other times, the re-experience occurs in nightmares that are so powerful the person awakens screaming in terror, as if he or she were re-enacting the trauma in sleep. In young children, distressing dreams of the traumatic event evolve into generalized nightmares of monsters, of rescuing others or of threats to self or others.

At times, the re-experience comes as a sudden, painful onslaught of emotions that seem to have no cause. These emotions, often those of grief that bring tears and a tight throat, can also be of anger or fear. Individuals say these emotional experiences occur repeatedly, much like memories or dreams about the traumatic event.

Symptoms of Avoidance

Another set of symptoms involves what is called avoidance phenomena. This affects the person's relationships with others, because he or she often avoids close emotional ties with family, colleagues and friends. At first, the person feels numb, has diminished emotions and can complete only routine, mechanical activities. Later, when re-experiencing the event begins, the individual alternates between the flood of emotions caused by re-experiencing and the inability to feel or express emotions at all. People who suffer post-traumatic stress disorder frequently say they can't feel emotions, especially toward those who are closest. Even if they can feel emotions, they often can't express them. As the avoidance continues, the person seems to be bored, cold or preoccupied. Family members often feel rebuffed by the person because he or she lacks affection and acts mechanically.

For children, emotional numbness and diminished interest in significant activities may be difficult concepts to explain to a therapist. For this reason, the reports of parents, teachers and other observers are particularly important.

The person with PTSD also avoids situations that are reminders of the traumatic event because the symptoms worsen when a situation or activity occurs that resembles, even in part, the original trauma. For example, a person who survived a prisoner-of-war camp might overreact to seeing people wearing uniforms similar to those of the camp guards. Over time, the person can become so fearful of particular situations that his or her daily life is ruled by attempting to avoid them.

Others, particularly war veterans, avoid accepting responsibility for others because they think they failed in ensuring the safety of those killed or injured during battle. As a result of this, many with PTSD have poor work records, trouble with their bosses and poor relationships with their family and friends. Children suffering from PTSD may show a marked change in orientation toward the future. A child may, for example, not expect to marry or have a career. Or he or she may exhibit "omen formation," the belief in an ability to predict future untoward events.

PTSD sufferers' inability to work out grief and anger over injury or loss during the traumatic event mean the trauma will continue to control their behavior without their being aware of it. Depression is a common product of this inability to resolve painful feelings. Some people also feel guilty because they survived a disaster while others—particularly friends or family—did not. In combat, veterans or survivors of civilian disasters, this guilt may be worse if they witnessed or participated in behavior that was necessary to survival but unacceptable to society. Such guilt can deepen depression as the person begins to look on him or herself as unworthy, a failure, a person who violated his or her pre-disaster values.

Symptoms of Hyperarousal

PTSD can cause those who suffer with it to act as if they were constantly threatened by the trauma that caused their illness. People with PTSD can often become suddenly irritable or explosive, even when they are not being provoked. They may have trouble concentrating or remembering current information, and, due to the terrifying nightmares that afflict them, they may develop insomnia.

This constant feeling that danger is near causes exaggerated startle reactions. War veterans may revert to their war behavior, diving for cover when they hear a car backfire or a string of firecrackers exploding. At times, those with PTSD suffer panic attacks, which result from the extreme fear they felt during the trauma, which has remained unresolved during later events in life. During the attack, their throats tighten, breathing and heart rate increase, and they feel dizzy and nauseated. Children may exhibit physical symptoms, including stomachaches and headaches, in addition to symptoms of increased arousal.

Associated Features

Finally, many who suffer with PTSD also attempt to rid themselves of their painful re-experiences, loneliness, and panic attacks by abusing alcohol or other drugs as a "self-medication" that helps them to blunt their emotions and forget the trauma. A person with PTSD may also show poor control over his or her impulses, and may be at risk for suicide.

Treatment

Psychiatrists and other mental health professionals today have good success in treating the very real and painful effects of PTSD. Using a variety of treatment methods, they help people who suffer with PTSD to work through their trauma and pain to resolve their unexpressed grief.

One important form of therapy for those who struggle with post-traumatic stress disorder is behavior therapy. This treatment approach focuses on correcting the PTSD sufferer's painful and intrusive patterns of behavior and thought by teaching him or her relaxation techniques, and examining (and challenging) his or her mental processes. A therapist using behavior therapy to treat a person with PTSD might, for example, help a patient who is provoked into panic attacks by loud street noises by setting a schedule that gradually exposes the patient to such noises in a controlled setting until he or she becomes "desensitized" and thus no longer so prone to terror. Using other such techniques, patient and therapist explore the patient's environment to determine what might aggravate the PTSD symptoms and work with the patient to reduce sensitivity or to teach them new skills for coping.

Psychiatrists and other mental health professionals also treat cases of PTSD by using psychodynamic psychotherapy. Post-traumatic stress disorder results, in part, from the difference between the individual's personal values or view of the world and the reality that he or she witnessed or lived during the traumatic event. Psychodynamic psychotherapy, then, focuses on helping the individual examine personal values and how behavior and experience during the traumatic event violated them. The goal is resolution of the conscious and unconscious conflicts that were thus created. In addition, the individual works to build self-esteem and self-control, develops a good and reasonable sense of personal accountability and renews a sense of integrity and personal pride.

In addition, therapists may recommend family therapy because the behavior of spouse and children may result from and affect the individual suffering post-traumatic stress disorder. Spouses and children report their loved one doesn't communicate, show affection, or share in family life. By working with the family, the therapist can work to bring about change within the family. Its members can learn to recognize and cope with the range of emotions each feels. They do this by learning good communication, parenting and stress management techniques.

Therapy involving rap groups or peer-counseling groups is another effective treatment for many suffering from post-traumatic stress disorder. This method encourages survivors of similar traumatic events to share their experiences and reactions to them. In doing so, group members help each other realize that many people would have done the same thing and felt the same emotions. That, in turn, helps the individual realize that he is not uniquely unworthy or guilty. Over time, individuals change opinions of themselves and others and can build a new view of the world and redefine a positive sense of self.

Generally, such treatments can be completed on an outpatient basis. But if the disorder is so severe that the person is dangerous to himself or others, inpatient treatment might be recommended.

With most patients, medication can help to control the symptoms of PTSD. While medication or psychotherapy alone are rarely sufficient to resolve the illness, the symptom relief medication provides enables most patients to participate more effectively in psychotherapy when their condition may otherwise prohibit it. Antidepressant medications are particularly helpful in treating the core symptoms of PTSD—especially intrusive symptoms.

Controlled studies of treatment for PTSD are only beginning to take place. Research into the effects of medication has been spurred by the growing awareness of the long-term physiological changes that appear to accompany PTSD, such as increased sympathetic arousal. Medication appears to alleviate these symptoms of hyperarousal, although it is ineffective against symptoms of avoidance such as alienation, detachment and emotional numbness.

The most thorough study of the use of medications for PTSD was reported in the American Journal of Psychiatry in March 1988. The study concluded that tricyclic antidepressants as well as some monoamine oxidase inhibitors are effective in the treatment of PTSD. Some success with lithium has been reported in the treatment of rage and affective (mood-related) symptoms. Benzodiazepines may be particularly effective for crises, although their addictive potential warrants caution. And beta-blockers and the alpha-2 agonist, clonidine, have been found effective for symptoms such as intrusive thoughts and explosive outbursts of emotion.

Bibliography

General Information

Burgess, Ann Wolbert. Rape: Victims of Crisis. Bowie, Maryland: Robert J. Brady, Co., 1984.

Burgess, Ann Wolbert. The Sexual Victimization of Adolescents. Rockville, Maryland: National Institute of Mental Health, National Center for the Prevention and Control of Rape, 1985.

Egendorf, A. Healing from the War: Trauma and Transformation After Vietnam. New York: Houghton Mifflin, 1985. (non-clinical)

Eitinger, Leo, and Robert Krell with Miriam Rieck. The Psychological and Medical Effects of Concentration Camps and Related Persecutions on Survivors of the Holocaust. Vancouver: University of British Columbia Press, 1985.

Eth, S. and R.S. Pynoos. Post-Traumatic Stress Disorder in Children. Washington, D.C.: American Psychiatric Press, Inc., 1985.

Friedman, Matthew, J. "Toward Rational Pharmacotherapy for Posttraumatic Stress Disorder: An Interim Report." The American Journal of Psychiatry, Vol. 145: No. 3 (March 1988), 281285.

Lindy, Jacob D. Vietnam: A Casebook. New York: Brunner/Mazel, 1987.

Sonnenberg, S. M., A.S. Blank and J.A. Talbott, editors. The Trauma of War: Stress and Recovery in Vietnam Veterans. Washington, D.C.: American Psychiatric Press, Inc., 1985.

Van der Kolk, B.A., editor. Post-Traumatic Stress Disorder: Psychological and Biological Sequelae. Washington, D.C.: American Psychiatric Press, Inc., 1984.

Other Resources

Anxiety Disorders Association of America, Inc.
6000 Executive Blvd.
Rockville, MD 20852-3801
(301) 831-8350

International Society for Traumatic Stress Studies
435 N. Michigan Ave., Suite 1717
Chicago, IL 60611-4067
(312) 644-0828

National Center for Post-traumatic Stress Disorder
VAM & ROC 116D
Rural Route 5
White River Junction, VT 05009
(802) 296-5132

National Institute of Mental Health
5600 Fishers Lane
Rockville, Maryland 20857
(301) 443-2403

U.S. Veterans Administration
Mental Health and Behavioral Sciences Services
810 Vermont Avenue, N.W., Room 915
Washington, D.C. 20410
(202) 389-3416

U.S. Veterans Administration
Readjustment Counseling Service (IOB/RC)
810 Vermont Avenue, N.W.
Washington, D.C. 20410
(202) 233-3317

Section 13.5

Posttraumatic Stress Disorder or Midlife Crisis in Vietnam Veterans?

©1994 National Association of Social Workers. *Social Work*. 36:3, May 1994. Reprinted with permission.

In October 1980 the Veterans Administration recognized posttraumatic stress disorder (PTSD) as a compensable disorder (Bitzer, 1980). An estimated 500,000 to 1.5 million combat and noncombat veterans suffer from the disorder (Sierles, Chen, McFarland, & Taylor, 1983). In one state, more than 40 claimants per month were being evaluated for PTSD by the Department of Veterans Benefits (Atkinson, Henderson, Sparr, & Deale, 1982).

PTSD occurs in a cluster of interrelated symptoms (American Psychiatric Association, 1980). The individual must have at least one of the following: persistent intrusive distressing recollections of the trauma, recurrent distressing dreams of the event, or feelings that the event is recurring (American Psychiatric Association, 1987).

Researchers Egendorf, Kadushin, and Laufer (1981) and Kadushin, Boulanger, and Martin (1981) developed a Stress Reaction Scale to more accurately measure symptoms particular to Vietnam veterans. Attempting to use most of the symptoms of PTSD contained in the Diagnostic and Statistical Manual of Mental Disorders, Third Edition, (American Psychiatric Association, 1980), they developed the following criteria for stress reaction: memory trouble, loss of interest, thought confusion, nightmares, feelings of loss of control, and panic attacks.

In contrast, the symptoms most commonly found in Vietnam veterans diagnosed as having PTSD are substance abuse, depression, jumpiness, sleep disturbances, marital and legal problems, emotional confusion, guilt, anger, alienation, and physical and psychosomatic illnesses (LaGuardia, Smith, Francois, & Bachman, 1983; Langley, 1982; Walker, 1981; Walker&Nash, 1981).

Although these symptoms suggest a diagnosis of PTSD in Vietnam veterans, the same symptoms are prevalent in middle-age men in crisis who are non-veterans (Downey, 1983; Keal & Hoag, 1984; Levinson, 1978; Medinger & Varghese, 1981; Peplau, 1975).

When comparing the incidence of depressive symptoms and syndromes of Vietnam veterans to that of non-veterans, studies have shown little difference between the two groups (Helzer, Robins, Wish, & Hesselbock, 1979; Starr, Henry, & Bonner, 1973). The high rate of emotionally disturbed backgrounds of Vietnam veterans suggests that emotional problems would have surfaced during middle age regardless of their war experiences (LaGuardia et al., 1983). In some cases, PTSD in veterans could be predicted with the use of childhood behavioral assessments (Helzer, Robins, & McEvoy, 1987).

Midlife Crisis

Although no single event indicates middle age, definite physiological, behavioral, social, and psychological changes occur (Langley, 1982; Zacks, 1980). Next to facing his own death, a man's realization that he is aging may be the most profound shock of his life (Levinson, 1978).

Middle age brings a sense of desperation to make the most out of what is left of one's life. A man may become confused, lose touch with his inner self, neglect his responsibilities, make a drastic career change, quit his job, or even abandon his family (Levinson, 1978; Medinger & Varghese, 1981; Peplau, 1975; Strickler, 1975).

Levinson (1977) warned that such men are not "sick," but in a normal developmental period that "must involve emotional turmoil, despair, the sense of not knowing where to turn or being stagnant and unable to move at all" (p. 107). Perhaps it is this normal transitional period, and not PTSD, that many Vietnam veterans are experiencing.

PTSD has become known as a "unique problem" among Vietnam veterans with psychological problems (Thienes-Hontos, Watson, & Kucala, 1982). When symptoms of PTSD and another syndrome overlap, PTSD generally becomes the primary target, taking the "either/or . . . position of excessive diagnostic parsimony" (Atkinson et al., 1982, p. 1120). Never before have so many labels been placed on war veterans. The following are a few:

- **Emotional conflict:** Withholding feelings and emotions is a common characteristic among American men who adhere to the masculine role stereotype (Downey, 1983; Goldberg, 1979;

Harrison, 1978). Even so, the absence of emotional expression by Vietnam veterans has been labeled "frozen mourning" (Shatan, 1973).

- **Marital conflict:** The high divorce rate among Vietnam veterans is also attributed to their war experiences (Langley, 1982). But Berman (1975) and Cuber and Haroff (1965) suggested that in the general population marital conflict peaks in couples between ages 30 and 50.

- **Depression, sleep disturbances, and violence:** Long-term alcohol abuse and illegal drug use are prevalent among Vietnam veterans (LaGuardia et al., 1983; Nace, Meyers, O'Brien, Ream, & Mintz, 1977; Sierles et al., 1983; Walker & Nash, 1981). Studies have shown that depression, sleep disturbances, violence, and nightmares are all closely linked to substance abuse (Leaton, 1978).

Clinical Evaluation for PTSD

Regrettably, few guidelines exist for the appropriate psychological assessment of PTSD (Fairbank, Keane, & Malloy, 1983). Clinical reports suggest that the most frequent symptoms of PTSD are psychosomatic ailments (DeFazio, Rustin, & Diamond, 1975; Lifton, 1973; Van & Emory, 1973). Hogben and Cornfeld (1981) warned that PTSD symptoms mimic other disorders including alcohol and drug abuse, schizophrenia, and hallucinogenic disorders, as well as phobic and depressive states.

Claimants are well informed of the symptoms of PTSD from brochures distributed by veterans groups and organizations (Atkinson et al., 1982). Sparr and Pankratz (1983) cautioned that a large number of veterans with fictitious symptoms are seeking treatment for war-related PTSD. PTSD has become so widely discussed and diagnosed that some veterans have used it as an excuse for murder (Ressler & Shadhtman, 1992).

Therefore, social workers and other counselors must conduct careful clinical evaluation of the veteran's military history. A veteran's claim of service in a combat theater can be verified by obtaining a copy of the veteran's discharge (DD214) and by requesting a copy of the veteran's military records from the Military Personnel Records Center.

A veteran's DD214 will verify whether the person served in Vietnam, in what capacity, and the number of months of foreign service.

The veteran's military records provide more detailed information than that on the discharge. Veterans Outreach Centers are also available to answer questions regarding veterans.

Conclusion

This article in no way discounts the existence, or the seriousness, of PTSD in Vietnam veterans. But it encourages therapists to look beyond a single diagnosis when treating Vietnam veterans and to stop viewing them as "psychiatric casualties" (Thienes-Hontos et al., 1982). More research is necessary to determine if the veteran's emotional distress is indeed a result of PTSD, if it is caused by age-related difficulties, or if it is caused by a combination of the two.

—Janet S. Pierson and Raymond F. Pierson

Janet S. Pierson, MA, SC-HIV/AIDS, is psychotherapist, HIV/AIDS counselor and tester, P.O. Box 39423, St. Louis, MO 63139. Raymond F. Pierson, LCSW, MSW, is clinical coordinator, Veterans Outreach Center, St. Louis.

References

American Psychiatric Association. (1980). Diagnostic and statistical manual of mental disorders (3rd ed.). Washington, D.C.: Author.

American Psychiatric Association. (1987). Diagnostic and statistical manual of mental disorders (3rd ed., rev.) Washington, D.C.: Author.

Atkinson, R. A., Henderson, R. G., Sparr, L. F., & Deale, S. (1982). Assessment of Viet Nam veterans for posttraumatic stress diverter in Veterans Administration disability claims. American Journal of Psychiatry, 139,1118-1121.

Berman, E. M. (1975). Marital therapy from a psychiatric perspective: An overview. American Journal of Psychiatry, 132, 585.

Bitzer, R. (1980). Caught in the middle: Mentally disabled veterans and the Veterans Administration. In C. R. Figley & C. Leventman (Eds.), Strangers at home: Vietnam veterans since the war (pp. 305-323). New York: Praeger.

Cuber, J. F., & Haroff, P. B. (1965). The significant Americans. New York Appleton-Century-Crofts.

DeFazio, V. J., Rustin, S., & Diamond, A. (1975). Symptoms development in Vietnam era veterans. American Journal of Orthopsychiatry, 45(1), 158-163.

Downey, A. M. (1983). The relationship of sex-role orientation to death anxiety in middle-aged males. Omega, 4, 355-367.

Egendorf, A., Kadushin, C., & LauEer, R. S. (Eds.). (1981). Legacies of Vietnam: Comparative adjustment of veterans and their peers. Washington, D.C.: U.S. Government Printing Office.

Fairbank, J. A., Keane, T. M., & Malloy, P. F. (1983). Some preliminary data on the psychological characteristics of Vietnam veterans with postraumatic stress disorders. Journal of Consulting and Clinical Psychology, 51, 912-919.

Goldberg, H. (1979). The new man. New York: William Morrow.

Harrison, J. (1978). Warning: The male sex role may be dangerous to your health. Journal of Social Issues, 34(1), 64-85.

Helzer, J. E., Robins, L. N., & McEvoy, L. (1987). Posttraumatic stress disorder in the general population. New England Journal of Medicine, 317(26), 16301634.

Helzer, J. E., Robins, L. N., Wish, E., & Hesselbrock, M. (1979). Depression in Viet Nam veterans and civilian controls. American Journal of Psychiatry, 136, 526-529.

Hogben, G. I., & Cornfeld, R. B. (1981). Treatment of traumatic war neurosis with phenelzine. Archives of General Psychiatry, 38, 440-445.

Kadushin, C., Boulanger, G., & Martin, J. (1981). Long-term stress reactions: Some causes, consequences, and naturally occurring support systems. In A. Egendorf, C. Kadushin, & R. S. Laufer, (Eds.), Legacies of Vietnam: Comparative adjustment of veterans and their peers (pp. 134ff). Washington, D.C.: U. S. Government Printing Office.

Keal, M. C., & Hoag, L. J. (1984). The social construction of the mid-life crisis: A case study in the temporalities of identity. Sociological Inquiries, 54, 279-300.

LaGuardia, R. L., Smith, G., Francois, R., & Bachman, L. (1983). Incidence of delayed stress disorder among Vietnam era veterans: The effects of priming on response set. American Journal of Orthopsychiatry, 53(1), 18-26.

Langley, K. M. (1982). Post-traumatic stress disorder among Vietnam combat veterans. Social Casework, 61 593-598.

Leaton, K. (1978). Loosening the grip. St. Louis: C. V. Mosby.

Levinson, D. J. (1977). The mid-life transition: A period in adult psychosocial development. Psychiatry, 40,99-112.

Levinson, D. J. (1978). The seasons of a man's life. New York: Ballantine Books.

Lifton, R. (1973). Home from the war. New York: Simon & Schuster.

Medinger, F., & Varghese, R. (1981). Psychological growth and the impact of stress in middle-aged males. International Journal of Aging and Human Development, 13(4), 247-263.

Nace, E., Meyers, A., O'Brien, C., Ream, N., & Mintz, J (1977). Depression in veterans two years after Viet Nam. American Journal of Psychiatry, 134, 167-170.

Peplau, H. (1975). Mid-life crisis. American Journal of Nursing, 75, 1761-1765.

Ressler, R. K., & Shachtman, T. (1992). Whoever fights monsters. New York: St. Martin's Press.

Shatan, C. (1973). The grief of soldiers: Vietnam combat veterans'self-help movement. American Journal of Orthopsychiatry, 43, 640 653.

Sierles, F. S., Chen, J. J., McFarland, R. E., & Taylor, M. A. (1983). Posttraumatic stress disorder and concurrent psychiatric illness: A preliminary report. American Journal of Psychiatry, 140, 1177-1179.

Sparr, L., & Pankratz, L. D. (1983). Factitious posttraumatic stress disorder. American Journal of Psychiatry, 140, 101-1019.

Starr, P., Henry, J., & Bonner, R. (1973). The discarded army: Veterans after Vietnam. New York: Charter House.

Stickler, M. (1975). Crisis intervention and the climacteric man. Social Casework, 56, 85-89.

Thienes-Hontos, P., Watson, C. G., & Kucala, T. (1982). Stress disorder symptoms in Vietnam veterans and Korean War veterans. Journal of Consulting and Clinical Psychology, 50, 558-561.

Van, P. T., & Emory, W. (1973). Traumatic neurosis in Vietnam returnees: A forgotten diagnosis? Archives of General Psychiatry, 29, 695-698.

Walker, J. I. (1981). The psychological problems of Viet Nam veterans. Journal of the American Medical Association, 246, 781-782.

Walka, J. I., & Nash, J. (1981). Group therapy in the treatment of Vietnam combat veterans. International Journal of Group Psychotherapy, 31, 379-389.

Zacks, H. (1980). Self-actualization: A mid-life problem. Social Casework, 61, 223-233.

Chapter 14

Homicide

Chapter Contents

Section 14.1

Victimization

NIH Publication No. 97-1232. Extracted from
Health United States 1996-97 and Injury Chartbook.
From Web Site: (http:www.cec.gov/nchswww/data/hus96_97.pdf).

In 1994 U. S. residents 12 years of age and over reported being victims in an estimated 10.9 million violent crimes at a rate of 51 per 1,000 persons. Nearly one-quarter of all violent victimizations, 2.7 million, resulted in an injury to the victim. These range in severity from bruises, black eyes, and broken teeth to rape, firearm, stabbing, and other injuries requiring hospitalization. One-third of all robberies resulted in an injury as did a quarter of all assaults. Nearly three-quarters of sexual assault victims were rape (including attempted rape).

These data, from the National Crime Victimization Survey, show that the likelihood of being an injured victim in a violent crime generally decreases with increasing family income. The victimization rate for persons in households with annual family incomes less than $7,500 was 1.7 times the rate for persons in households with incomes of $25,000–$35,000, and was 2.1 times the rate in households with incomes of $75,000 or more.

The rate of victimization resulting in injury among persons in the lowest income household (less than $7,500) was also higher compared with rates in higher income households. The rate of victimization resulting in injury in the lowest family income group (26 per 1,000 persons) was 1.6 times the rate in the next income group, and it was 2.7 and 3.9 times the rates in the two highest income groups.

In households where the annual family income was at least $25,000, there were no significant differences in criminal victimization rates among white and black persons. At the lowest end of the family income distribution, however, victimization rates were higher for white persons than for black persons, 90 compared with 68 per 1,000 persons 12 years of age and over. Virtually all of this difference is in the level of the rates for "simple" rather than "aggravated assault" rates. Simple assaults accounted for 64 percent and 46 percent, respectively of crimes against white and black persons.

On the other hand where the family income was $15,000–$24,999, the victimization rate was higher for black persons than for white persons, 71 compared with 47 per 1,000 persons, with higher rates of aggravated assaults for black persons than for white persons (20 compared with 12 per 1,000 persons). Nearly a quarter of violent crimes against white and black persons were aggravated assaults.

In 1993–94 an estimated average annual 58 million episodes of injury, occurring at a rate of 23 episodes per 100 people, were reported in household interviews of the civilian noninstitutionalized population of the United States. The rate was higher for persons under 45 years of age than for older persons. An injury episode was more likely to be reported by males ages 15–24 years and 25–44 years than by females of those ages. On the other hand, for persons 65 years of age and over, females were more likely than males to report an injury.

For infants and young children under 5 years of age and for people over age 65 years, the majority of injuries (53 percent and 56 percent) occurred in the home.

For the population aged 15–24 years and 45–64 years, 8–9 percent of all injury episodes involved a moving motor vehicle.

Among all currently employed persons ages 18–44 years, about a third of all reported injuries happened at work, 43 percent for males compared with 21 percent among females.

Injury episodes were more likely to be reported by persons who lived alone rather than by those who lived with others. At ages 15–24 years through 65–74 years, the rate of injury episodes for people who lived alone was 2 times the rate for those who lived with other people.

It is important to realize that the number of episodes of injury is equal to or less than the incidence of injury conditions because a person may incur more than one injury in a single episode. In 1994 there were an estimated 62 million reported injury conditions in the United States at a rate of 23.8 per 100 persons per year. Ninety-two percent of reported injuries were medically attended. The most often reported injury conditions were sprains and strains, contusions and superficial injuries, open wounds and lacerations, and fractures and dislocations, all accounting for about three-fourths of current injuries.

Figure 14.1. *Violent crime victimization rates among persons 12 years of age and over by family income and race: United States, 1994 SOURCE: Bureau of Justice Statistics, National Crime Victimization Survey.*

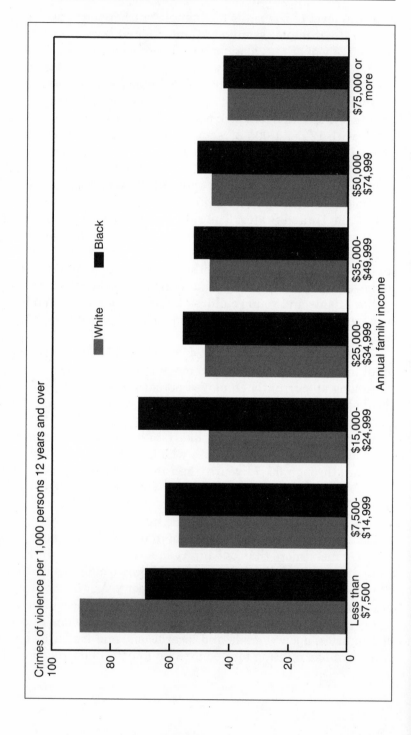

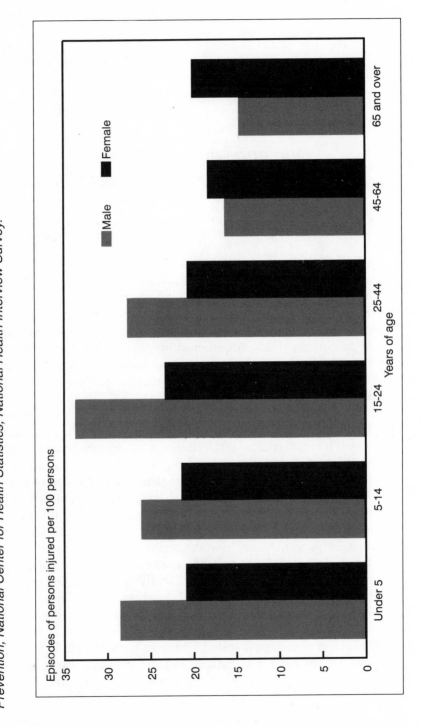

Figure 14.2. Episodes of injury by age and sex: United States, 1993–94. SOURCE: Centers for Disease Control and Prevention, National Center for Health Statistics, National Health Interview Survey.

Section 14.2

Violence and Work Injury: A Revealing Look at Turbulent Times

Violence in America is on the rise.

Violence has spanned the history of humankind. It has formed a common link between cultures and ethnic groups. We do not know whether aggression is genetic or learned, but we do know that all animals acquire this trait to ensure survival, territorial rights, and sexual dominance. However, in most animals except humans aggressive behavior ceases with victory or resolution of threat. The causes of human violence can be ascribed to endogenous (biological) or exogenous (psychosocial) factors (Table 14.1).[1]

Violence is endemic throughout American society and usually occurs between individuals or groups who know each other, often coworkers. The statistics about violence at work are staggering. The National Institute of Occupational Safety and Health found that homicide accounted for 12 percent of deaths in the workplace between 1980 and 1988, a figure exceeded only by transportation and machine-related work injuries.[2] In 1992, there were 110,000 incidents of workplace violence in the United States, and 1,004 worker deaths, of which 24 percent were in managerial or administrative support personnel.[3] In both 1992 and 1993, homicide was the second leading cause of workplace death.[4] In 1993, traffic accidents and workplace violence were the leading causes of death in North Carolina (Table 14.2)[2]; 54 of 214 fatal occupational injuries were due to homicide or suicide, second only to transportation as a cause of death.[5]

Workers in commercial settings were at highest risk, but "a sizable proportion of the victims of nonfatal violence were caregivers in nursing homes and hospitals" who were assaulted by patients.[6] In 1992, workplace violence cost American business approximately $4.2 billion.[7]

Usually violence is the result of outside problems spilling over into the workplace-for example, the nighttime robbery of a convenience store. However, workplace conflict can turn into real violence such as the shooting sprees of angry postal workers in California and Michigan. The senseless bombing of the federal building in Oklahoma City has made it apparent that our homes and workplaces are no longer safe. Americans are concerned. Though such events are not yet commonplace, employers and employees must recognize the potential for violent responses created by a changing economy, corporate downsizing, reinventing jobs, and the evolving character of our modern workforce.

Job terminations, whether due to economic factors or performance issues, may lead to acts of anger or workplace violence by disgruntled former employees. Companies that are downsizing or restructuring are well advised to use consultants and mediators to minimize the adverse effects on workers who are laid off and the morale of workers who remain.

"Post-mortem" evaluation of workplace incidents often reveals that management has responded poorly to employees' needs and concerns. Causes of violent acts in the workplace should be assessed and ways sought to prevent repetition. Education, debriefing, and counseling programs can help workers who have experienced physically or emotionally traumatic events.[3]

Currently, North Carolina has an increasing number of foreign-born workers. There are factories in Charlotte where workers speak five different languages. Employee relations must pay attention to cross-cultural issues, including attitudes about ethnicity, interpersonal relations, and the prevalence of violent and aggressive behaviors. Management must not only understand these issues, but secure the workplace for its employees.[5]

Workplace Security: Limiting Exposure[5, 8]

Four axioms relate to security in the workplace:

1. **Communication.** When threats are made, employers and supervisors must listen. Employee frustration and anger must be recognized and communication established. In North Carolina, most employers can fire employees at will. Summary dismissal can affect employees emotionally and even threaten the survival of some. Employee assistance programs and other forms of employee mental health assistance should be available as a matter of protocol. These programs should provide

education and counseling about the recognition and management of stress and substance abuse, prevention of personal crises, and the recovery from trauma.

2. **Architecture and policy design.** Ample outside lighting secures pedestrian and parking areas. Access to parking lots and buildings should be monitored by guards or pass-card so that workers are protected from the potential for outside disputes overflowing into the workplace. Entrances and walk areas should be clear of obstructions. Escorts and security patrols should be used when indicated. A "buddy system" for employees at risk assigns personal responsibility and may alleviate some employer liability. Also, employees should be reminded of their responsibility to notify security of any potential for violence. A lockable "safe room" equipped with a cellular telephone can provide a secure location where threatened workers can wait for help.

3. **Hire well.** Pre-employment checks regarding previous unacceptable behavior, violence, or a migratory work history can identify potential risks. All character references should be checked. Applicants should be told they will be drug tested if hired, and that employee security is a corporate priority.

4. **Deal with bad behavior.** Safety directors, plant managers, and employers must be accessible to be effective. Management's prompt response to inappropriate worker behaviors will emphasize the importance of safety and harmony in the workplace culture.

War Games: The Injured Worker in an Adversarial Health Care System

Times have changed. Workers can no longer rely on local companies to provide lifelong employment and eventual retirement within the community. Today's generation of workers are likely to face job changes or layoffs. When employees find themselves economically cornered and threatened, animal instincts for survival may resurface. A sense of entitlement or of employer wrongdoing may lead to aggressive behavior, perhaps stoked by the idea that violence will lead to "justice."

Furthermore, we know that both physical and psychosocial issues surround work injuries whose symptoms last more than three months.[9, 10] In such cases, the potential for assault or violent behavior may extend into the physician's workplace. Without doubt, violent assaults on physicians have become more common in recent years (witness the attacks on physicians who perform abortions). Angry patients and family members have attacked both hospitals and health care providers. In 1993, a Los Angeles County physician was killed and two other doctors were held hostage by a man who stated "I want doctors, not nurses." The assailant held his hostages for five hours, telling negotiators that he was in no hurry to surrender because he "wanted to let them know how it felt to wait [for health care]."[11] In June 1994, a gunman entered the hospital grounds at Fairchild Air Force Base near Spokane spraying bullets. He killed four people and wounded 19, 10 seriously.[12]

Illness and injury may lead to serious physical disability, prolonged suffering, and even death. Despite knowing this, consumers' expectations about medical care have steadily risen so that incomplete recovery, medical complications, even the development of an anticipated medical outcome may lead to an aggressive, emotional response by the patient or his or her family. In modern America this often takes the form of legal redress. Plaintiff lawyers advertise their availability, and many advocate an adversarial response. Injured workers who find themselves unemployed and without control over their condition usually turn to the health care system for help. If the system responds slowly, or the injury resolves slowly, those workers may seek the advice of attorneys or solicitous family members.

Ideally, employers should identify injured workers so that they may express their concern: "You are valued. We need you. Please come back to work as soon as possible." The employer should be the first to establish communication, not a solicitous relative or local attorney. As the worker recovers, light duty should be made available in order to reduce lost productivity and the potential that the injured worker will develop a disability lifestyle.[10] Management should foster empathy and concern toward injured workers, not misunderstanding or ambivalence because of the company's losses. When communication from the workplace is not forthcoming or maintained, return to work is impeded. When workers feel traumatized, emotional factors inevitably lead to anger, blame, and variable degrees of conflict.

Insurance carriers are for-profit businesses. Many adjusters are medically uneducated, but often assert great control over case management. The receipt of financial reimbursement and other income guaranteed to the injured worker may be delayed while mortgage, utility, and car payments pile up. Insurance adjusters often ignore the inevitable psychosocial fall-out associated with work injury, preferring to blame the individual or identify the problem as pre-existing.

Lawyers see another side of the truth, seeking payment from the dwindling financial resources of the injured worker and family at the same time that they seek total and permanent disability status for their client. The defense attorney wants closure and will recommend ways in which the client can save money. The injured worker, by this time, wants "justice."

Physicians are often the source of much conflict. Most physicians do not know how to manage injured workers or how to navigate within the workers' compensation system. Physicians may see themselves as patient advocates, leading to criticism from insurers or employers. On the other hand, physicians may choose not to be advocates for the worker but for the system. They act as agents of social control, like police in the criminal justice system. They speak of "tough love" and become enforcers instead of healers.

Profiles of Individuals Prone to Violence[1, 8]

Psychologists and sociologists stress that the causes of violence are multifactorial, but point out that the typical perpetrator of violence is a white male between the ages of 30 and 40. Individuals involved in work injury often have a heavy investment in job-related self-esteem, but some have a history of oppositional behavior frequent disputes with management or violations of company policy. Violence-prone individuals may be emotionally disturbed. They may suffer from extreme stress in their personal life or job. They may be loners with minimal outside support systems and few interests who tend to externalize blame for disappointments. The workplace may serve as their surrogate family.

When medically evaluating injured workers, health care personnel should be concerned about any individual who expresses fear of losing outward control (threats of assault or homicide) or inward control (suicidal ideation or intent). Clues that the patient is looking for help include acts such as doctor shopping, gun purchases, reckless driving, or frequent temperamental outbursts.

The patient's medical history may reveal episodes of altered consciousness or dissociative states leading to violent behavior. Caregivers should seek possible organic causes such as an underlying brain lesion or previous psychiatric problems (Table 14.1). Past violent acts toward animals, children, or women suggest chronically low thresholds for anxiety, anger, and frustration, and difficulty controlling aggressive behavior. Previous fire-setting, assault, and homicide

360

are important clues, especially if the individual has worked within systems where violent behavior is frequently encountered, such as the military or police. Previous suicide attempts indicate a low threshold of impulse control and a proclivity to violence. Early developmental history may indicate severe emotional deprivation or rejection (such as abandonment by one or both parents), acts of sexual or physical abuse, witnessing violence in the home, or irresponsible behaviors by parents (such as drug and alcohol abuse). Unfortunately, the 1990s have made the graphic depiction of violence, including murder and sexual assault, generally available to children.[13]

Stress may trigger desire for vengeance toward those who are thought to have damaged a worker's self-esteem. The impulses may be deflected toward the workplace if the injured worker feels humiliated by job termination, particularly after a physical injury. Financial collapse and inability to maintain the family can invoke animal-like protective instincts. Violence in the health care workplace may result from such mechanisms.

Managing Injured Workers at Risk for Violent Behavior

Case presentation: A 38-year-old man had worked since age 14 when he was abandoned by his parents. He was raised by his disabled grandmother, and completed a ninth-grade education. He had undergone multiple surgeries as a child, including removal of a testicle at age 12. His longest period of employment was five years as a squad leader in the military where he specialized in demolition. Subsequently, he had a migratory work history and had been involved in altercations with several of his supervisors. In 1991, after three months of employment in a textile mill, he slipped while trying to support a 500-pound roll of cloth, twisting and injuring his back. A physician prescribed conservative care and relieved him of work duty.

Six months after the injury, he underwent lumbar decompression at L1-2 and L2-3, but his pain was worse after surgery. A recurrent disc herniation was discovered and a surgeon offered to operate, but the insurance carrier would not approve further surgery until at least six months had passed. The patient gained 30 pounds and became deconditioned. He smoked three packs of cigarettes and drank three pots of coffee per day. A second surgeon was consulted and felt that further surgery was not indicated; the patient was cleared for sedentary work. He was not able to do this because of perceived worsening of his pain. He spent most of his time in bed, adopting a disability lifestyle. Twice divorced, he lived alone with two dogs.

Almost two years after his injury, a psychological evaluation was approved. Depression was diagnosed, but no treatment offered. Finally, a spine surgeon performed a kyphoreduction with decompression of L1-2, L2-3, and fusion from L9 to L3. Unfortunately, his pain persisted.

During rehabilitation after surgery, the patient began to make angry comments, blaming the operating surgeon. He said: "If the lawsuit does not go through, I will end his career personally so he can't do this to anyone else. " He complained about the rehabilitation specialist: "All she does is make problems for me. Going to physical therapy is harassment. She knows therapy makes me worse and that is why she sends me here." He admitted that medical providers incited feelings of rage, and he made physical threats against all members of the treatment team. He frequently threatened suicide, and on one occasion came into the medical office with a gun. He was angry, depressed, and could not sleep, but no treatment was prescribed for these problems. The patient was sent to a multidisciplinary pain-rehabilitation treatment program but he did not follow the discharge recommendations and prescriptions.

Finally, in 1994, a complete diagnostic reevaluation revealed that the surgery had been technically in order. The patient was tapered off analgesic narcotics and released from treatment. He has continued to make violent threats, including homicide, toward the doctor, rehabilitation specialist, insurance carrier, and others.

This case points out the premorbid biological and psychological matrix of an individual at risk for violent behavior. This patient endured injury and pain within a "system of care" that provided minimal communication and support and responded slowly with appropriate medical management. Despite eventually receiving appropriate care, the patient experienced delays in implementation and communication which produced irreversible and permanent consequences, including dissatisfaction and hostility toward his doctors and care providers.

Ideally, the treatment of an injured worker[1, 14] begins at the workplace where employers and supervisors offer immediate support. Generally patients get frustrated and angry when workplace interventions have been absent or ineffective. Dissatisfaction with care and prognostic uncertainty may lead to threats of violence toward health care providers. If this occurs the physician should act first to protect himself or herself and surrounding staff. Afterward, the patient must be controlled using techniques ranging from the support of family members to physical restraints and seclusion.

The appropriate place in which to continue medical care will depend on the potential danger and difficulty in securing safe communication with the patient. Medical or other mediation experts should be used. A calm, facilitating manner and clear, non-judgmental verbalization by the clinician will often establish communication. If the patient's mental capacity or judgment are questionable, assistance from security or police, even hospital admission may be necessary.

The physician must assess the patient's ability to think and talk about his or her problem, so that any distorted perceptions and ideas can be identified. Appropriate treatment of depression or anxiety are important, as are assessments of organic brain dysfunction. Secluding patients who suffer from an acute organic cause such as drug intoxication or metabolic encephalopathy, or those with a potential for self-mutilation is contraindicated. Acute care is summarized in Table 14.1, below. Often the best initial intervention for an acutely disturbed patient consists of neuroleptic medication (usually thorazine or haloperidol) by intramuscular injection. Benzodiazepines or barbiturates may provide adjunctive benefit. Once psychiatric intervention is completed, all parties involved in the injured worker's care and case management must come together in arbitration. Unfortunately, such vital communication often does not occur.

Table 14.1 Acute care of the violent patient

1. Ensure safety of health care personnel.

2. Establish control and setting for interview.

3. Summon psychiatrist or mediation expert.

4. Establish calm non-threatening environment to facilitate patient communication.

5. Establish differential diagnosis.

6. Emergency medication management: parenteral thorazine or haloperidol; adjunctive brazepam, if needed.

7. Diagnostic and laboratory evaluation.

8. Psychiatry intervention.

A Final Word

Violence pervades modern society. Whether we like it or not, the human propensity for aggressive behavior has invaded the workplace, the school, and the home. Physicians and other health care providers must learn to manage this affliction along with other diseases characteristic of modern American society and culture. As with all medical disorders, prevention is the most cost-effective treatment. However, unlike infectious conditions vaccination does not seem to be an option.

Authors' note: This manuscript represents, in part, a synopsis of an Industrial Symposium sponsored by Charlotte Orthopedic Specialists on December 2, 1994. Speakers included Drs. Wheeler and Ruth and The Honorable Harry E. Payne, Jr., Commissioner, Department of Labor, State of North Carolina.

—Anthony H. Wheeler, MD, and Robed D. Ruth, PhD

Dr. Wheeler is an Orthopedic Neurologist at Charlotte Orthopedic Specialists, 1915 Randolph Road, Charlotte 28207. Dr. Ruth is Associate Professor of Sociology at Davidson College.

References

1. Tardiff K. Assessment and management of violent patients. Washington, DC: American Psychiatric Press, Inc., 1989.

2. Wall Street Journal, June 15,1993, A-1.

3. Stenberg CR, Gammon PJ. Occupational mental health: evolving strategies for a rapidly changing world. NC Med J 1995;59:228-33.

4. US Department of Labor, Bureau of Labor Statistics. Census of fatal occupational injuries, 1992 and 1993.

5. Payne HE. Violence and work-related injury: the facts. Industrial Symposium: Exploring the Issues...Defining the Solutions. Charlotte, NC: December 2, 1994.

6. US Department of Labor, Bureau of Labor Statistics. Violence in the workplace comes under closer scrutiny. Summary 94-10. August 1994.

7. Braverman M. Violence: the newest worry on the job. New York Times, December 12, 1993, Fell.

8. Ruth RD. The risk of violence in the healthcare provider system. Industrial Symposium: Exploring the Issues... Defining the Solutions. Charlotte, NC: December 2, 1994.

9. Polatin PB, Kenny RK, Gatchel RJ, Lillo E, Mayer TJ. Psychiatric illness in chronic low back pain. The mind and the spine. Which goes first? Spine 1993;18:66-71.

10. Wheeler AH. Evolutionary mechanisms on chronic low back pain and rationale for treatment Am J Pdn Management 1995;5 62-66.

11. King PH. Who would shoot a doctor? Los Angeles Time', February 10, 1993, A-3.

12. New York Times, June 21, 1994, A-10.

13. Lacayo R, Zoglin R. America's cultural revulsion. Time, June 12, 1995;145:24-39.

14. Roth LH, ed. Clinical Treatment of the Violent Person. New York: The Guilford Press, 1989.

Part Three

Family Planning Decisions

Chapter 15

Impotence and Infertility

Chapter Contents

Section 15.1

Understanding Impotence

NIH Publication No. 95-3923 September 1995.
National Institute of Diabetes and Digestive and Kidney Diseases.

What is impotence?

Impotence is a consistent inability to sustain an erection sufficient for sexual intercourse. Medical professionals often use the term "erectile dysfunction" to describe this disorder and to differentiate it from other problems that interfere with sexual intercourse, such as lack of sexual desire and problems with ejaculation and orgasm. This section focuses on impotence defined as erectile dysfunction.

Impotence can be a total inability to achieve erection, an inconsistent ability to do so, or a tendency to sustain only brief erections. These variations make defining impotence and estimating its incidence difficult. Experts believe impotence affects between 10 and 15 million American men. In 1985, the National Ambulatory Medical Care Survey counted 525,000 doctor-office visits for erectile dysfunction.

Impotence usually has a physical cause, such as disease, injury, or drug side-effects. Any disorder that impairs blood flow in the penis has the potential to cause impotence. Incidence rises with age: about 5 percent of men at the age of 40 and between 15 and 25 percent of men at the age of 65 experience impotence. Yet, it is not an inevitable part of aging.

Impotence is treatable in all age groups, and awareness of this fact has been growing. More men have been seeking help and returning to near-normal sexual activity because of improved, successful treatments for impotence. Urologists, who specialize in problems of the urinary tract, have traditionally treated impotence—especially complications of impotence.

How does an erection occur?

The penis contains two chambers, called the *corpora cavernosa*, which run the length of the organ (see Figure 15.1). A spongy tissue fills the chambers. The *corpora cavernosa* are surrounded by a membrane, called the *tunica albuginea*. The spongy tissue contains smooth muscles, fibrous tissues, spaces, veins, and arteries. The urethra, which is the channel for urine and ejaculate, runs along the underside of the *corpora cavernosa*.

Erection begins with sensory and mental stimulation. Impulses from the brain and local nerves cause the muscles of the *corpora cavernosa* to relax, allowing blood to flow in and fill the open spaces. The blood creates pressure in the *corpora cavernosa*, making the penis expand. The *tunica albuginea* helps to trap the blood in the *corpora cavernosa*, thereby sustaining erection. Erection is reversed when muscles in the penis contract, stopping the inflow of blood and opening outflow channels.

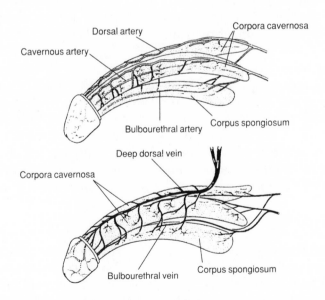

Figure 15.1. *Arteries (top) and veins (bottom) penetrate the long, filled cavities running the length of the penis—the* corpora cavernosa *and the cor-*
pus spongiosum. *Erection occurs when relaxed muscles allow the* corpora cavernosa *to fill with excess blood fed by the arteries, while drainage of blood through the veins is blocked.*

What causes impotence?

Since an erection requires a sequence of events, impotence can occur when any of the events is disrupted. The sequence includes nerve impulses in the brain, spinal column, and area of the penis, and response in muscles, fibrous tissues, veins, and arteries in and near the *corpora cavernosa*.

Damage to arteries, smooth muscles, and fibrous tissues, often as a result of disease, is the most common cause of impotence. Diseases— including diabetes, kidney disease, chronic alcoholism, multiple sclerosis, atherosclerosis, and vascular disease—account for about 70 percent of cases of impotence. Between 35 and 50 percent of men with diabetes experience impotence.

Surgery (for example, prostate surgery) can injure nerves and arteries near the penis, causing impotence. Injury to the penis, spinal cord, prostate, bladder, and pelvis can lead to impotence by harming nerves, smooth muscles, arteries, and fibrous tissues of the *corpora cavernosa*.

Also, many common medicines produce impotence as a side effect. These include high blood pressure drugs, antihistamines, antidepressants, tranquilizers, appetite suppressants, and cimetidine (an ulcer drug).

Experts believe that psychological factors cause 10 to 20 percent of cases of impotence. These factors include stress, anxiety, guilt, depression, low self-esteem, and fear of sexual failure. Such factors are broadly associated with more than 80 percent of cases of impotence, usually as secondary reactions to underlying physical causes.

Other possible causes of impotence are smoking, which affects blood flow in veins and arteries, and hormonal abnormalities, such as insufficient testosterone.

How is impotence diagnosed?

Patient History. Medical and sexual histories help define the degree and nature of impotence. A medical history can disclose diseases that lead to impotence. A simple recounting of sexual activity might distinguish between problems with erection, ejaculation, orgasm, or sexual desire.

A history of using certain prescription drugs or illegal drugs can suggest a chemical cause. Drug effects account for 25 percent of cases of impotence. Cutting back on or substituting certain medications often can alleviate the problem.

Physical Examination. A physical examination can give clues for systemic problems. For example, if the penis does not respond as expected to certain touching, a problem in the nervous system may be a cause. Abnormal secondary sex characteristics, such as hair pattern, can point to hormonal problems, which would mean the endocrine system is involved. A circulatory problem might be indicated by, for example, an aneurysm in the abdomen. And unusual characteristics of the penis itself could suggest the root of the impotence—for example, bending of the penis during erection could be the result of Peyronie's disease.

Laboratory Tests. Several laboratory tests can help diagnose impotence. Tests for systemic diseases include blood counts, urinalysis, lipid profile, and measurements of creatinine and liver enzymes. For cases of low sexual desire, measurement of testosterone in the blood can yield information about problems with the endocrine system.

Other Tests. Monitoring erections that occur during sleep (nocturnal penile tumescence) can help rule out certain psychological causes of impotence. Healthy men have involuntary erections during sleep. If nocturnal erections do not occur, then the cause of impotence is likely to be physical rather than psychological. Tests of nocturnal erections are not completely reliable, however. Scientists have not standardized such tests and have not determined when they should be applied for best results.

Psychosocial Examination. A psychosocial examination, using an interview and questionnaire, reveals psychological factors. The man's sexual partner also may be interviewed to determine expectations and perceptions encountered during sexual intercourse.

How is impotence treated?

Most physicians suggest that treatments for impotence proceed along a path moving from least invasive to most invasive. This means cutting back on any harmful drugs is considered first. Psychotherapy and behavior modifications are considered next, followed by vacuum devices, oral drugs, locally injected drugs, and surgically implanted devices (and, in rare cases, surgery involving veins or arteries).

Psychotherapy. Experts often treat psychologically based impotence using techniques that decrease anxiety associated with intercourse.

The patient's partner can help apply the techniques, which include gradual development of intimacy and stimulation. Such techniques also can help relieve anxiety when physical impotence is being treated.

Drug Therapy. Drugs for treating impotence can be taken orally or injected directly into the penis. Oral testosterone can reduce impotence in some men with low levels of natural testosterone. Patients also have claimed effectiveness of other oral drugs, including yohimbine hydrochloride, dopamine and serotonin agonists, and trazodone — but no scientific studies have proved the effectiveness of these drugs in relieving impotence. Some observed improvements following their use may be examples of the placebo effect, that is, a change that results simply from the patient's believing that an improvement will occur.

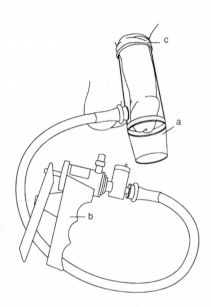

Figure 15.2. *A vacuum-constrictor device causes an erection by creating a partial vacuum around the penis which draws blood into the* corpora cavernosa. *Pictured here are the necessary components: (a) a plastic cylinder, which covers the penis; (b) a pump, which draws air out of the cylinder; and (c) an elastic ring, which, when fitted over the base of the penis, traps the blood and sustains the erection after the cylinder is removed.*

Many men gain potency by injecting drugs into the penis, causing it to become engorged with blood. Drugs such as papaverine hydrochloride, phentolamine, and prostaglandin E1 widen blood vessels. These drugs may create unwanted side effects, however, including persistent erection (known as priapism) and scarring. Nitroglycerin, a muscle relaxant, sometimes can enhance erection when rubbed on the surface of the penis.

Research on drugs for treating impotence is expanding rapidly. Patients should ask their doctors about the latest advances.

Vacuum Devices. Mechanical vacuum devices cause erection by creating a partial vacuum around the penis, which draws blood into the penis, engorging it and expanding it. The devices have three components: a plastic cylinder, in which the penis is placed; a pump, which draws air out of the cylinder; and an elastic band, which is placed around the base of the penis, to maintain the erection after the cylinder is removed and during intercourse by preventing blood from flowing back into the body (see Figure 15.2).

One variation of the vacuum device involves a semirigid rubber sheath that is placed on the penis and remains there after attaining erection and during intercourse.

Surgery. Surgery usually has one of three goals:

1. to implant a device that can cause the penis to become erect;
2. to reconstruct arteries to increase flow of blood to the penis; or
3. to block off veins that allow blood to leak from the penile tissues.

Implanted devices, known as prostheses can restore erection in many men with impotence. Possible problems with implants include mechanical breakdown and infection. Mechanical problems have diminished in recent years because of technological advances.

Malleable implants usually consist of paired rods, which are inserted surgically into the *corpora cavernosa*, the twin chambers running the length of the penis. The user manually adjusts the position of the penis and, therefore, the rods. Adjustment does not affect the width or length of the penis.

Inflatable implants consist of paired cylinders, which are surgically inserted inside the penis and can be expanded using pressurized fluid (see Figure 15.3). Tubes connect the cylinders to a fluid reservoir and pump, which also are surgically implanted. The patient inflates the cylinders by pressing on the small pump, located under the skin in the scrotum. Inflatable implants can expand the length and width of the penis somewhat. They also leave the penis in a more natural state when not inflated.

Surgery to repair arteries can reduce impotence caused by obstructions that block the flow of blood to the penis. The best candidates for such surgery are young men with discrete blockage of an artery because of an injury to the crotch area or fracture of the pelvis. The procedure is less successful in older men with widespread blockage.

Surgery to veins that allow blood to leave the penis usually involves an opposite procedure—intentional blockage. Blocking off veins (ligation) can reduce the leakage of blood that diminishes rigidity of the penis during erection. However, experts have raised questions about this procedure's long-term effectiveness.

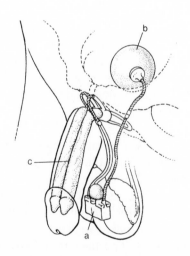

Figure 15.3. With an inflatable implant, erection is produced by squeezing a small pump (a) implanted in the scrotum. The pump causes fluid to flow from a reservoir (b) residing in the lower pelvis to two cylinders (c) residing in the penis. The cylinders expand to create the erection.

What will the future bring?

Advances in injectable medications, implants, and vacuum devices have expanded the options for men seeking treatment for impotence. These advances also have helped increase the number of men seeking treatment.

One possible new treatment, currently in experimental stages, is a small pellet that a man can insert in the end of his penis. The pellet releases a drug that migrates into the erectile tissue and causes a temporary erection. There is no need for a needle. Whether or not this method proves to be safe and effective, ongoing improvements in traditional methods should continue to create more successful and widespread treatment of impotence.

Points to Remember

- Impotence is a consistent inability to sustain an erection sufficient for sexual intercourse.

- Impotence affects 10 to 15 million American men.

- Impotence usually has a physical cause.

- Impotence is treatable in all age groups.

- Treatments include psychotherapy, drug therapy, vacuum devices, and surgery.

Resources for More Information

Impotence Information Center
P.O. Box 9
Minneapolis, MN 55440
(800) 843-4315

Impotence Institute of America
8201 Corporate Drive Suite
320 Landover, MD 20785
(301) 577-0650

Sexual Function Health Council
American Foundation for Urologic Disease
300 West Pratt Street
Suite 401 Baltimore, MD 21201
(800) 242-2383

The Geddings Osbon, Sr. Foundation
P.O. Drawer 1593
Augusta, GA 30903-1593
(800) 433-4215

Section 15.2

The Hows and Ys of Male Infertility

NCRR Reporter, November/December 1996.

When a couple is unable to conceive, attention often focuses first on the woman because she is most likely to seek medical advice. But statistics show that men and women contribute equally to the problem. Male infertility is something of an enigma, however, because physicians are unable to pinpoint its cause in more than half of infertile men. In initial attempts to understand male infertility, researchers now have shown that previously undetected genetic defects on the Y chromosome, which is present only in men, may be a significant contributor in 15 to 20 percent of unexplained cases of male infertility.

Supported by a recent NCRR effort to stimulate patient-oriented research at minority institutions known as the Research Centers in Minority Institutions Clinical Research Infrastructure Initiative, Dr. Shalender Bhasin at Charles R. Drew University of Medicine and Science in Los Angeles is using molecular genetics to study defects on the Y chromosome. Dr. Bhasin, professor of medicine and chief of the division of endocrinology, metabolism, and molecular medicine at Drew, has found that in some men the Y chromosome contains small genetic errors called microdeletions that might affect genes involved in sperm production.

The research grew out of an earlier observation that a section of the Y chromosome in a region known as interval 6 is missing in a small percentage of men who have low sperm counts. The Y chromosome is divided into two sections. One, known as the short arm, contains genes regulating development of the testes and male sexual characteristics. The other, called the long arm, contains genes controlling sperm production and also contains interval 6.

Conventional technology—visual examination of chromosomes under a light microscope—can detect only very large chromosomal deletions. But Dr. Bhasin and his colleagues hypothesized that microdeletions, too small to be seen under a microscope, might be present in interval 6 of some infertile men. To detect these smaller deletions and test their hypothesis, the Bhasin team turned to a molecular biological technique known as sequence-tagged site (STS) mapping.

STS mapping detects multiple, evenly spaced sites on a chromosome. If a specific site is missing, researchers assume that the piece of chromosome containing that site has been deleted. "A sequence-tagged site is really a marker, or flag, that allows the researcher to identify the presence or absence of a portion of the genome," explains Dr. Bhasin. Comparing the markers to milestones placed every 10 miles on a road along a river, he explains that someone wanting to see if part of the road had been flooded could look for these milestones. "If some of them are submerged, one could assume that those portions of the road are flooded," he says.

To detect chromosomal "milestones," researchers use short strands of DNA called primers, designed to pair with specific DNA building blocks, or bases, at the milestone sites. If the chromosome is intact at a particular site, the primer for that site binds to it. But if the chromosome has a microdeletion, some of the bases are missing and the primer does not bind. Dr. Bhasin and his colleagues used STS mapping to examine 26 milestone sites within interval 6.

Each STS in interval 6 is only a few hundred bases in length; the distance between sites is much longer, averaging 75,000 bases. Microdeletions can be detected because they are usually even longer, some of them as large as 500,000 bases. In contrast, macrodeletions visible by light microscopy are usually several million bases long.

In one recently completed study, Dr. Bhasin and his colleagues used STS mapping to detect microdeletions in 50 men with zero sperm counts and 10 men with low sperm counts. Among these men, 18 percent had microdeletions in interval 6. In contrast, the researchers found no microdeletions in 16 normal fertile men or in patients with other genetic disorders.

Dr. Bhasin says his findings could be used to develop a screening test for infertile men to detect microdeletions in the Y chromosome.

But he cautions that the discovery of Y chromosome deletions poses important ethical questions for reproductive specialists. Currently, possible causes of low sperm count are not considered when assisted reproductive technology (ART) is used to help an infertile couple conceive. Instead, with newer techniques for ART, a single sperm can be isolated and microinjected into the woman's egg in a laboratory dish. Even in men with zero sperm count, an individual sperm can sometimes be found in testicular tissue removed by biopsy. Subsequently the fertilized egg is implanted in the womb.

Before the advent of ART, men with these microdeletions were infertile or subfertile and had little chance of conceiving and passing on defective genes to a new generation. But now, Dr. Bhasin says, "because fertility can be achieved by ART, these men pass their genes on to their children. The father's genetic disorder on the Y chromosome may are transmitted to a male baby." To avoid transmission of defective genes from one generation to the next, Dr. Bhasin suggests that infertile men might wish to be tested for Y chromosome microdeletions. The results of these tests could be used to counsel infertile couples considering ART in the same way that couples are offered genetic counseling for cystic fibrosis or other inherited disorders. Although screening of infertile men using STS mapping would be an added expense, Dr. Bhasin notes that tests for Y microdeletions would provide essential information for counseling infertile couples.

The Drew University researchers are now trying to target the genes affected by microdeletions. Dr. Bhasin says, "Most of the questions still remain unanswered, such as 'What are the genes in this region of the Y chromosome that cause infertility, what is their role in germ cell development, and how do they regulate sperm production?'" Future experiments will involve cloning and characterizing these genes to understand their function in animal models. The scientists note, however, that their results suggest that when with these microdeletions usually have severe defects in sperm production. In addition to low sperm counts, some of the men also had smaller-than-normal testes.

Dr. Bhasin explains that there may be other genes, not only on the Y chromosome but on other chromosomes as well, that may cause infertility. "There are many different subtypes of infertility. We are trying to categorize these patients and understand the genetic defects involved," he says. "I think microdeletions are just the beginning."

— William Oldendorf

This research is supported by the Research Infrastructure area of the National Center for Research Resources and by the National Institute of Diabetes and Digestive and Kidney Diseases.

Additional Reading

Najmabadi, H.. Huang, V., Yen, P., et al., Substantial prevalence of microdeletions of the Y chromosome in infertile men with idiopathic azoospermia and oligozoospermia detected using a sequence-tagged site-based mapping strategy. *Journal of Clinical Endocrinology and Metabolism* 81:1347-1352. 1996.

Section 15.3

Overcoming Infertility

FDA Consumer online archives at (http://www.fda.gov/fdac/fdacfeatures/ 1997/197_fert.html). This article originally appeared in the January-February 1997 *FDA Consumer*. The version below is from a reprint of the original article and contains revisions made in February 1997. (Illustrations in this article drawn by Renée Gordon.) Publication No. (FDA) 97-1269.

Myth or fact: If a couple is having trouble conceiving a child, the man should try wearing loose underwear? That's a fact, according to a study on "Tight-fitting Underwear and Sperm Quality" published June 29, 1996, in the scientific journal *The Lancet*. Tight-fitting underwear—as well as hot tubs and saunas—is not recommended for men trying to father a child because it may raise testes temperature to a point where it interferes with sperm production.

But couples having difficulty getting pregnant can tell you the solution is almost never as simple as wearing boxers instead of briefs. Lisa (who asked that her last name not be used) tried for more than two years to get pregnant without success. "Everyone gave me advice," she says. "My mother said I should just go to church and pray more.

381

My friends said, 'Try to relax and not think about it' or 'You're just overstressed. You work too much.'"

Actually, psychological stress is more likely a result of infertility than the cause, according to Resolve, a nonprofit consumer organization specializing in infertility.

"Fertility problems are a huge psychological stressor, a huge relationship stressor," says Lisa Rarick, M.D., director of the Food and Drug Administration's division of reproductive and urologic drug products.

So, while going on a relaxing vacation may temporarily relieve the stress that comes with fertility problems, a solution may require treatment by a health-care professional. Treatment with drugs such as Clomid or Serophene (both clomiphene citrate) or Pergonal, Humegon, Metrodin, or Fertinex (all menotropins) are used in some cases to correct a woman's hormone imbalance. (See "Drug Supply Restored.") Surgery is sometimes used to repair damaged reproductive organs. And in about 10 percent of cases, less conventional, high-tech options like *in vitro* fertilization are used.

Will the therapies work? "Talking about the success rate for fertility treatments is like saying, 'What's the chance of curing a headache?'" according to Benjamin Younger, M.D., executive director of the American Society for Reproductive Medicine. "It depends on many things, including the cause of the problem and the severity." Overall, Younger says, about half of couples that seek fertility treatment will be able to have babies.

A Year Without Pregnancy

Infertility is defined as the inability to conceive a child despite trying for one year. The condition affects about 5.3 million Americans, or 9 percent of the reproductive age population, according to the American Society for Reproductive Medicine.

Ironically, the best protection against infertility is to use a condom while you are not trying to get pregnant. Condoms prevent sexually transmitted diseases, a primary cause of infertility.

Even a completely healthy couple can't expect to get pregnant at the drop of a hat. Only 20 percent of women who want to conceive become pregnant in the first ovulation cycle they try, according to Younger.

To become pregnant, a couple must have intercourse during the woman's fertile time of the month, which is right before and during ovulation. Because it's tough to pinpoint the exact day of ovulation, having intercourse often during the approximate time maximizes the chances of conception.

After a year of frequent intercourse without contraception that doesn't result in pregnancy, a couple should go to a health-care professional for an evaluation. In some cases, it makes sense to seek help for fertility problems even before a year is up.

A woman over 30 may wish to get an earlier evaluation. "At age 30, a woman begins a slow decline in her ability to get pregnant," says Younger. "The older she gets, the greater her chance of miscarriage, too." But a woman's fertility doesn't take a big drop until around age 40.

"A man's age affects fertility to a much smaller degree and 20 or 30 years later than in a woman," Younger says. Despite a decrease in sperm production that begins after age 25, some men remain fertile into their 60s and 70s.

A couple may also seek earlier evaluation if:

- The woman isn't menstruating regularly, which may indicate an absence of ovulation that would make it impossible for her to conceive without medical help.

- The woman has had three or more miscarriages (or the man had a previous partner who had had three or more miscarriages).

- The woman or man has had certain infections that sometimes affect fertility (for example, pelvic infection in a woman, or mumps or prostate infection in a man).

- The woman or man suspects there may be a fertility problem (if, for example, attempts at pregnancy failed in a previous relationship).

The Man or the Woman?

Impairment in any step of the intricate process of conception can cause infertility. For a woman to become pregnant, her partner's sperm must be healthy so that at least one can swim into her fallopian tubes. An egg, released by the woman's ovaries, must be in the fallopian tube ready to be fertilized. Next, the fertilized egg, called an embryo, must make its way through an open-ended fallopian tube into the uterus, implant in the uterine lining, and be sustained there while it grows.

It is a myth that infertility is always a "woman's problem." Of the 80 percent of cases with a diagnosed cause, about half are based at least partially on male problems (referred to as male factors); usually that the man produces no sperm, a condition called azoospermia, or that he produces too few sperm, called oligospermia.

Lifestyle can influence the number and quality of a man's sperm. Alcohol and drugs including marijuana, nicotine, and certain medications, can temporarily reduce sperm quality. Also, environmental toxins, including pesticides and lead, may be to blame for some cases of infertility.

The causes of sperm production problems can exist from birth or develop later as a result of severe medical illnesses, including mumps and some sexually transmitted diseases, or from a severe testicle injury, tumor, or other problem. Inability to ejaculate normally can prevent conception, too, and can be caused by many factors, including diabetes, surgery of the prostate gland or urethra, blood pressure medication, or impotence.

The other half of explained infertility cases are linked to female problems (called female factors), most commonly ovulation disorders. Without ovulation, eggs are not available for fertilization. Problems with ovulation are signaled by irregular menstrual periods or a lack of periods altogether (called amenorrhea). Simple lifestyle factors—including stress, diet, or athletic training—can affect a woman's hormonal balance. Much less often, a hormonal imbalance can result from a serious medical problem such as a pituitary gland tumor.

Other problems can also lead to female infertility. If the fallopian tubes are blocked at one or both ends, the egg can't travel through the tubes into the uterus. Such blockage may result from pelvic inflammatory disease, surgery for an ectopic pregnancy (when the embryo implants in the fallopian tube rather than in the uterus), or other problems, including endometriosis (the abnormal presence of uterine lining cells in other pelvic organs).

A medical evaluation may determine whether a couple's infertility is due to these or other causes. If a medical and sexual history doesn't reveal an obvious problem, like improperly timed intercourse or absence of ovulation, specific tests may be needed.

Tests for Both

The man's evaluation focuses on the number and health of his sperm. The laboratory first examines a sperm sample under a microscope to check sperm number, shape and movement. Further tests may be needed to look for infection, hormonal imbalance, or other problems.

Male tests include:

- **X-ray:** If damage to one or both of the vas deferens (the ducts in the male that transport the sperm to the penis) is known or suspected, an x-ray is taken to examine the organs.

- **Mucus penetrance test:** Test of whether the man's sperm are able to swim through a drop of the woman's fertile vaginal mucus on a slide (also used to test the quality of the woman's mucus).

- **Hamster-egg penetrance assay:** Test of whether the man's sperm will penetrate hamster egg cells with their outer cells removed, indicating somewhat their ability to fertilize human eggs.

For the woman, the first step in testing is to determine if she is ovulating each month. This can be done by charting changes in morning body temperature, by using an FDA-approved home ovulation test kit (which is available over the counter), or by examining cervical mucus, which undergoes a series of hormone-induced changes throughout the menstrual cycle.

Checks of ovulation can also be done in the physician's office with simple blood tests for hormone levels or ultrasound tests of the ovaries. If the woman is ovulating, further testing will need to be done.

Common female tests include:

- **Hysterosalpingogram:** An x-ray of the fallopian tubes and uterus after they are injected with dye, to show if the tubes are open and to show the shape of the uterus.

- **Laparoscopy:** An examination of the tubes and other female organs for disease, using a miniature light-transmitting tube called a laparoscope. The tube is inserted into the abdomen through a one-inch incision below the navel, usually while the woman is under general anesthesia.

- **Endometrial biopsy:** An examination of a small shred of uterine lining to see if the monthly changes in the lining are normal.

Some tests require participation of both partners. Samples of cervical mucus taken after intercourse can show whether sperm and mucus have properly interacted. Also, a variety of tests can show if the man or woman is forming antibodies that are attacking the sperm.

Drugs and Surgery

Depending on what the tests turn up, different treatments are recommended. Eighty to 90 percent of infertility cases are treated with drugs or surgery.

Therapy with the fertility drug Clomid or with a more potent hormone stimulator—Pergonal, Metrodin, Humegon, or Fertinex—is often recommended for women with ovulation problems. The benefits of each drug and the side effects, which can be minor or serious but rare, should be discussed with the doctor. Multiple births occur in 10 to 20 percent of births resulting from fertility drug use.

Other drugs, used under very limited circumstances, include Parlodel (bromocriptine mesylate), for women with elevated levels of a hormone called prolactin, and a hormone pump that releases gonadotropins necessary for ovulation.

If drugs aren't the answer, surgery may be. Because major surgery is involved, operations to repair damage to the woman's ovaries, fallopian tubes, or uterus are recommended only if there is a good chance of restoring fertility.

In the man, one infertility problem often treated surgically is damage to the vas deferens, commonly caused by a sexually transmitted disease, other infection, or vasectomy (male sterilization).

Other important tools in the battle against infertility include artificial insemination and the so-called assisted reproductive technologies. (See "Science and Art.")

Fulfillment Regardless

Lisa became pregnant without assisted reproductive technologies, after taking ovulation-promoting medication and undergoing surgery to repair her damaged fallopian tubes. Her daughter is now 4 years old.

"It was definitely worth it. I really appreciate having my daughter because of what I went through," she says. But Lisa and her husband won't try to have a second child just yet. "At some point you have to stop trying to have a baby, stop obsessing over what might be an unreachable goal," she says.

When having a genetically related baby seems unachievable, a couple may decide to stop treatment and proceed with the rest of their lives. Some may choose to lead an enriched life without children. Others may choose to adopt.

And no, according to Resolve, you're not more likely to get pregnant if you adopt a baby.

To get more information about infertility, send a self-addressed stamped envelope to:

Resolve
1310 Broadway
Somerville MA 02144-1731, or
call their National Helpline at (617) 623-0744.

Science and ART

Sometimes it may be necessary or preferable to get pregnant without intercourse. A woman may choose to get pregnant with the sperm of someone who is not her partner.

In some cases, a woman may not be able to become pregnant with her partner because his sexual problems make it impossible for him to ejaculate normally during sex, or because the sperm have to bypass the vagina if the vaginal mucus cannot support them, or for other reasons. In these cases, through artificial insemination, the semen is placed into the woman's uterus or vaginal canal using a hollow, flexible tube called a catheter.

New, more complex assisted reproductive technologies, or ART, procedures, including in vitro fertilization (IVF), have been available since the birth 18 years ago of Louise Brown, the world's first "test tube baby." IVF makes it possible to combine sperm and eggs in a laboratory for a baby that is genetically related to one or both partners.

IVF is often used when a woman's fallopian tubes are blocked. First, medication is given to stimulate the ovaries to produce multiple eggs. Once mature, the eggs are suctioned from the ovaries and placed in a laboratory culture dish with the man's sperm for fertilization. The dish is then placed in an incubator. About two days later, three to five embryos are transferred to the woman's uterus. If the woman does not become pregnant, she may try again in the next cycle.

Other ART procedures, based on many of the same principles, include:

- **Gamete intrafallopian transfer, or GIFT:** Similar to IVF, but used when the woman has at least one normal fallopian tube. Three to five eggs are placed in the fallopian tube, along with the man's sperm, for fertilization inside the woman's body.

387

- **Zygote intrafallopian transfer, or ZIFT (also called tubal embryo transfer):** A hybrid of IVF and GIFT. The eggs retrieved from the woman's ovaries are fertilized in the lab and replaced in the fallopian tubes rather than the uterus.

- **Donor egg IVF:** For women who, for example, have impaired ovaries or carry a genetic disease that can be transferred to the offspring. Eggs are donated by another healthy woman and fertilized in the lab with the male partner's sperm before being transferred to the female partner's uterus.

- **Frozen embryos:** Excess embryos are frozen, to be thawed in the future if the woman doesn't get pregnant on the first cycle or wants another baby in the future.

New treatments for male factors are fast-evolving. Intracytoplasmic sperm injection is one of the most exciting new procedures, according to Benjamin Younger, M.D., executive director of the American Society for Reproductive Medicine. A single egg is injected with a single sperm to produce an embryo that can implant and grow in the uterus.

About two-thirds of births from ART procedures are single births. Of the rest, almost all are twins, with about 6 percent resulting in the birth of triplets or more.

Drug Supply Restored

The availability of sufficient supplies of the FDA-approved fertility drugs Pergonal, Metrodin, and Humegon, and the recent FDA apppoval of the fertility drug Fertinex have ended a shortage of these types of drugs in the United States. Since the drugs are not in short supply anymore, FDA will no longer allow the importation of unapproved versions of fertility drugs, even for personal use.

In February 1995, FDA became aware of a shortage of the approved fertility drugs Pergonal and Metrodin, both manufactured by Serono Laboratories Inc of Switzerland.

Because of the shortage, FDA has allowed people to temporarily import unapproved foreign versions of fertility drugs for their own use. "FDA used its enforcement discretion to allow the importation of unapproved versions of fertility drugs on a personal use basis," says Thomas Gardine, director of the agency's division of import operations and policy.

FDA asked doctors to wait until the supply of approved drugs increased unless a patient was in the midst of therapy. "There's always a danger in taking unapproved drugs because they are of unknown quality and haven't been shown to FDA to be safe, effective, and adequately labeled," Gardine says.

The Serono manufacturing plant in Switzerland is again supplying adequate amounts of Pergonal and Metrodin for U.S. patients. Also, other products are now available for the same use.

"The drug shortage no longer exists to merit our allowing importation of the unapproved products," Gardine says. After a reasonalbe time to make the public aware of the change in FDA's position, the agency will no longer allow the unapproved versions of these drugs to enter the country.

The following fertility drugs are approved by FDA and can be obtained with a doctor's prescription:

Clomid (clomiphene citrate), Hoechst Marion Roussel—(816) 966-5170

Serophene (clomiphene citrate), Serono—(800) 283-8088

Clomiphene citrate (clomiphene citrate), Milex—(312) 631-6484

Pergonal (menotropins), Serono—(800) 283-8088

Humegon (menotropins), Organon—(800) 631-1253

Metrodin (urofollitropin), Serono—(800) 238-8088

Fertinex (urofollitropin highly purified), Serono—(800) 283-8088

Chorionic gonadotropin (chorionic gonadotropin), Steris—(602) 278-1400

A.P.L. (chorionic gonadotropin), Wyeth Ayerst—(601) 341-2239

Chorionic gonadotropin (chorionic gonadotropin), Fujisawa—(847) 317-8800

Pregnyl (chorionic gonadotropin), Organon—(800) 631-1253

Some of these drug products may be sold under other brand names by distributors who buy the products from the listed manufacturers.

Chorionic gonadotropin is not normally used alone as a fertility drug; it is normally administered after administration of menotropins or urofollitropin.

—Tamar Nordenberg

Tamar Nordenberg is a staff writer for FDA Consumer.

Section 15.4

Looking for a Libido Lift:
The Facts about Aphrodisiacs

FDA Consumer, June 1996.

The moon is nothing
But a circumambulating aphrodisiac
Divinely subsidized to provoke the world
Into a rising birth-rate
           —from A Sleep of Prisoners by Christopher Fry

In the pursuit of sexual success and fertility, the moon, and every-thing under it, has been touted as an aphrodisiac by some person or culture. Love potion peddlers stop at nothing to sell their sexual wares. "I'll make you the same promise that my wife made to me," says Theodore Maximillian in the provocative brochure for his "Maxim" product. "I'm going to cure your impotence immediately!" Maxim "acts as a potent aphrodisiac," according to the advertisement.

An aphrodisiac is a food, drink, drug, scent, or device that, pro-moters claim, can arouse or increase sexual desire, or libido. A broader definition includes products that improve sexual performance. Named after Aphrodite, the Greek goddess of sexual love and beauty, the list of supposed sexual stimulants includes anchovies and adrenaline, lico-rice and lard, scallops and Spanish fly, and hundreds of other items.

According to the Food and Drug Administration, the reputed sexual effects of so-called aphrodisiacs are based in folklore, not fact. In 1989, the agency declared that there is no scientific proof that any over-the-counter aphrodisiacs work to treat sexual dysfunction.

Countering Cultural Views

FDA's findings clash with a 5,000-year tradition of pursuing sexual betterment through use of plants, drugs and magic. Despite FDA's determination that OTC aphrodisiacs are ineffective—and sometimes even dangerous—people continue the optimistic quest for drug-induced sexual success.

Several principles help demystify some cultural views about aphrodisiacs. Sometimes the reason for an item's legendary reputation is obvious. It's easy to imagine how the sex organs of animals such as goats and rabbits, known for their procreativeness, have achieved their esteemed status as love aids in some cultures.

Chilies, curries, and other spicy foods have been viewed as aphrodisiacs because their physiological effects—a raised heart rate and sometimes sweating—are similar to the physical reactions experienced during sex. And some foods were glorified as aphrodisiacs based on their rarity and mystery. While chocolate was once considered the ultimate aphrodisiac, the reputation wore off as it became commonly available.

Many ancient peoples believed in the so-called "law of similarity," reasoning that an object resembling genitalia may possess sexual powers. Ginseng, rhinoceros horn, and oysters are three classical examples.

The word ginseng means "man root," and the plant's reputation as an aphrodisiac probably arises from its marked similarity to the human body. Ginseng has been looked on as an invigorating and rejuvenating agent for centuries in China, Tibet, Korea, Indochina, and India. The root may have a mild stimulant action, like coffee. There have been some experiments reporting a sexual response in animals treated with ginseng, but there is no evidence that ginseng has an effect on human sexuality.

The similarity of the shape of the rhinoceros horn to the penis is credited for its worldwide reputation as a libido enhancer. The horn contains significant amounts of calcium and phosphorus. The addition of the food to a deficient diet could improve general physical vigor and possibly lead to an increased sexual interest. But in most Americans' diets, which are usually not lacking calcium or phosphorus, the small quantities usually consumed would not affect physical performance.

Because Aphrodite was said to be born from the sea, many types of seafood have reputations as aphrodisiacs. Oysters are particularly esteemed as sex aids, possibly gaining their reputation at a time when their contribution of zinc to the nutritionally deficient diets of the day could improve overall health and so lead to an increased sex drive.

Shortage of Studies

There is no proof that ginseng, rhinoceros horn, or oysters have an effect on human sexual reaction. But might some foods and OTC drugs eventually be proven to affect sexual appetite? Some big obstacles exist to answering this question. The placebo effect is one scientific stumbling block.

"The mind is the most potent aphrodisiac there is," says John Renner, founder of the Consumer Health Information Research Institute (CHIRI). "It's very difficult to evaluate something someone is taking because if you tell them it's an aphrodisiac, the hope of a certain response might actually lead to an additional sexual reaction."

Because the psychological complications are absent in animals, some studies have been done on the effect of certain drugs on animals' sexual activity. One substance that was tested extensively in animals is yohimbine. Obtained from the bark of an African tree, yohimbine has been used for centuries in Africa and West India for its supposed aphrodisiac properties. It supposedly works by stimulating the nerve centers in the spine that control erection. FDA called the results of preliminary animal studies "encouraging," but animal studies cannot be relied on to show the effectiveness of the drug in humans.

In people, the only available evidence is anecdotal and subjective. To scientifically measure sexual stimulation, a valid human study would have to be performed in the laboratory, comparing a placebo (an inert pill with no active ingredients) to the test aphrodisiac. Preferably, neither the researchers nor the patients would know who was getting the test substance. Because of cultural taboos, few such studies have been undertaken.

A second obstacle to obtaining proof of aphrodisiac effects is that some drugs may not actually have specific sexual effects, but may change a person's mood and therefore seem to be an aphrodisiac. For example, alcohol has been called a "social lubricant." People drink for many reasons, including to relax, reduce anxiety, gain self-confidence, and overcome depression. Because sexual problems can be caused or worsened by psychological stress, moderate drinking might seem like a sexual enhancer. In fact, it merely lessens inhibitions.

Alcohol is actually a depressant, and so, as the porter in Shakespeare's Macbeth observed, it "provokes the desire, but it takes away the performance." And drinking too much actually decreases desire.

No Quick Fix

Despite the lack of scientific evidence of safety and effectiveness, the fraudulent OTC love potion industry thrives to this day. Marketers use a "blatant snake-oil approach," according to CHIRI's Renner.

He estimates that the aphrodisiac sellers, who do much of their business by mail-order, take in revenues in the hundreds of millions of dollars a year.

FDA sends warning letters to companies that make aphrodisiac claims, stating that the agency may take further regulatory action if the violations continue. "In the health fraud area, when they get a warning letter, most people take their profits and run," says Joel Aronson, director of FDA's division of nontraditional drugs. "They don't want to get into a legal battle with the agency because it could involve protracted, expensive litigation."

Aphrodisiac experimentation isn't just a rip-off—it can be deadly. Spanish fly, or cantharides, is probably the most legendary aphrodisiac—and the most dangerous. Made from dried beetle remains, the reported sexual excitement from Spanish fly comes from the irritation to the urogenital tract and a resultant rush of blood to the sex organs. But Spanish fly is a poison that burns the mouth and throat and can lead to genitourinary infections, scarring of the urethra, and even death.

To avoid being taken for their money or their lives, individuals with sexual problems should seek a physician's advice. A lack of sexual energy or ability in men or women could be caused by something as simple as stress or a medication one is taking, or as serious as an underlying condition like diabetes or high blood pressure.

A doctor can diagnose a sexual problem and recommend treatment. If necessary, a doctor can prescribe a drug to treat sexual dysfunction. Testosterone replacement therapy is one prescription option for men whose natural testosterone level is not within the normal range, but its serious potential side effects call for a physician's supervision. For those with an impotence problem that isn't caused by low testosterone levels, the new injection may be the answer.

"People will continue to have false hopes of finding easy ways of resolving their problems," says Aronson. And so the hunt for the elusive love drug persists. A universal aphrodisiac may never be found, but experts agree that what's good for your overall health is probably good for your sex life too.

A good diet and a regular exercise program are a more dependable path to better sex than are goats' eyes, deer sperm, and frogs' legs. A good mental state is equally important.

Maybe the wishful search for a cure-all drug should be abandoned in favor of an easier, more reliable mechanism: the erotic stimulation of one's own imagination. To quote renowned sex expert "Dr. Ruth" Westheimer, Ed.D.: "The most important sex organ lies between the ears."

First Impotence Drug

For the 10 million to 20 million American men who suffer from impotence, the Food and Drug Administration's July 6, 1995, approval of Upjohn Company's prescription drug Caverject (alprostadil) may prove to be life-altering. Caverject is the first prescription drug approved for impotence, and is expected to successfully treat 70 to 80 percent of patients.

The drug provides an alternative to devices previously approved by FDA. A vacuum device involves placing a cylinder-like device and attached pump over the penis. By using the pump, blood is drawn into the penis, creating an erection. A constriction band is then placed at the base of the penis to maintain erection. A second treatment option, the penile implant, involves the surgical placement of cylinders in the penis and is available in a variety of designs. (See "Inflatable Penile Implants Under Scrutiny" in the January-February 1994 *FDA Consumer.*)

FDA approved Caverject to treat impotence caused by neurological, vascular or psychological dysfunction. While psychological factors such as anxiety and depression can lead to sexual dysfunction, more than 85 percent of impotence cases have a physical cause, according to the Impotence Institute of America. A complete physical examination is important so that any underlying condition can be diagnosed and treated. Some common causes of impotence are diabetes, arteriosclerosis (hardening of the arteries), and high blood pressure. Also, impotence has reportedly been caused by 16 of the 200 most commonly prescribed drugs, including drugs for high blood pressure, heart disease, and depression.

Caverject is self-injected into the penis shortly before sexual intercourse. The drug creates an erection by relaxing the smooth muscle tissue and dilating the major artery in the penis, which enhances the blood flow to the penis.

The drug's most common side effect is penile pain. Other side effects include bleeding at the injection site and an unhealthy, prolonged erection of four to six hours.

— Tamar Nordenberg

Tamar Nordenberg is a lawyer with the Office of the Director in FDA's Center for Drug Evaluation and Research.

Section 15.5

Understanding Klinefelter Syndrome

NIH Publication No. NIH Pub. No. 93–3202, August 1993. U.S. Department of Health and Human Services, Public Health Service, National Institutes of Health, National Institute of Child Health and Human Development.

What is Klinefelter Syndrome?

In 1942, Dr. Harry Klinefelter and his coworkers at the Massachusetts General Hospital in Boston published a report about nine men who had enlarged breasts, sparse facial and body hair, small testes, and an inability to produce sperm.

By the late 1950s, researchers discovered that men with Klinefelter syndrome, as this group of symptoms came to be called, had an extra sex chromosome, XXY instead of the usual male arrangement, XY.

Chromosomes and Klinefelter Syndrome. Chromosomes, the spaghetti–like strands of hereditary material found in each cell of the body, determine such characteristics as the color of our eyes and hair, our height, and whether we are male or female.

Women usually inherit two X chromosomes—one from each parent. Men tend to inherit an X chromosome from their mothers, and a Y chromosome from their fathers. Most males with the syndrome Dr. Klinefelter described, however, have an additional X chromosome—a total of two X chromosomes and one Y chromosome.

In the early 1970s, researchers around the world sought to identify males having the extra chromosome by screening large numbers of newborn babies. One of the largest of these studies, sponsored by the National Institute of Child Health and Human Development (NICHD), checked the chromosomes of more than 40,000 infants.

Based on these studies, the XXY chromosome arrangement appears to be one of the most common genetic abnormalities known, occurring as frequently as 1 in 500 to 1 in 1,000 male births. Although the syndrome's cause, an extra sex chromosome, is widespread, the syndrome itself—the set of symptoms and characteristics that may result from having the extra chromosome—is uncommon. Many men live out their lives without ever even suspecting that they have an additional chromosome.

"I never refer to newborn babies as having Klinefelter's, because they don't have a syndrome," said Arthur Robinson, M.D., a pediatrician at the University of Colorado Medical School in Denver and the director of the NICHD–sponsored study of XXY males "Presumably, some of them will grow up to develop the syndrome Dr. Klinefelter described, but a lot of them won't."

For this reason, the term "Klinefelter syndrome" has fallen out of favor with medical researchers. Most prefer to describe men and boys having the extra chromosome as "XXY males."

In addition to occasional breast enlargement, lack of facial and body hair, and a rounded body type, XXY males are more likely than other males to be overweight, and tend to be taller than their fathers and brothers.

For the most part, these symptoms are treatable. Surgery, when necessary, can reduce breast size. Regular injections of the male hormone testosterone, beginning at puberty, can promote strength and facial hair growth—as well as bring about a more muscular body type.

A far more serious symptom, however, is one that is not always readily apparent. Although they are not mentally retarded, most XXY males have some degree of language impairment. As children, they often learn to speak much later than do other children and may have difficulty learning to read and write. And while they eventually do learn to speak and converse normally, the majority tend to have some degree of difficulty with language throughout their lives. If untreated, this language impairment can lead to school failure and its attendant loss of self esteem.

Fortunately, however, this language disability usually can be compensated for. Chances for success are greatest if begun in early childhood. Sections that follow describe possible strategies for meeting the special educational needs of many XXY males.

Causes

No one knows what puts a couple at risk for conceiving an XXY child. Advanced maternal age increases the risk for the XXY chromosome count, but only slightly. Furthermore, recent studies conducted by NICHD grantee Terry Hassold, a geneticist at Case Western Reserve University in Cleveland, OH, show that half the time, the extra chromosome comes from the father.

Dr. Hassold explained that cells destined to become sperm or eggs undergo a process known as meiosis. In this process, the 46 chromosomes in the cell separate, ultimately producing two new cells having 23 chromosomes each. Before meiosis is completed, however, chromosomes pair with their corresponding chromosomes and exchange bits of genetic material. In women, X chromosomes pair; in men, the X and Y chromosome pair. After the exchange, the chromosomes separate, and meiosis continues.

In some cases, the Xs or the X chromosome and Y chromosome fail to pair and fail to exchange genetic material. Occasionally, this results in their moving independently to the same cell, producing either an egg with two Xs, or a sperm having both an X and a Y chromosome. When a sperm having both an X and a Y chromosome fertilizes an egg having a single X chromosome, or a normal Y-bearing sperm fertilizes an egg having two X chromosomes, an XXY male is conceived.

Diagnosis

Because they often don't appear any different from anyone else, many XXY males probably never learn of their extra chromosome. However, if they are to be diagnosed, chances are greatest at one of the following times in life: before or shortly after birth, early childhood, adolescence, and in adulthood (as a result of testing for infertility).

In recent years, many XXY males have been diagnosed before birth, through amniocentesis or chorionic villus sampling (CVS). In amniocentesis, a sample of the fluid surrounding the fetus IS withdrawn. Fetal cells in the fluid are then examined for chromosomal abnormalities. CVS is similar to amniocentesis, except that the procedure is done in the first trimester, and the fetal cells needed for examination are taken from the placenta. Neither procedure is used routinely, except when there is a family history of genetic defects, the pregnant woman is older than 35, or when other medical indications are present.

"If I were going to say something to parents who have had a prenatal diagnosis, it would be 'You are so lucky that you know,'" said Melissa, the mother of one XXY boy. "Because there are parents who don't know that their sons have this problem. And they will never be able to help them lead a normal life. But you can."

The next most likely opportunity for diagnosis is when the child begins school. A physician may suspect a boy is an XXY male if he is delayed in learning to talk and has difficulty with reading and writing. XXY boys may also be tall and thin and somewhat passive and shy. Again, however, there are no guarantees. Some of the boys who fit this description will have the XXY chromosome count, but many others will not.

A few XXY males are diagnosed at adolescence, when excessive breast development forces them to seek medical attention. Like some chromosomally normal males, many XXY males undergo slight breast enlargement at puberty. Of these, only about a third—10 percent of XXY males in all—will develop breasts large enough to embarrass them.

The final chance for diagnosis is at adulthood, as a result of testing for infertility. At this time, an examining physician may note the undersized testes characteristic of an XXY male. In addition to infertility tests, the physician may order tests to detect increased levels of hormones known as gonadotropins, common in XXY males.

A karyotype is used to confirm the diagnosis. In this procedure, a small blood sample is drawn. White blood cells are then separated from the sample, mixed with tissue culture medium, incubated, and checked for chromosomal abnormalities, such as an extra X chromosome.

What to Tell Families, Friends, and XXY Boys

Expectant parents awaiting the arrival of their XXY baby have difficult choices to make: whom to tell—and how much to tell— about their son's extra chromosome. Fortunately, however, there are some guidelines that new parents can take into account when making their decisions.

One school of thought holds that the best course is to go on slowly, waiting at least 1 year before telling anyone—grandparents included—about the child's extra chromosome. Many people are frightened by the diagnosis, and their fears will color their perceptions of the child. For example, some people may confuse the term Klinefelter syndrome with Down syndrome, a condition resulting in mild to moderate mental retardation.

Others may prefer to reveal the diagnosis early. Some parents have found that grandparents, aunts, uncles—and even extended family members—are more supportive when given accurate information. Another important decision parents must make is when to tell their son about his diagnosis. Some experts recommend telling the child early. When the truth is withheld, children often suspect 's that their parents are hiding something and may imagine a condition that is worse than their actual diagnosis.

This school of thought maintains that by the time he is 10 or 11 years old, the child can be told that his cells differ slightly from those of other people. Soon after, he can be filled in on the details: that the cell difference is due to an additional X chromosome, which is responsible for his undersized testes and any reading difficulties he may have. At this time, the child can be reassured that he does not have a disease and will not become sick. The child should also be told that some people may misunderstand this information and that he should exercise discretion in sharing it with others.

By roughly the age of 12, depending on the child's emotional maturity, he can be told that he will most probably be infertile. Parents should stress that neither the X chromosome nor the infertility associated with it mean that he is in any way less masculine than other males his age. The child's parents or his physician can explain that although he may not be able to make a baby, he can consider adopting one. Parents may also need to reassure an XXY boy that his small testes will in no way interfere with his ability to have a normal sex life.

Adherents of this school of thought believe that learning about possible infertility in such a gradual manner will be less of a shock than finding out about it all at once, late in the teen years.

Conversely, other experts believe that holding back the information does not appear to do any harm. Instead, telling an XXY boy about his extra chromosome too early may have some unpleasant consequences. An 11 or 12-year-old, for example, may associate infertility with sexual disorders and other concepts he may not yet understand

Moreover, children, when making friends, tend to share secrets. But childhood friendships may be fleeting, and early confidences are sometimes betrayed. A malicious or thoughtless child may tell all the neighborhood children that his former companion is a "freak" because he has an extra chromosome.

For this reason, the best time to reveal the information may be mid-to-late adolescence, when an XXY male is old enough to understand his condition and better able to decide with whom he wishes to share this knowledge.

Childhood

According to Dr. Robinson, the director of the NICHD-funded study, XXY babies differ little from other children their age. They tend to start life as what many parents call "good" babies—quiet, undemanding, and perhaps even a little passive. As toddlers, they may be somewhat shy and reserved. They usually learn to walk later than most other children, and may have similar delays in learning to speak.

In some, the language delays may be more severe, with the child not fully learning to talk until about age 5. Others may learn to speak at a normal rate, and not meet with any problems until they begin school, where they may experience reading difficulties. A few may not have any problems at all—in learning to speak or in learning to read.

XXY males usually have difficulty with expressive language— the ability to put thoughts, ideas, and emotions into words. In contrast, their faculty for receptive language—understanding what is said—is close to normal.

"It's one of the conflicts they have," said Melissa, the mother of an XXY boy. "My son can understand the conversations of other 10-year olds. But his inability to use the language the way other 10-year olds use it makes him stand out."

In addition to academic help, XXY boys, like other language-disabled children, may need help with social skills. Language is essential not only for learning the school curriculum, but also for building social relationships. By talking and listening, children make friends— in the process, sharing information, attitudes, and beliefs. Through language, they also learn how to behave—not just in the schoolroom, but also on the playground. If their sons' language disability seems to prevent them from fitting in socially, the parents of XXY boys may want to ask school officials about a social skills training program.

Throughout childhood—perhaps, even, for the rest of their lives— XXY boys retain the same temperament and disposition they first displayed as infants and toddlers. As a group, they tend to be shy, somewhat passive, and unlikely to take a leadership role. Although they do make friends with other children, they tend to have only a few friends at a time. Researchers also describe them as cooperative and eager to please.

Detecting Language Problems Early

The parents of XXY babies can compensate for their children's language disability by providing special help in language development, beginning at an early age. However, there is no easy formula to meet the language needs of all XXY boys. Like everyone else, XXY males are unique individuals. A few may not have any trouble learning to read and write, while the rest may have language impairments ranging from mild to severe.

If their son's speech seems to be lagging behind that of other children, parents should ask their child's pediatrician for a referral to a speech pathologist for further testing. A speech pathologist specializes in the disorders of voice, speech, and language. (The American Speech, Language and Hearing Association, listed in the reference section, distributes a free pamphlet on the stages of language development during the first 5 years of life.)

Parents should also pay particular attention to their children's hearing. Like other small children, XXY infants and toddlers may suffer from frequent ear infections. With any child, such infections may impair hearing and delay the acquisition of language. Such a hearing impairment may be a further setback for an XXY child who is already having language difficulties.

Guidelines for Detecting Language Problems

Shortly after the first birthday, children should be able to make their wishes known with simple one word utterances. For example, a child may say "milk" to mean "I want more milk." Gradually, children begin to combine words to produce two-word sentences, such as "More milk." By age three, most children use an average of about four words per sentence.

If a child is not communicating effectively with single words by 18 to 24 months, then parents should seek a consultation with a speech and language pathologist.

The XXY Boy in the Classroom

Although there are exceptions, XXY boys are usually well behaved in the classroom. Most are shy, quiet, and eager to please the teacher. But when faced with material they find difficult, they tend to withdraw into quiet daydreaming. Teachers sometimes fail to realize they have a language problem, and dismiss them as lazy, saying they could do the work if they would only try. Many become so quiet that teachers forget they're even in the room. As a result, they fall farther and farther behind, and eventually may be held back a grade.

Help under the Law

According to Dr. Robinson, XXY boys do best in small, uncrowded classrooms where teachers can give them a lot of individual attention. He suggests that parents who can meet the expense consider sending their sons to a private school offering special educational services.

Parents who cannot afford private schools should become familiar with Public Law 94-142, the Education of the Handicapped Act—now called the Individuals with Disabilities Education Act. This law, adopted by Congress in 1975, states that all children with disabilities have a right to a free, appropriate public education. The law cannot ensure that every child who needs special educational services will automatically get them. But the law does allow parents to take action when they suspect their child has a learning disability.

Chances for success are greatest for parents who are well informed and work cooperatively with the schools to plan educational and related service programs for their sons. For in-depth information on Public Law 94-142, parents may contact the National Information Center for Children and Youth with Disabilities (NICHCY), listed in the Resources section.

Parents may also wish to contact their local and state boards of education for information on how the law has been implemented in their area. in addition, local educational groups may be able to provide useful information on working with school systems. Parents should also consider taking a course in educational advocacy. The local public school system, the state board of education, or local parents groups may be able to tell parents where they can enroll in such a course.

For information on learning disabilities, parents can contact the Learning Disabilities Association of America and the Orton Dyslexia Society, both listed in the reference section.

Services for Infants, Toddlers and Preschoolers

The chances for reducing the impact of a learning disability are greatest in early childhood. Public Law 99-457 is an amendment to Public Law 94-142 that assists states in providing special educational services for infants, toddlers, and preschoolers. Eligibility requirements and entrance procedures vary from state to state. To learn the agencies to contact in their area, parents may call the Federation for Children with Special Needs (listed in the Resources section). The NICHCY (also listed in the Resources section) distributes the brochure "A Parent's Guide to Accessing Programs for Infants, Toddlers, and Preschoolers with Handicaps."

Teaching Tips

XXY males often have decreased immediate auditory recall they have trouble remembering what they have just heard. Parents and teachers can help them remember by approaching memory through visual channels. Illustrating words with pictures may help. Gesturing is another useful technique. For example, a teacher might accompany the word "yes" with a nod of the head. Similarly, shaking the head from side to side is the universal gesture for "no." Other useful gestures include waving goodbye, showing the child an upraised palm to indicate "stop," and holding the arms outstretched to mean "so big."

XXY males frequently have trouble finding the right word to describe an object or a situation. Parents and teachers can help them build vocabulary through a variety of techniques. One way is to provide them with synonyms, such as pointing out that a car is also called an automobile. Another important teaching tool is categorizing—showing the child that an item belongs to a larger class of items. With this technique, a child could be told that cars, buses, trucks, and bicycles are all vehicles, machines that carry people and things from place to place.

Because XXY boys have difficulty expressing themselves, they may do poorly on essay-style test questions. Multiple choice questions will give teachers a better idea of what an XXY child has learned—and prove less stressful for him as well. Similarly, rather than asking an open-ended question, parents and teachers may wish to present alternatives. Instead of asking "What would you like to do now?" they may wish to offer a choice: "Would you rather work on your spelling or work on your math?"

Parents and teachers can help XXY boys develop the ability to express themselves through solicited dialogue—engaging them in conversation through a series of questions. The same technique can be used to get the child to develop his narrative (storytelling) abilities. For example, a parent might begin by asking a child what he did at recess that day, and by following up with questions that get the child to talk about his activities: "Did you go down the slide? Were you afraid when you climbed all the way to the top of the ladder? And then what? Did you go on the seesaw? Who sat on the other end?"

Parents can also help XXY boys develop their expressive language abilities simply by providing good examples. Through a technique known as modeling, they can help organize their children's thoughts and provide them with examples of how to express oneself. For instance, if a younger child indicated that he wanted a toy fire engine by pointing at it and grunting, the parent could hand it to him while saying "Here you are. This is a fire engine." Similarly, if an older child asked "Are we going to put the stuff in the thing?", the parent might reply "Yes, we're going to put the oranges in the shopping cart."

Research indicates that XXY boys may do poorly in an open class-room situation and seem to prefer a structured, tightly organized environment centered around familiar routines. First, teachers can reduce distraction by placing them in front row seats. Teachers also should present information slowly and repeat key points—several times, if necessary. XXY boys should not be given tasks that have many small steps. Rather, each step should be presented individually. On completion, the child may then be asked to work on the next item in the series.

As mentioned above, XXY boys may withdraw from material they find difficult and retreat into day dreaming. A teacher or parent should gently regain the child's attention and help him to focus again on the task at hand. Similarly, XXY boys may have difficulty putting one task aside and beginning another one. Again, the parent or teacher should gently shift the child's attention, by saying something like "Drawing time is over. Let's put away the crayons and take out the math book."

—adapted from John Graham et al., "Oral and Written Language Abilities of XXY Boys: Implications for Anticipatory Guidance, " Pediatrics, Vol. 81(6), June 1988.

Adolescence

In general, XXY boys enter puberty normally, without any delay of physical maturity. But as puberty progresses, they fail to keep pace with other males. In chromosomally normal teenaged boys, the testes gradually increase in size, from an initial volume of about 2 ml, to about 15 ml. In XXY males, while the penis is usually of normal size, the testes remain at 2 ml, and cannot produce sufficient quantities of the male hormone testosterone. As a result, many XXY adolescents, although taller than average, may not be as strong as other teenaged boys, and may lack facial or body hair.

As they enter puberty, many boys will undergo slight breast enlargement. For most teenaged males, this condition, known as gynecomastia, tends to disappear in a short time. About one-third of XXY boys develop enlarged breasts in early adolescence)slightly more than do chromosomally normal boys. Furthermore, in XXY boys, this condition may be permanent. However, only about 10 percent of XXY males have breast enlargement great enough to require surgery.

Most XXY adolescents benefit from receiving an injection of testosterone every 2 weeks, beginning at puberty. The hormone increases strength and brings on a more muscular, masculine appearance. More information about testosterone and XXY males can be found in the section titled "Testosterone Treatment."

Adolescence and the high school years can be difficult for XXY boys and their families, particularly in neighborhoods and schools where the emphasis is on athletic ability and physical prowess.

"They're usually tall, good-looking kids, but they tend to be awkward," Dr. Robinson said of the XXY teenagers he has met through his study. "They don't necessarily make good football players or good basketball players."

Lack of strength and agility, combined with a history of learning disabilities, may damage self-esteem. Unsympathetic peers, too, sometimes may make matters worse, through teasing or ridicule.

"Lots of kids have a tough time during adolescence," Dr. Robinson said. "But a higher proportion of XXY boys have a tough time. High school is very competitive, and these kids are not very good competitors, in general."

Dr. Robinson again stressed, however, that while XXY males share many characteristics, they cannot be pigeonholed into rigid categories. Several of his patients have played football, and one, in particular, is an excellent tennis player.

Damage to self esteem may be more severe in XXY teenagers who are diagnosed in early or late adolescence. Teachers—and even parents—may have dismissed their scholastic difficulties as laziness. Lack of athletic prowess and the inability to use language properly in social settings may have helped to isolate them from their peers. Some may react by sliding quietly into depression and withdraw from contact with other people. Others may find acceptance in a dangerous crowd

For these reasons, XXY males diagnosed as teenagers may need psychological counseling as well as help in overcoming their learning disabilities. Help with learning disabilities is available through public school systems for XXY males high-school age and under. Referrals to qualified mental health specialists may be obtained from family physicians.

Testosterone Treatment

Ideally, XXY males should begin testosterone treatment as they enter puberty. XXY males diagnosed in adulthood are also likely to benefit from the hormone. A regular schedule of testosterone injections will increase strength and muscle size, and promote the growth of facial and body hair.

In addition to these physical changes, testosterone injections often bring on psychological changes as well. As they begin to develop a more masculine appearance, the self-confidence of XXY males tends to increase. Many become more energetic and stop having sudden, angry changes in moods.

What is not clear is whether these psychological changes are a direct result of testosterone treatment or are a side benefit of the increased self confidence that the treatment may bring. As a group, XXY boys tend to suffer from depression, principally because of their scholastic difficulties and problems fitting in with other males their age. Sudden, angry changes in mood are typical of depressed people.

Other benefits of testosterone treatment may include decreased need for sleep, an enhanced ability to concentrate, and improved relations with others. But to obtain these benefits an XXY male must decide, on his own, that he is ready to stick to a regular schedule of injections.

Sometimes, younger adolescents, who may be somewhat immature, seem not quite ready to take the shots. It is an inconvenience, and many don't like needles.

Most physicians do not push the young men to take the injections. Instead, they usually recommend informing XXY adolescents and their parents about the benefits of testosterone injections and letting them take as much time as they need to make their decision Individuals may respond to testosterone treatment in different ways. Although the majority of XXY males ultimately will benefit from testosterone, a few will not.

To ensure that the injections will provide the maximum benefit, XXY males who are ready to begin testosterone injections should consult a qualified endocrinologist (a specialist in hormonal interactions) who has experience treating XXY males.

Side effects of the injections are few. Some individuals may develop a minor allergic reaction at the injection site, resulting in an itchy welt resembling a mosquito bite. Applying a non-prescription hydrocortisone cream to the area will reduce swelling and itching.

In addition, testosterone injections may result in a condition known as benign prostatic hyperplasia (BPH). This condition is common in chromosomally normal males as well, affecting more than 50 percent of men in their sixties, and as many as 90 percent in their seventies and eighties. In XXY males receiving testosterone injections, this condition may begin sometime after age 40.

The prostate is a small gland about the size of a walnut, which helps to manufacture semen. The gland is located just beneath the bladder and surrounds the urethra, the tube through which urine passes out of the body.

In BPH, the prostate increases in size, sometimes squeezing the bladder and urethra and causing difficulty urinating, "dribbling" after urination, and the need to urinate frequently.

XXY males receiving testosterone injections should consult their physicians about a regular schedule of prostate examinations. BAH can often be detected early by a rectal exam. If the prostate greatly interferes with the flow of urine, excess prostate tissue can be trimmed away by a surgical instrument that is inserted in the penis, through the urethra.

Chromosomal Variations

Occasionally, variations of the XXY chromosome count may occur, the most common being the XY/XXY mosaic. In this variation, some of the cells in the male's body have an additional X chromosome, and the rest have the normal XY chromosome count. The percentage of cells containing the extra chromosome varies from case to case. In some instances, XY/XXY mosaics may have enough normally functioning cells in the testes to allow them to father children.

A few instances of males having two or even three additional X chromosomes have also been reported in the medical literature. In these individuals, the classic features of Klinefelter syndrome may be exaggerated, with low I.Q. or moderate to severe mental retardation also occurring.

In rare instances, an individual may possess both an additional X and an additional Y chromosome. The medical literature describes XXYY males as having slight to moderate mental retardation. They may sometimes be aggressive or even violent. Although they may have a rounded body type and decreased sex drive, experts disagree whether testosterone injections are appropriate for all of them.

One group of researchers reported that after receiving testosterone injections, an XXYY male stopped having violent sexual fantasies and ceased his assaults on teenaged girls. In contrast, Dr. Robinson found that testosterone injections seemed to make an XXYY boy he had been treating more aggressive.

Scientists admit, however, that because these cases are so rare, not much is known about them. Most of the XXYY males who have been studied were referred to treatment because they were violent and got into trouble with the law. It is not known whether XXYY males are inherently aggressive by nature, or whether only a few extreme individuals come to the attention of researchers precisely because they are aggressive.

Sexuality

The parents of XXY boys are sometimes concerned that their sons may grow up to be homosexual. This concern is unfounded, however, as there is no evidence that XXY males are any more inclined toward homosexuality than are other men.

In fact, the only significant sexual difference between XXY men and teenagers and other males their age is that the XXY males may have less interest in sex. However, regular injections of the male sex hormone testosterone can bring sex drive up to normal levels.

In some cases, testosterone injections lead to a false sense of security: After receiving the hormone for a time, XXY males may conclude they've derived as much benefit from it as possible and discontinue the injections. But when they do, their interest in sex almost invariably diminishes until they resume the injections.

Infertility

The vast majority of XXY males do not produce enough sperm to allow them to become fathers. If these men and their wives wish to become parents, they should seek counseling from their family physician regarding adoption and infertility.

However, no XXY male should automatically assume he is infertile without further testing. In a very small number of cases, XXY males have been able to father children.

In addition, a few individuals who believe themselves to be XXY males may actually be XY/XXY mosaics. Along with having cells with the XXY chromosome count, these males may also have cells with the normal XY chromosome count. If the number of XY cells in the testes is great enough, the individual should be able to father children

Karyotyping, the method traditionally used to identify an individual's chromosome count, may sometimes fail to identify XY/XXY mosaics. For this reason, a karyotype should never be used to predict whether an individual will be infertile or not.

Health Considerations

Compared with other males, XXY males have a slightly In creased risk of autoimmune disorders. In this group of diseases, the immune system, for unknown reasons, attacks the body's organs or tissues. The most well known of these diseases are type I (insulin dependent) diabetes, autoimmune thyroiditis, and lupus erythematosus. Most of these conditions can be treated with medication. XXY males with enlarged breasts have the same risk of breast cancer as do women— roughly 50 times the risk XY males have. For this reason, these XXY adolescents and men need to practice regular breast self examination. The free booklet *Breast Exams: What You Should Know* is available from the National Cancer Institute, listed in the Resources section. The last page of the booklet is a pullout chart listing the instructions for breast self examination. Although the booklet was written primarily for women, the breast self examination technique also can be used by XXY males. XXY males may also wish to consult their physicians about the need for more thorough breast examinations by medical professionals.

In addition, XXY males who do not receive testosterone injections may have an increased risk of developing osteoporosis in later life. In this condition, which usually afflicts women after the age of menopause, the bones lose calcium, becoming brittle and more likely to break.

Adulthood

Unfortunately, comparatively little is known about XXY adults. Studies in the United States have focused largely on XXY males identified in infancy from large random samples. Only a few of these individuals have reached adulthood; most are still in adolescence. At this time, researchers simply do not know what kind of adults they will become.

"Some of them have really struggled through adolescence," said Dr. Bruce Bender, the psychologist for the NICHD-sponsored study of XXY males. "But we don't know whether they'll have serious problems in adulthood, or, like many troubled teenagers, overcome their problems and lead productive lives."

Comparatively few studies of XXY males diagnosed in adulthood have been conducted. By and large, the men who took part in these studies were not selected at random but identified by a particular characteristic, such as height. For this reason, it is not known whether these individuals are truly representative of XXY men as a whole or represent a particular extreme.

One study found a group of XXY males diagnosed between the ages of 27 and 37 to have suffered a number of setbacks, in comparison to a similar group of XY males. The XXY men were more likely to have had histories of scholastic failure, depression and other psychological problems, and to lack energy and enthusiasm.

But by the time the XXY men had reached their forties, most had surmounted their problems. The majority said that their energy and activity levels had increased, that they were more productive on the job, and that their relationships with other people had improved. In fact, the only difference between the XY males and the XXY males was that the latter were less likely to have been married.

That these men eventually overcame their troubled pasts is encouraging for all XXY males and particularly encouraging for those diagnosed in childhood. Had they received counseling, support, and testosterone treatments beginning in childhood, these men might have avoided the difficulties of their twenties and thirties. Although a supportive environment through childhood and adolescence appears to offer the greatest chance for a well-adjusted adulthood, it is not too late for XXY men diagnosed as adults to seek help. Research has shown that testosterone injections, begun in adulthood, can be beneficial. Psychological counseling also offers the best hope of overcoming depression and other psychological problems. For referrals to endocrinologists qualified to administer testosterone or to mental health specialists, XXY men should consult their physicians. The Orton Dyslexia Society and the Learning Disabilities Association of America, listed in the Resources section, can provide information on overcoming a reading disability.

Resources

The American Speech Language and Hearing Association
10801 Rockville Pike
Rockville, MD 20852
1-800-638-TALK (301) 897-8682

Distributes a pamphlet parents may consult to determine if their children's communication abilities are developing at a normal rate.

The Federation for Children with Special Needs
95 Berkely Street, Suite 104
Boston, MA 02116
(617) 482-2915

Maintains a listing of local and state agencies providing special educational services for infants, toddlers, and preschoolers under Public Law 99-457

Learning Disabilities Association of America
4156 Library Road
Pittsburgh, PA 15234
(412) 341-1515

Provides information on dyslexia and other learning disabilities. Has local chapters throughout the country

K.S. and Associated
P.O. Box 119
Roseville, CA 95678

Support group for XXY males as well as males with other sex chromosome disorders. Operated by "Melissa," mother of a 12-year-old XXY boy. Provides literature on XXY males and other chromosome disorders, periodic newsletter.

The National Cancer Institute
Building 31, Room 10A16
9000 Rockville Pike
Bethesda, MD 20982

Offers the free booklet *Breast Exams: What You Should Know*. The last page of the booklet is a pull-out chart listing the instructions for breast self examination. Although the booklet was written primarily for women, the breast self examination technique also can be used by XXY males.

The National Information Center for Children and Youth With Disabilities (NICHCY)
P.O. Box 1492
Washington, DC 20013
1-800-999-5599; (703) 893-6061

Distributes information on Public Law 94-142, the Individuals with Disabilities Education Act.

The Orton Dyslexia Society
Chester Building, Suite 382
8600 La Salle Road
Baltimore, MD 21286
(410) 296-0232

Provides information on dyslexia. Has local chapters throughout the country.

—Robert Bock

Office of Research Reporting, NICHD

Section 15.6

Peyronie's Disease

NIH Publication No. 95-3902 May 1995, U.S. Department of Health and Human Services, Public Health Service, National Institutes of Health.

Peyronie's disease, a condition of uncertain cause, is characterized by a plaque, or hard lump, that forms on the penis. The plaque develops on the upper or lower side of the penis in layers containing erectile tissue. It begins as a localized inflammation and can develop into a hardened scar.

Peyronie's disease often occurs in a mild form that heals without treatment in 6 to 15 months. But in severe cases, the hardened plaque reduces flexibility, causing pain and forcing the penis to bend or arc during erection.

The plaque itself is benign, or noncancerous. A plaque on the top of the shaft (most common) causes the penis to bend upward; a plaque on the underside causes it to bend downward. In some cases, the plaque develops on both top and bottom, leading to indentation and shortening of the penis. At times, pain, bending, and emotional distress prohibit sexual intercourse.

One study found Peyronie's disease occurring in 1 percent of men. Although the disease occurs mostly in middle-aged men, younger and older men can acquire it. About 30 percent of people with Peyronie's disease develop fibrosis (hardened cells) in other elastic tissues of the body, such as on the hand or foot. A common example is a condition known as Dupuytren's contracture of the hand. In some cases, men who are related by blood tend to develop Peyronie's disease, which suggests that familial factors might make a man vulnerable to the disease.

Men with Peyronie's disease usually seek medical attention because of painful erections and difficulty with intercourse. Since the cause of the disease and its development are not well understood, doctors treat the disease empirically; that is, they prescribe and continue methods that seem to help. The goal of therapy is to keep the Peyronie's patient sexually active. Providing education about the disease and its course often is all that is required. No strong evidence shows that any treatment other than surgery is effective. Experts usually recommend surgery only in long-term cases in which the disease is stabilized and the deformity prevents intercourse.

A French surgeon, Francois de la Peyronie, first described Peyronie's disease in 1743. The problem was noted in print as early as 1687. Early writers classified it as a form of impotence. Peyronie's disease can be associated with impotence; however, experts now recognize impotence as one factor associated with the disease—a factor that is not always present.

Course of the Disease

Many researchers believe the plaque of Peyronie's disease develops following trauma (hitting or bending) that causes localized bleeding inside the penis. A chamber (actually two chambers known as the corpora cavernosa) runs the length of the penis. The inner-surface membrane of the chamber is a sheath of elastic fibers. A connecting tissue, called a septum, runs along the center of the chamber and attaches at the top and bottom (see Figure 15.4).

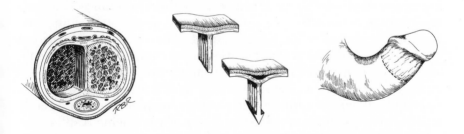

Figure 15.4. *A cross-section of the penis (left) displays the internal cavity that runs the length of the penis and is divided into two chambers (*corpora cavernosa*) by a vertical connecting tissue known as a septum. It is believed that, during trauma such as bending bleeding might occur at a point of attachment of the septum to tissue lining the chamber wall (center). The bleeding results in a hard scar, which is characteristic of Peyronie's disease. The scar reduces flexibility on one side of the penis during erection, leading to curvative (right). Illustrations by Robin Franklin.*

413

If the penis is abnormally bumped or bent, an area where the septum attaches to the elastic fibers may stretch beyond a limit, injuring the lining of the erectile chamber and, for example, rupturing small blood vessels. As a result of aging, diminished elasticity near the point of attachment of the septum might increase the chances of injury.

The damaged area might heal slowly or abnormally for two reasons: repeated trauma and a minimal amount of blood-flow in the sheath-like fibers. In cases that heal within about a year, the plaque does not advance beyond an initial inflammatory phase. In cases that persist for years, the plaque undergoes fibrosis, or formation of tough fibrous tissue, and even calcification, or formation of calcium deposits.

While trauma might explain acute cases of Peyronie's disease, it does not explain why most cases develop slowly and with no apparent traumatic event. It also does not explain why some cases disappear quickly, and why similar conditions such as Dupuytren's contracture do not seem to result from severe trauma.

Treatment

Because the plaque of Peyronie's disease often shrinks or disappears without treatment, medical experts suggest waiting one to two years or longer before attempting to correct it surgically. During that wait, patients often are willing to undergo treatments that have unproven effectiveness. Some researchers have given men with Peyronie's disease vitamin E orally in small-scale studies and have reported improvements. Yet, no controlled studies have established the effectiveness of vitamin E therapy. Similar inconclusive success has been attributed to oral application of para-aminobenzoate, a substance belonging to the family of B-complex molecules.

Researchers have injected chemical agents such as collagenase, dimethyl sulfoxide, steroids, and calcium channel blockers directly into the plaques. None of these has produced convincing results. Steroids, such as cortisone, have produced unwanted side effects, such as atrophy, or death of healthy tissues. Perhaps the most promising directly injected agent is collagenase, an enzyme that attacks collagen, the major component of Peyronie's plaques.

Radiation therapy, in which high-energy rays are aimed at the plaque, also has been used. Like some of the chemical treatments, radiation appears to reduce pain, yet it has no effect on the plaque itself and can cause unwelcome side effects. Currently, none of the treatments mentioned here has equalled the body's natural ability to eliminate Peyronie's disease. The variety of agents and methods used points to the lack of a proven, effective treatment.

Peyronie's disease has been treated with some success by surgery. The two most common surgical methods are: removal or expansion of the plaque followed by placement of a patch of skin or artificial material, and removal or pinching of tissue from the side of the penis opposite the plaque, which cancels out the bending effect. The first method can involve partial loss of erectile function, especially rigidity. The second method, known as the Nesbit procedure, causes a shortening of the erect penis.

Some men choose to receive an implanted device that increases rigidity of the penis. In some cases, an implant alone will straighten the penis adequately. In other cases, implantation is combined with a technique of incisions and grafting or plication (pinching or folding the skin) if the implant alone does not straighten the penis.

Most types of surgery produce positive results. But because complications can occur, and because many of the phenomena associated with Peyronie's disease (for example, shortening of the penis) are not corrected by surgery, most doctors prefer to perform surgery only on the small number of men with curvature so severe that it prevents sexual intercourse.

Sources of More Information

American Foundation for Urologic Diseases
30 West Pratt Street Suite 401
Baltimore, MD 21201
Tel: (203) 764-6518 or (800) 828-7866

National Organization for Rare Disorders
P.O. Box 8923
New Fairfield, CT 06812-1783
Tel: (800) 999-6673

**National Kidney and Urologic Diseases
Information Clearinghouse**
3 Information way
Bethesda, MD 20892-3580
(301) 654-4415

Chapter 16

Contraception

Chapter Contents

Section 16.1

A Guide to Contraceptive Choices: Barrier, Hormonal, Traditional and Surgical Methods

FDA Consumer, June 1997. This article originally appeared in the April 1997 *FDA Consumer*. The version below is from a reprint of the original article and contains revisions made in June 1997.

I am 20 and have never gone to see a doctor about birth control. My boyfriend and I have been going together for a couple of years and have been using condoms. So far, everything is fine. Are condoms alone safe enough, or is something else safe besides the Pill? I do not want to go on the Pill.

—Letter to the Kinsey Institute for Research in Sex, Gender, and Reproduction

This young woman is not alone in her uncertainty about contraceptive options. A 1995 report by the National Academy of Sciences' Institute of Medicine, The Best Intentions: Unintended Pregnancy and the Well-being of Children and Families, attributed the high rate of unintended pregnancies in the United States, in part, to Americans' lack of knowledge about contraception. About 6 of every 10 pregnancies in the United States are unplanned, according to the report.

Being informed about the pros and cons of various contraceptives is important not only for preventing unintended pregnancies but also for reducing the risk of illness or death from sexually transmitted diseases (STDs), including AIDS.

The Food and Drug Administration has approved a number of birth control methods, ranging from over-the-counter male and female condoms and vaginal spermicides to doctor-prescribed birth control pills, diaphragms, intrauterine devices (IUDs), injected hormones, and hormonal implants. Other contraceptive options include fertility awareness and voluntary surgical sterilization.

"On the whole, the contraceptive choices that Americans have are very safe and effective," says Dennis Barbour, president of the Association of Reproductive Health Professionals, "but a method that is very good for one woman may be lousy for another."

The choice of birth control depends on factors such as a person's health, frequency of sexual activity, number of partners, and desire to have children in the future. Effectiveness rates, based on statistical estimates, are another key consideration. (See the Birth Control Guide) FDA has developed a more consumer-friendly effectiveness table, which the agency will encourage all contraceptives marketers to add to their products' labeling. A copy of the table can be obtained by sending a request to FDA's Office of Women's Health, 5600 Fishers Lane (HF-8), Room 15-61, Rockville, MD 20857.

Barrier Methods

Male Condom

The male condom is a sheath placed over the erect penis before penetration, preventing pregnancy by blocking the passage of sperm.

A condom can be used only once. Some have spermicide added, usually nonoxynol-9 in the United States, to kill sperm. Spermicide has not been scientifically shown to provide additional contraceptive protection over the condom alone. Because they act as a mechanical barrier, condoms prevent direct vaginal contact with semen, infectious genital secretions, and genital lesions and discharges.

Most condoms are made from latex rubber, while a small percentage are made from lamb intestines (sometimes called "lambskin" condoms). Condoms made from polyurethane have been marketed in the United States since 1994.

Except for abstinence, latex condoms are the most effective method for reducing the risk of infection from the viruses that cause AIDS, other HIV-related illnesses, and other STDs.

Some condoms are prelubricated. These lubricants don't provide more birth control or STD protection. Non-oil-based lubricants, such as water or K-Y jelly, can be used with latex or lambskin condoms, but oil-based lubricants, such as petroleum jelly (Vaseline), lotions, or massage or baby oil, should not be used because they can weaken the material.

Female Condom

The Reality Female Condom, approved by FDA in April 1993, consists of a lubricated polyurethane sheath shaped similarly to the male condom. The closed end, which has a flexible ring, is inserted into the vagina, while the open end remains outside, partially covering the labia.

The female condom, like the male condom, is available without a prescription and is intended for one-time use. It should not be used together with a male condom because they may not both stay in place.

Diaphragm

Available by prescription only and sized by a health professional to achieve a proper fit, the diaphragm has a dual mechanism to prevent pregnancy. A dome-shaped rubber disk with a flexible rim covers the cervix so sperm can't reach the uterus, while a spermicide applied to the diaphragm before insertion kills sperm.

The diaphragm protects for six hours. For intercourse after the six-hour period, or for repeated intercourse within this period, fresh spermicide should be placed in the vagina with the diaphragm still in place. The diaphragm should be left in place for at least six hours after the last intercourse but not for longer than a total of 24 hours because of the risk of toxic shock syndrome (TSS), a rare but potentially fatal infection. Symptoms of TSS include sudden fever, stomach upset, sunburn-like rash, and a drop in blood pressure.

Cervical Cap

The cap is a soft rubber cup with a round rim, sized by a health professional to fit snugly around the cervix. It is available by prescription only and, like the diaphragm, is used with spermicide.

It protects for 48 hours and for multiple acts of intercourse within this time. Wearing it for more than 48 hours is not recommended because of the risk, though low, of TSS. Also, with prolonged use of two or more days, the cap may cause an unpleasant vaginal odor or discharge in some women.

Sponge

The vaginal contraceptive sponge has not been available since the sole manufacturer, Whitehall Laboratories of Madison, NJ, voluntarily stopped selling it in 1995. It remains an approved product and could be marketed again.

The sponge, a donut-shaped polyurethane device containing the spermicide nonoxynol-9, is inserted into the vagina to cover the cervix. A woven polyester loop is designed to ease removal.

The sponge protects for up to 24 hours and for multiple acts of intercourse within this time. It should be left in place for at least six hours after intercourse but should be removed no more than 30 hours after insertion because of the risk, though low, of TSS.

Vaginal Spermicides Alone

Vaginal spermicides are available in foam, cream, jelly, film, suppository, or tablet forms. All types contain a sperm-killing chemical.

Studies have not produced definitive data on the efficacy of spermicides alone, but according to the authors of Contraceptive Technology, a leading resource for contraceptive information, the failure rate for typical users may be 21 percent per year.

Package instructions must be carefully followed because some spermicide products require the couple to wait 10 minutes or more after inserting the spermicide before having sex. One dose of spermicide is usually effective for one hour. For repeated intercourse, additional spermicide must be applied. And after intercourse, the spermicide has to remain in place for at least six to eight hours to ensure that all sperm are killed. The woman should not douche or rinse the vagina during this time.

Hormonal Methods

Combined Oral Contraceptives

Typically called "the pill," combined oral contraceptives have been on the market for more than 35 years and are the most popular form of reversible birth control in the United States. This form of birth control suppresses ovulation (the monthly release of an egg from the ovaries) by the combined actions of the hormones estrogen and progestin.

If a woman remembers to take the pill every day as directed, she has an extremely low chance of becoming pregnant in a year. But the pill's effectiveness may be reduced if the woman is taking some medications, such as certain antibiotics.

Besides preventing pregnancy, the pill offers additional benefits. As stated in the labeling, the pill can make periods more regular. It also has a protective effect against pelvic inflammatory disease, an infection of the fallopian tubes or uterus that is a major cause of infertility in women, and against ovarian and endometrial cancers.

The decision whether to take the pill should be made in consultation with a health professional. Birth control pills are safe for most women—safer even than delivering a baby—but they carry some risks.

Current low-dose pills have fewer risks associated with them than earlier versions. But women who smoke—especially those over 35—and women with certain medical conditions, such as a history of blood clots or breast or endometrial cancer, may be advised against taking the pill. The pill may contribute to cardiovascular disease, including high blood pressure, blood clots, and blockage of the arteries.

One of the biggest questions has been whether the pill increases the risk of breast cancer in past and current pill users. An international study published in the September 1996 journal, *Contraception* concluded that women's risk of breast cancer 10 years after going off birth control pills was no higher than that of women who had never used the pill. During pill use and for the first 10 years after stopping the pill, women's risk of breast cancer was only slightly higher in pill users than non-pill users.

Side effects of the pill, which often subside after a few months' use, include nausea, headache, breast tenderness, weight gain, irregular bleeding, and depression.

Doctors sometimes prescribe higher doses of combined oral contraceptives for use as "morning after" pills to be taken within 72 hours of unprotected intercourse to prevent the possibly fertilized egg from reaching the uterus. On June 28, 1996, FDA's Advisory Committee for Reproductive Health Drugs concluded that certain oral contraceptives are safe and effective for this use. At press time in January, no drug firm had submitted an application to FDA to label its pills for this use, and the agency had not yet acted on the committee's recommendation.

Minipills

Although taken daily like combined oral contraceptives, minipills contain only the hormone progestin and no estrogen. They work by reducing and thickening cervical mucus to prevent sperm from reaching the egg. They also keep the uterine lining from thickening, which prevents a fertilized egg from implanting in the uterus. These pills are slightly less effective than combined oral contraceptives.

Minipills can decrease menstrual bleeding and cramps, as well as the risk of endometrial and ovarian cancer and pelvic inflammatory disease. Because they contain no estrogen, minipills don't present the risk of blood clots associated with estrogen in combined pills. They are a good option for women who can't take estrogen because they are breast-feeding or because estrogen-containing products cause them to have severe headaches or high blood pressure.

Side effects of minipills include menstrual cycle changes, weight gain, and breast tenderness.

Injectable Progestins

Depo-Provera, approved by FDA in 1992, is injected by a health professional into the buttocks or arm muscle every three months. Depo-Provera prevents pregnancy in three ways: It inhibits ovulation, changes the cervical mucus to help prevent sperm from reaching the egg, and changes the uterine lining to prevent the fertilized egg from implanting in the uterus. The progestin injection is extremely effective in preventing pregnancy, in large part because it requires little effort for the woman to comply: She simply has to get an injection by a doctor once every three months.

The benefits are similar to those of the minipill and another progestin-only contraceptive, Norplant. Side effects are also similar and can include irregular or missed periods, weight gain, and breast tenderness.

(See "Depo-Provera: The Quarterly Contraceptive" in the March 1993 *FDA Consumer.*)

Implantable Progestins

Norplant, approved by FDA in 1990, and the newer Norplant 2, approved in 1996, are the third type of progestin-only contraceptive. Made up of matchstick-sized rubber rods, this contraceptive is surgically implanted under the skin of the upper arm, where it steadily releases the contraceptive steroid levonorgestrel.

The six-rod Norplant provides protection for up to five years (or until it is removed), while the two-rod Norplant 2 protects for up to three years. Norplant failures are rare, but are higher with increased body weight.

Some women may experience inflammation or infection at the site of the implant. Other side effects include menstrual cycle changes, weight gain, and breast tenderness.

Intrauterine Devices

An IUD is a T-shaped device inserted into the uterus by a health-care professional. Two types of IUDs are available in the United States: the Paragard CopperT 380A and the Progestasert Progesterone T. The Paragard IUD can remain in place for 10 years, while the Progestasert IUD must be replaced every year.

It's not entirely clear how IUDs prevent pregnancy. They seem to prevent sperm and eggs from meeting by either immobilizing the sperm on their way to the fallopian tubes or changing the uterine lining so the fertilized egg cannot implant in it.

IUDs have one of the lowest failure rates of any contraceptive method. "In the population for which the IUD is appropriate—for those in a mutually monogamous, stable relationship who aren't at a high risk of infection—the IUD is a very safe and very effective method of contraception," says Lisa Rarick, M.D., director of FDA's division of reproductive and urologic drug products.

The IUD's image suffered when the Dalkon Shield IUD was taken off the market in 1975. This IUD was associated with a high incidence of pelvic infections and infertility, and some deaths. Today, serious complications from IUDs are rare, although IUD users may be at increased risk of developing pelvic inflammatory disease. Other side effects can include perforation of the uterus, abnormal bleeding, and cramps. Complications occur most often during and immediately after insertion.

Traditional Methods

Fertility Awareness

Also known as natural family planning or periodic abstinence, fertility awareness entails not having sexual intercourse on the days of a woman's menstrual cycle when she could become pregnant or using a barrier method of birth control on those days.

Because a sperm may live in the female's reproductive tract for up to seven days and the egg remains fertile for about 24 hours, a woman can get pregnant within a substantial window of time—from seven days before ovulation to three days after. Methods to approximate when a woman is fertile are usually based on the menstrual cycle, changes in cervical mucus, or changes in body temperature.

"Natural family planning can work," Rarick says, "but it takes an extremely motivated couple to use the method effectively."

Withdrawal

In this method, also called *coitus interruptus*, the man withdraws his penis from the vagina before ejaculation. Fertilization is prevented because the sperm don't enter the vagina.

Effectiveness depends on the male's ability to withdraw before ejaculation. Also, withdrawal doesn't provide protection from STDs, including HIV. Infectious diseases can be transmitted by direct contact with surface lesions and by pre-ejaculatory fluid.

Surgical Sterilization

Surgical sterilization is a contraceptive option intended for people who don't want children in the future. It is considered permanent because reversal requires major surgery that is often unsuccessful.

Female Sterilization

Female sterilization blocks the fallopian tubes so the egg can't travel to the uterus. Sterilization is done by various surgical techniques, usually under general anesthesia.

Complications from these operations are rare and can include infection, hemorrhage, and problems related to the use of general anesthesia.

Male Sterilization

This procedure, called a vasectomy, involves sealing, tying or cutting a man's vas deferens, which otherwise would carry the sperm from the testicle to the penis.

Vasectomy involves a quick operation, usually under 30 minutes, with possible minor postsurgical complications, such as bleeding or infection.

Research continues on effective contraceptives that minimize side effects. One important research focus, according to FDA's Rarick, is the development of birth control methods that are both spermicidal and microbicidal to prevent not only pregnancy but also transmission of HIV and other STDs.

Preventing HIV and Other STDs

Some people mistakenly believe that by protecting themselves against pregnancy, they are automatically protecting themselves from HIV, the virus that causes AIDS, and other sexually transmitted diseases (STDs). But the male latex condom is the only contraceptive method considered highly effective in reducing the risk of STDs.

Unlike latex condoms, lambskin condoms are not recommended for STD prevention because they are porous and may permit passage of viruses like HIV, hepatitis B and herpes. Polyurethane condoms are an alternative method of STD protection for those who are latex-sensitive.

Because it is a barrier method that works in much the same way as the male condom, the female condom may provide some protection against STDs. Both condoms should not be used together, however, because they may not both stay in place.

According to an FDA advisory committee panel that met Nov. 22, 1996, it appears, based on several published scientific studies, that some vaginal spermicides containing nonoxynol-9 may reduce the risk of gonorrhea and chlamydia transmission. However, use of nonoxynol-9 may cause tissue irritation, raising the possibility of an increased susceptibility to some STDs, including HIV.

As stated in their labeling, birth control pills, Norplant, Depo-Provera, IUDs, and lambskin condoms do not protect against STD infection. For STD protection, a male latex condom can be used in combination with non-condom methods. The relationship of the vaginal barrier methods—the diaphragm, cap and sponge—to STD prevention is not yet clear.

Birth Control Guide

Efficacy rates in this chart are based on Contraceptive Technology (16th edition, 1994). They are yearly estimates of effectiveness in typical use, which refers to a method's reliability in real life, when people don't always use a method properly. For comparison, about 85 percent of sexually active women using no contraception would be expected to become pregnant in a year.

This chart is a summary; it is not intended to be used alone. All product labeling should be followed carefully, and a health-care professional should be consulted for some methods.

Male Condom

- *Estimated Effectiveness:* 88 percent (a)

- *Some Risks (d):* Irritation and allergic reactions (less likely with polyurethane)

- *Protection from Sexually Transmitted Diseases (STDs):* Except for abstinence, latex condoms are the best protection against STDs, including herpes and AIDS.

- *Convenience:* Applied immediately before intercourse; used only once and discarded.

- *Availability:* Nonprescription

Female Condom

- *Estimated Effectiveness:* 79 percent

- *Some Risks (d):* Irritation and allergic reactions

- *Protection from Sexually Transmitted Diseases (STDs):* May give some STD protection; not as effective as latex condom.

- *Convenience:* Applied immediately before intercourse; used only once and discarded.

- *Availability:* Nonprescription

Diaphragm with Spermicide

- *Estimated Effectiveness:* 82 percent

- *Some Risks (d):* Irritation and allergic reactions, urinary tract infection

- *Protection from Sexually Transmitted Diseases (STDs):* Protects against cervical infection; spermicide may give some protection against chlamydia and gonorrhea; otherwise unknown.

- *Convenience:* Inserted before intercourse and left in place at least six hours after; can be left in place for 24 hours, with additional spermicide for repeated intercourse.

- *Availability:* Prescription

Cervical Cap with Spermicide

- *Estimated Effectiveness:* 64-82 percent (b)

- *Some Risks (d):* Irritation and allergic reactions, abnormal Pap test

- *Protection from Sexually Transmitted Diseases (STDs):* Spermicide may give some protection against chlamydia and gonorrhea; otherwise unknown.

- *Convenience:* May be difficult to insert; can remain in place for 48 hours without reapplying spermicide for repeated intercourse.

- *Availability:* Prescription

Sponge with Spermicide *(not currently marketed)*

- *Estimated Effectiveness:* 64-82 percent (b)

- *Some Risks (d):* Irritation and allergic reactions, difficulty in removal

- *Protection from Sexually Transmitted Diseases (STDs):* Spermicide may give some protection against chlamydia and gonorrhea; otherwise unknown.

- *Convenience:* Inserted before intercourse and protects for 24 hours without additional spermicide; must be left in place for at least six hours after intercourse; must be removed within 30 hours of insertion; used only once and discarded.

- *Availability:* Nonprescription; not currently marketed.

Spermicides Alone

- *Estimated Effectiveness:* 79 percent

- *Some Risks (d):* Irritation and allergic reactions

- *Protection from Sexually Transmitted Diseases (STDs):* May give some protection against chlamydia and gonorrhea; otherwise unknown.

- *Convenience:* Instructions vary; usually applied no more than one hour before intercourse and left in place at least six to eight hours after.

- *Availability:* Nonprescription

Oral Contraceptives—combined pill

- *Estimated Effectiveness:* Over 99 percent (c)

- *Some Risks (d):* Dizziness; nausea; changes in menstruation, mood, and weight; rarely cardiovascular disease, including high blood pressure, blood clots, heart attack, and strokes

- *Protection from Sexually Transmitted Diseases (STDs):* None, except some protection against pelvic inflammatory disease.

- *Convenience:* Must be taken on daily schedule, regardless of frequency of intercourse.

- *Availability:* Prescription

Oral Contraceptives—progestin-only minipill

- *Estimated Effectiveness:* Over 99 percent (c)
- *Some Risks (d):* Ectopic pregnancy, irregular bleeding, weight gain, breast tenderness
- *Protection from Sexually Transmitted Diseases (STDs):* None, except some protection against pelvic inflammatory disease.
- *Convenience:* Must be taken on daily schedule, regardless of frequency of intercourse.
- *Availability:* Prescription

Injection (Depo-Provera)

- *Estimated Effectiveness:* Over 99 percent
- *Some Risks (d):* Irregular bleeding, weight gain, breast tenderness, headaches
- *Protection from Sexually Transmitted Diseases (STDs):* None
- *Convenience:* One injection every three months
- *Availability:* Prescription

Implant (Norplant)

- *Estimated Effectiveness:* Over 99 percent
- *Some Risks (d):* Irregular bleeding, weight gain, breast tenderness, headaches, difficulty in removal
- *Protection from Sexually Transmitted Diseases (STDs):* None
- *Convenience:* Implanted by health-care provider—minor outpatient surgical procedure; effective for up to five years.
- *Availability:* Prescription

IUD (Intrauterine Device)

- *Estimated Effectiveness:* 98-99 percent
- *Some Risks (d):* Cramps, bleeding, pelvic inflammatory disease, infertility, perforation of uterus
- *Protection from Sexually Transmitted Diseases (STDs):* None

- *Convenience:* After insertion by physician, can remain in place for up to one or 10 years, depending on type.

- *Availability:* Prescription

Periodic Abstinence

- *Estimated Effectiveness:* About 80 percent (variable, based on method)

- *Some Risks (d):* None

- *Protection from Sexually Transmitted Diseases (STDs):* None

- *Convenience:* Requires frequent monitoring of body functions (for example, body temperature for one method).

- *Availability:* Instructions from health-care provider

Surgical Sterilization—female or male

- *Estimated Effectiveness:* Over 99 percent

- *Some Risks (d):* Pain, bleeding, infection, other minor postsurgical complications

- *Protection from Sexually Transmitted Diseases (STDs):* None

- *Convenience:* One-time surgical procedure

- *Availability:* Surgery

Footnotes

(a) Effectiveness rate for polyurethane condoms has not been established.

(b) Less effective for women who have had a baby because the birth process stretches the vagina and cervix, making it more difficult to achieve a proper fit.

(c) Based on perfect use, when the woman takes the pill every day as directed.

(d) Serious medical risks from contraceptives are rare.

—Tamar Nordenberg

Tamar Nordenberg is a staff writer for FDA Consumer.

Section 16.2

Vasectomy: Your Sterilization Operation

U.S. Department of Health and Human Services
Pamphlet "Information for Men."

YOUR DECISION AT ANY TIME NOT TO BE STERILIZED WILL NOT RESULT IN THE WITHDRAWAL OR WITHHOLDING OF ANY BENEFITS PROVIDED BY PROGRAMS OR PROJECTS RECEIVING FEDERAL FUNDS.

Why this Section Is Important to You

Sterilization is an operation that is intended to be permanent. This section describes the sterilization operation for men—vasectomy—its benefits, discomforts, and risks. Other family planning methods that are not permanent are also described. You should feel free to ask your doctor any questions after you have read the section completely.

Both men and women can be sterilized. (Ask your doctor or clinic for the pamphlet on sterilization for women.) The man's operation is easier, safer, and less expensive than the woman's operation.

If the Federal government is to pay for your sterilization, certain conditions must be met. They are listed at the end of this section. See "Rules for Sterilization Operations Funded by the Federal Government." The purpose of these conditions is to ensure that you understand sterilization and that you choose freely to have this operation.

Making up Your Mind

Sterilization must be considered permanent. Some doctors try to undo a vasectomy with surgery. This is a difficult and expensive operation which frequently does not work. So it's not a good idea to think your vasectomy can be undone.

Some men have heard about storing their sperm in banks to use later to father children. Men should not count on stored sperm because it rarely achieves pregnancy.

431

Make sure you do not want to father children under any circumstances before you decide to be sterilized. Are you sure you would not want to father children even if one of your present children died? Or your wife died? Or you got divorced and remarried? Be sure of your decision before you decide to be sterilized. Talk it over with your family or others you trust.

No one can force you to be sterilized. Don't let anyone push you into it. If you do not want to be sterilized, no one can take away any of your Federal benefits such as welfare, Social Security, or health care—including sterilization at a later date.

To have this operation paid for with Federal funds, you must be at least 21 years old. If you are married, discuss the operation with your wife. However, her consent is not required if Medicaid or any other Federal government program is going to pay for your operation. Your consent to sterilization cannot be obtained if you are under the influence of alcohol or other substances that affect your state of awareness.

You must sign the consent form at least 30 days before you plan to have the operation. This is so you will have at least 30 days to think it over and discuss it with your family and others. You may change your mind any time before the operation and cancel your appointment.

Other Methods of Family Planning

There are many other ways to avoid fathering children. Before you decide to be sterilized, think about other methods of family planning.

Temporary Methods of Family Planning

The following methods of family planning are temporary. This means that when you or your partner do not use them you can father children. Temporary methods of family planning are effective only if you use them correctly. If you think you might want to father children later, you should use a temporary method of family planning instead of sterilization. Ask your doctor or clinic for pamphlets and counseling on any of these temporary methods of family planning.

Condom, Rubber, Prophylactic. A thin sheath of rubber the man places over his penis each time before intercourse. In general use, it is 88 percent effective in preventing pregnancy. There are no serious side effects. A condom can be used with contraceptive foam, cream or gel, or with a diaphragm for extra protection. Condoms give protection against sexually transmitted diseases including HIV/AIDS.

Birth Control Pill. A pill a woman takes regularly which is 97 percent effective in preventing pregnancy. It is usually safe. In some women the pill causes minor side effects such as darkening of the skin of the face, nausea, spotting, missed periods or tender breasts. More serious complications which occur infrequently include depression, increased tendency for abnormal blood clotting, increased risk of heart attack and stroke (especially in women over age 35 who smoke), and a small increased risk of liver or gall bladder disease.

Intrauterine Device (IUD). A small piece of plastic is inserted into a woman's uterus (womb) by a doctor or family planning clinician. It is 94 percent effective in pre venting pregnancy. IUD use can cause heavier periods and cramps. A serious complication in couples who are not mutually faithful is increased risk of sexually transmitted infection which can cause infertility.

Diaphragm, Cervical Cap, or Contraceptive Sponge. A rubber cup or sponge a woman places in her vagina over her cervix before intercourse. The diaphragm or cap must be used with contraceptive gel or cream for it to be effective. The diaphragm or cap is 82 percent effective in preventing pregnancy. The sponge contains a contraceptive already. The effectiveness rate of the sponge is 82 percent for women who have not had children and 72 percent for women who have had children. There is little risk of serious complications, but minor side effects such as vaginal and urinary tract infections may occur. Benefits include some protection against sexually transmitted diseases.

Contraceptive Foam, Cream, Gel, Tablet or Film (Spermicide). Spermicidal preparations a woman places in her vagina each time before intercourse. They are 79 percent effective in preventing pregnancy. They occasionally cause minor side effects such as allergic reactions. Benefits include some protection against sexually transmitted diseases.

Natural Family Planning. A type of family planning in which intercourse is avoided on the days each month when a woman is likely to get pregnant. In general use, it is 80 percent effective in preventing pregnancy. Natural family planning consists of several methods, all of which require instruction. Different methods involve some combination of:

- charting the menstrual periods;
- charting the woman's body temperature;
- checking the cervical mucus;
- checking the position and texture of the cervix.

Effectiveness requires cooperation between partners. There is no risk of complications. No drugs or devices are necessary. Natural family planning teaches a woman about her own fertility patterns.

Norplant—A set of six hormone-containing capsules which are inserted beneath the skin of the inner upper arm and can remain effective for five years. It is over 99 percent effective in preventing pregnancy. Its effectiveness is decreased in women who weigh over 150 pounds. Most women using Norplant will have an abnormal bleeding pattern. Other minor side effects may occur, such as headache, nervousness, nausea, dizziness. A health care provider must insert or remove Norplant in a procedure which lasts 15-20 minutes. Norplant does not protect against sexually transmitted diseases including HIV/AIDS.

Sterilization for a Woman

A woman can be sterilized by an operation called a tubal sterilization. This operation is intended to prevent her from bearing children. Tubal sterilization is more complex and more expensive than the sterilization operation for a man. The risks of serious short-term and long-term complications are also much greater. Sterilization does not offer protection against sexually transmitted diseases, including HIV/AIDS. (Ask your doctor or clinic for the pamphlet on sterilization for a woman.)

What about Abortion?

Abortion does not prevent pregnancy. It is an operation to terminate a pregnancy which has already started.

This section does not address abortion; it only addresses ways to avoid pregnancy.

When Can a Man Have a Sterilization Operation?

A man may choose to have a sterilization operation at any time in his life. It doesn't matter if he is not married or doesn't have children.

It is up to him. Sterilizations done at too young an age or before a man has any children may result in regret later. Circumstances also can change in your life which might cause you to regret your decision to be sterilized.

Facts about the Operation

The surgical method of family planning for men is called a vasectomy. It is done in the doctor's office or clinic. Under local anesthesia, the doctor closes off the sperm ducts so that sperm cannot get through these ducts into the semen (the fluid ejected at orgasm). (See Figure 16.1.) When there are no sperm in the semen, you cannot cause a pregnancy. Only the sperm are blocked, not the liquid part of the semen. You will still ejaculate (eject fluid) as before. Vasectomy will not change your hormones.

(NOTE: Vasectomy is not castration. The testicles are not removed.) Sterilization does not offer protection against sexually transmitted diseases, including HIV/AIDS.

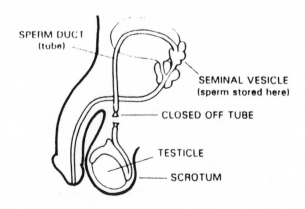

Figure 16.1. How a vasectomy is done.

How a vasectomy is done

First a local anesthetic is injected into your skin on each side of the scrotum to make it temporarily numb. You will feel mild pain, like a pin prick, for a few seconds.

Once the area is numb, the doctor makes one or two very small (one-half inch) incisions (cuts). Through these, the doctor reaches the sperm ducts, cuts them, and closes them off. The incisions in the skin are then closed with stitches. The scars can hardly be seen after a couple of weeks.

The operation, including anesthesia, usually takes about 15-20 minutes. You can usually go home shortly after the operation.

Is the operation guaranteed to work?

Vasectomy works almost all the time. This means that fewer than 1 out of 100 men who have the operation will still be able to get a woman pregnant. This is usually because the two ends of the ducts have grown back together. Vasectomy is more than 99 percent effective—higher than all other methods of family planning for men.

You are not immediately sterile after your vasectomy. There will still be some sperm in your ducts until you have ejaculated at least 15 times or at least 6 weeks have elapsed since your operation. During this time, you can still cause a pregnancy. So it is important that you and your partner use another method of family planning. The only certain way of knowing that you are sterile is to have your doctor do a simple test of your semen under a microscope at your follow-up appointment.

Benefits of Vasectomy

The benefits of vasectomy are:

- You don't have to worry about making a woman pregnant.
- You don't have to use a temporary method of family planning again.

Discomforts and Risks

Vasectomy is considered a safe and simple operation, but there is a small chance you will have some medical problems afterwards. You can expect some soreness after the operation. This is not serious and usually goes away after a few days.

Serious medical problems happen rarely. Most of the time they can be treated and cured by the doctor without further surgery; however, an operation may be necessary to correct some of them. Some of the medical problems you could have after a sterilization operation include:

1. You may have swelling around the incision on your skin. This happens right after the operation and is only temporary.

2. You may have bleeding under the skin which causes a bruise. This usually clears up by itself. Ice bags are often recommended to reduce the chance of this bleeding

3. You may get an infection either on the skin or inside the scrotum. It is important to follow the doctor's recommendation about the care and cleansing of the incision while it is healing.

4. The operation may not make you sterile. The operation cannot be guaranteed 100 percent to make you sterile. Less than 1 out of 100 men who have the operation will still be able to get a woman pregnant.

Go back to your doctor at once if swelling lasts for more than a few days, if you have a fever, or if you have severe pain.

Vasectomy will not alter your sexual drive; your erections and orgasms will be the same. A very few men who have had a vasectomy say they have sexual problems after the operation. There is no medical explanation for these rare symptoms, and they are believed to result from an emotional reaction to the operation. If you are concerned about how a vasectomy would affect you sexually, discuss your questions with the doctor.

Many studies have shown that men who have had vasectomies are just as healthy as other men. The long-term effects of vasectomy have been widely studied; there are no proven long-term health problems which result from having the procedure.

Summary

If you are sure you do not want to father children and you want to become permanently sterile, then vasectomy is a safe, effective option. The operation is done in a doctor's office or clinic, and problems are rare.

If You Have Questions

If there is anything that is not clear to you, or anything you are worried about, it is important that you ask these questions. All of your questions should be answered to your satisfaction before the operation.

Remember

You may change your mind at any time before the operation. Make sure you do not wish to father children under any circumstances before you decide to be sterilized.

Rules for Sterilization Operations Funded by the Federal Government

- You must be at least 21 years old.

- You must wait at least 30 days to have the operation after you sign the consent form.

- You may, if you choose, bring someone with you when you sign the consent form.

- Your consent is effective for 180 days from the date you sign the consent form.

- Your consent to sterilization cannot be obtained while you are under the influence of alcohol or other substances that affect your state of awareness.

Your consent to sterilization must be documented by signing a consent form available from U.S. Department of Health and Human Services.

Chapter 16.3

"No-Scalpel" Vasectomy

Effective Birth Control

Over 500,000 vasectomy procedures are done each year in the
United States. Vasectomy is a simple, safe surgical procedure for permanent male fertility control. The tube (called a "vas") which leads
from the testicle is cut and sealed in order to stop sperm from leaving. The procedure usually takes about 15 to 20 minutes. Since the
procedure simply interrupts the delivery of sperm it does not change
hormonal function—leaving sexual drive and potency unaffected.

The "No-Scalpel" Technique

The "No-Scalpel" technique is a technique to do the vasectomy
through one single puncture. This puncture is made into the scrotum
and requires no suturing or stitches.

It represents a significant improvement over conventional vasectomy
techniques in that it is less traumatic and shortens recovery time.

This procedure is done with the aid of a local anesthetic called
"Xylocaine" (similar to "Novocaine"). The actual interruption of the
vas which is done with the "No-Scalpel" technique is identical to the
interruption made with conventional techniques. The "No-Scalpel"
technique is simply a more elegant and less traumatic way for the
surgeon to control the vas and proceed with its interruption.

Risks, Complications, Important Information

As with any surgical procedure, the primary risks of vasectomy are
infection and bleeding. These risks are generally low for this procedure.

It is also important that each patient understand that vasectomy is approached as an irreversible procedure. While vasectomy can be reversed surgically at times, its successful reversal cannot be guaranteed. Also important is the fact that the vas deferens can grow back together. This is called recanalization and occurs only rarely—less than 1/2 to 1 percent of the time.

The Effects of a Vasectomy

A vasectomy leaves the patient unchanged except for the fact that the sperm cord (vas) is blocked. The testes still produce sperm, but they die and are absorbed by the body. The level of male hormone remains the same and all sexual characteristics remain the same. Ability to have an erection is also entirely unchanged.

Preparing for Your Vasectomy

Prior to coming to your doctor for vasectomy you should take a shower. Your doctor may request that you shave your scrotum. You will be asked to sign a permission form before your vasectomy.

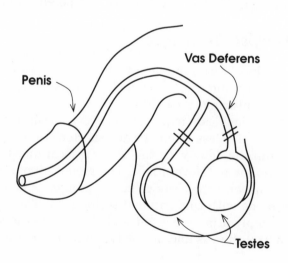

Figure 16.2. *A single puncture in the scrotum allows access for the surgeon to cut and seal the vas deferens.*

The Procedure

After you undress, the scrotum will be washed and a drape will be put on you. The anesthetic will be injected into the scrotum at the site of the vasectomy. This will not be an injection into the testicle. The anesthetic will prevent you from feeling pain as the doctor uses a special instrument to puncture the scrotum and grasp the vas deferens. The vas is then cut and sealed. Through the same puncture the other side is similarly done.

After Vasectomy

Following your procedure it is important that you remain off your feet as much as possible for 24 to 48 hours. This is important in order to minimize the chance of post-surgical complications. The anesthetic will wear off in approximately 1 to 2 hours after surgery. You should have someone else drive you home. You may shower at your leisure. Sexual activity may be resumed in approximately 3 to 4 days. (At this time you are not yet sterile and safe from pregnancy.)

Your doctor will ask you to bring a semen specimen in approximately 4 to 6 weeks after your vasectomy. ***This must be checked in order to be assured that the vasectomy worked and that you are sterile.***

More about the "No-Scalpel" Technique

The "No-Scalpel" technique is a technique that was first done in China in 1974. Over recent years it has become more and more popular in the United States. The vasectomy done is essentially the same as vasectomies done for many, many years. Its primary difference is that the vas deferens is controlled and grasped by the surgeon in a less traumatic manner. This results in less pain and fewer postoperative complications. As time continues more and more physicians will be using the technique.

Section 16.4

Vasectomy Safety

NIH Publication No. 96-4094. April 1996.

Vasectomy is a simple operation designed to make a man sterile, or unable to father a child. It is used as a means of contraception in many parts of the world. A total of about 50 million men have had a vasectomy–a number that corresponds to roughly 5 percent of all married couples of reproductive age. In comparison, about 15 percent of couples rely on female sterilization for birth control.

Approximately half a million vasectomies are performed in the United States each year. About one out of six men over age 35 has been vasectomized, the prevalence increasing along with education and income. Among married couples in this country, only female sterilization and oral contraception are relied upon more often for family planning.

Vasectomy involves blocking the tubes through which sperm pass into the semen. Sperm are produced in a man's testis and stored in an adjacent structure known as the epididymis. During sexual climax, the sperm move from the epididymis through a tube called the vas deferens and mix with other components of semen to form the ejaculate. All vasectomy techniques involve cutting or otherwise blocking both the left and right vas deferens, so the man's ejaculate will no longer contain sperm, and he will not be able to make a woman pregnant.

Vasectomy Techniques

In the conventional approach, a physician makes one or two small incisions, or cuts, in the skin of the scrotum, which has been numbed with a local anesthetic. The vas is cut, and a small piece may be removed. Next, the doctor ties the cut ends and sews up the scrotal incisions. The entire procedure is then repeated on the other side. Vasectomy is a simple operation designed to make a man sterile.

An improved method, devised by a Chinese surgeon, has been widely used in China since 1974. This so-called nonsurgical or no-scalpel vasectomy was introduced into the United States in 1988, and many doctors are now using the technique here.

In a no-scalpel vasectomy, the doctor feels for the vas under the skin of the scrotum and holds it in place with a small clamp. Then a special instrument is used to make a tiny puncture in the skin and stretch the opening so the vas can be cut and tied. This approach produces very little bleeding, and no stitches are needed to close the punctures, which heal quickly by themselves. The newer method also produces less pain and fewer complications than conventional vasectomy.

Post-vasectomy

Regardless of how it is performed, vasectomy offers many advantages as a method of birth control. Like female sterilization, it is a highly effective one-time procedure that provides permanent contraception. But vasectomy is medically much simpler than female sterilization, has a lower incidence of complications, and is much less expensive

After vasectomy, the patient will probably feel sore for a few days, and he should rest for at least one day. However, he can expect to recover completely in less than a week. Many men have the procedure on a Friday and return to work on Monday. Although complications such as swelling, bruising, inflammation, and infection may occur, they are relatively uncommon and almost never serious. Nevertheless, men who develop these symptoms at any time should inform their physician.

A man can resume sexual activity within a few days after vasectomy, but precautions should be taken against pregnancy until a test shows that his semen is free of sperm. Generally, this test is performed after the patient has had 10-20 post-vasectomy ejaculations. If sperm are still present in the semen, the patient is told to return later for a repeat test.

A major study of vasectomy side effects occurring within 8 to 10 years after the procedure was published in the British Medical Journal in 1992. This study, the Health Status of American Men, or HAM, was sponsored by the National Institute of Child Health and Human Development (NICHD). Investigators questioned 10,590 vasectomized men, and an equal number of nonvasectomized men, to see if they had developed any of 99 different disorders. After a total of 182,000 person-years of follow-up, only one condition, epididymitis/orchitis (defined as painful, swollen, and tender epididymis or testis), was found to be more common after vasectomy. This local inflammation most often occurs during the first year after surgery. Treated with heat, it usually clears up within a week.

Disadvantages of Vasectomy

The chief advantage of vasectomy—its permanence—is also its chief disadvantage. The procedure itself is simple, but reversing it is difficult, expensive, and often unsuccessful. Researchers are studying new methods of blocking the vas that may produce less tissue damage and scarring and might thus permit more successful reversal. But these methods are all experimental, and their effectiveness has not yet been confirmed. It is possible to store semen in a sperm bank to preserve the possibility of producing a pregnancy at some future date. However, doing this is costly, and the sperm in stored semen do not always remain viable (able to cause pregnancy). For all of these reasons, doctors advise that vasectomy be undertaken only by men who are prepared to accept the fact that they will no longer be able to father a child. The decision should be considered along with other contraceptive options and discussed with a professional counselor. Men who are married or in a serious relationship should also discuss the issue with their partners.

Although it is extremely effective for preventing pregnancy, vasectomy does not offer protection against AIDS or other sexually transmitted diseases. Consequently, it is important that vasectomized men continue to use condoms, preferably latex, which offer considerable protection against the spread of disease, in any sexual encounter that carries the risk of contracting or transmitting infection.

Masculinity and Sexuality

Vasectomy does not affect production or release of testosterone, the male hormone responsible for a man's sex drive, beard, deep voice, and other masculine traits. The operation also has no effect on sexuality. Erections, climaxes, and the amount of ejaculate remain the same.

Occasionally, a man may experience sexual difficulties after vasectomy, but these almost always have an emotional basis and can usually be alleviated with counseling. More often, men who have undergone the procedure, and their partners, find that sex is more spontaneous and enjoyable once they are freed from concerns about contraception and accidental pregnancy.

Immune Reactions to Sperm

After vasectomy, the testes continue to make sperm. When the sperm cells die, they are absorbed by the body, much like unused sperm in a nonvasectomized man. Nevertheless, many vasectomized men develop immune reactions to sperm, although current evidence indicates that these reactions do not cause any harm.

Ordinarily, sperm do not come in contact with immune cells, so they do not elicit an immune response. But vasectomy breaches the barriers that separate immune cells from sperm, and many men develop anti-sperm antibodies after undergoing the procedure. This has given rise to concern on the part of doctors and researchers, because immune reactions against parts of one's own body sometimes cause disease. Rheumatoid arthritis, juvenile diabetes, and multiple sclerosis are just some of the illnesses suspected or known to be caused by immune reactions of this type.

Immune reactions can also contribute to the development of atherosclerosis, the clogging of arteries that leads to heart attacks. In the late 1970s, after a study of 10 monkeys showed an increased risk of atherosclerosis in vasectomized animals, doctors became concerned that vasectomy might increase the risk of heart disease in men.

Other, more persuasive research results, however, indicated that these concerns were not warranted. In particular, the HAM study provided a high level of reassurance. Researchers conducting this study found no evidence that vasectomized men were more likely than others to develop heart disease or any other immune illnesses.

But just as concerns about heart disease and immune ailments following vasectomy were being laid to rest, worries about prostate cancer were taking their place. Although the HAM and a number of other studies showed no increase in cancer among vasectomized men, three separate hospital based studies published in 1990 reported positive correlations between vasectomy and prostate cancer. However, a well-regarded 1991 study found no such relationship.

Because of the importance of the issue, all of this research has been carefully analyzed, and scientists have identified several potential problems in the studies. It is possible, for example, that men who choose vasectomy for contraception have above average access to health care. In particular, these men may be more likely than others to visit urologists—physicians whose specialty includes the male reproductive organs, and they might thus be more likely to receive an accurate diagnosis of prostate cancer, a disease that often causes no symptoms and remains undiagnosed. If this were the case, vasectomy might falsely appear to increase the risk of this cancer.

In October 1991, the World Health Organization (WHO) sponsored a meeting of experts from around the world to evaluate the available evidence regarding a link between vasectomy and prostate cancer. Because additional concerns had been raised about a possible association between vasectomy and testicular cancer, evidence for such an association was also weighed at the meeting. The assembled experts concluded that a causal relationship between vasectomy and cancer of either the prostate or testis was unlikely. This conclusion was based in large measure on an overview of study results. But it was strengthened by the absence of a biological explanation of how vasectomy might produce any form of cancer.

Following the WHO meeting, two additional studies of vasectomized men found no increased risk of either prostate cancer or all cancers combined. Subsequently, a study conducted in three regions of the United States suggested that the subgroup of men who had a vasectomy before age 35 might have a slightly increased risk of developing prostate cancer. However, the size of this subgroup was not large enough to make the result conclusive. The study did not find any increased cancer risk in men who underwent vasectomy after age 35.

In 1993, a noted team of Harvard epidemiologists published findings from two large studies in the *Journal of the American Medical Association* (JAMA). One of these studies was retrospective (backward-looking), while the other was prospective and followed new patients. Both found vasectomy to be associated with a moderately elevated relative risk of prostate cancer that increased with time after the procedure. After more than 20 years, a vasectomized man appeared to be twice as likely to develop prostate cancer as a nonvasectomized man of the same age. Although this conclusion may seem startling, scientists generally consider risk findings of this magnitude to be of doubtful significance.

The studies were examined by experts in several professional organizations as well as in a JAMA article. The authors of this article concluded that the studies could neither be relied upon nor ignored and that further research was essential.

These authors pointed out that, since the causes of prostate cancer remain unknown, it had been impossible to assure that risk factors for the illness were equally distributed between the vasectomized and nonvasectomized men. In one of the studies, the men who had undergone vasectomy had a lower overall death rate than the men who had not, supporting the likelihood that the two groups had different characteristics. Differences of this type might have affected prostate cancer risk, producing study results that misleadingly implicated vasectomy as a cause of prostate cancer.

Like others before them, these scientists also noted the lack of evidence for any biological mechanism that could link vasectomy with prostate cancer.

In 1993, NICHD convened a meeting at which an expert panel considered published data, preliminary results from studies in progress, and an analysis of eight epidemiologic studies, including the two reports mentioned above. The panelists concluded that the positive associations between vasectomy and prostate cancer found in some studies might or might not be valid. Scientists agree, however, that if any increased risk is caused by vasectomy, it is relatively small.

WHO is currently conducting a major study of vasectomy and prostate cancer in several developing countries, and three other studies are ongoing in the United States and Canada. Scientists expect these investigations to help resolve the issue.

In the interim, most physicians will be guided by NICHD's expert panel of 1993 which concluded there is insufficient basis for recommending any change in current clinical or public health practice. Providers should continue to offer vasectomy and to perform the procedure, the panel said. Vasectomy reversal is not warranted to prevent prostate cancer, and screening for prostate cancer should not be any different for men who have had a vasectomy than for those who have not undergone the procedure.

Vasectomy has been used for about a century as a means of sterilization. It has a long track record as a safe and effective method of contraception and is relied upon by millions of people throughout the world. On the basis of much evidence, experts believe that vasectomy can safely continue to be used as it has been in the past, while further research is carried out.

Chapter 16.5

The Patient's Guide to Vasectomy Reversal

The Patient's Guide to Vasectomy Reversal has been written to assist men who want to restore their fertility through vasectomy reversal surgery. In practice, I have treated many individuals who have successfully undergone vasectomy reversal surgery and while each case is unique, I have found similar questions and concerns. The purpose of the Patient's Guide to Vasectomy Reversal is to familiarize men with the procedures that are involved, from the initial examination through surgery and the post-operative period, to help lessen the apprehension that can accompany the decision process.

This guide is designed in a simple question and answer format to address particular concerns, as well as to expand on other issues that also need to be understood before proceeding with vasectomy reversal.

1. **What is a vasectomy?**

A vasectomy is a safe, simple, quick and effective method of contraception.

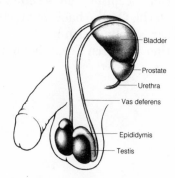

Figure 16.3.

To understand what a vasectomy is, a little knowledge of normal male anatomy is needed. As illustrated in Figure 16.3, the testicles are continually producing sperm even after a vasectomy. The sperm is stored in the epididymis, located directly above the testicles. Sperm moves from the epididymis through each vas deferens to the prostate, located in front of the bladder. When ejaculation occurs, sperm is expelled from the penis.

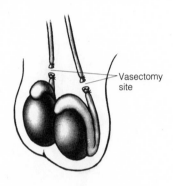

A vasectomy is a surgical procedure that disrupts the flow of sperm through the vas deferens as illustrated in Figure16.4. The surgeon actually cuts through the vas deferens and then places a clip or suture around the cut ends.

Figure 16.4.

2.   **What is a vasectomy reversal?**

A vasectomy reversal is, a surgical procedure that restores the flow of sperm through the vas deferens. It is usually performed by an experienced microsurgeon using specialized instruments, including an operating microscope. The sutures used in vasectomy reversal are finer than human hair.

There are two types of vasectomy reversals: *vasovasostomy and vasoepididymostomy.*

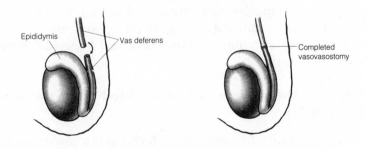

Figure 16.5. *Vasovasostomy*

449

A *vasovasostomy* is the operation most frequently performed for vasectomy reversal. It entails stitching the cut ends of the vas deferens together as illustrated in Figure 16.6.

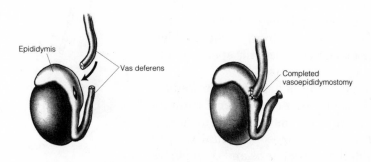

Figure 16.6. *Vasoepididymostomy*

A *vasovasostomy* is the surgery of choice for vasectomy reversal. However, if excessive inflammation or scarring has occurred in the epididymis, sperm may be blocked from getting to the vas deferens. If a blockage has occurred in the epididymis, merely connecting the two cut ends of the vas deferens (as is done in a vasovasostomy) will not solve the problem. To bypass the blockage in the epididymis, a *vasoepididymostomy* must be performed.

A *vasoepididymostomy* is performed by connecting the vas deferens directly to the epididymis as illustrated in Figure 16.6. One end of the vas deferens is stitched directly to the epididymis.

More information regarding vasovasostomy and vasoepididymostomy is provided in question 10.

3. **What are the success rates associated with vasectomy reversal?**

Before the advent of microsurgical techniques, vasectomy reversal procedures were only occasionally successful. With the relatively recent advances in microsurgical techniques, instruments and suture materials, success rates have greatly increased.

Results of recent studies indicate that following microsurgical vasovasostomy sperm appears in the semen in approximately 85 to 97 percent of men. Approximately 50 percent of couples subsequently achieve a pregnancy.

Following microsurgical *vasoepididymostomy,* sperm appears in the semen in approximately 65 percent of men. Approximately 20 percent of couples subsequently achieve a pregnancy.

4. Is vasectomy reversal a common procedure?

Current estimates are that about 1 percent of men who have undergone a vasectomy will eventually want reversal surgery.

About 500,000 men have vasectomies each year in the United States. While the number of men requesting vasectomy has remained approximately the same, the number of men requesting vasectomy reversal has increased.

5. Why do men want vasectomy reversals?

The leading reason that men elect to have vasectomy reversal is to father a child after remarriage following divorce or death of a spouse.

Others seek vasectomy reversal after the death of a child. A small percentage of men seek reversal for relief of scrotal pain attributed to the vasectomy, a desire to restore fertility independent of any change in marital status, or because of religious beliefs.

6. Can all vasectomies be reversed?

From a surgical standpoint, it is rare that a vasectomy cannot be reversed. In the past, if the epididymis was blocked or a large segment of the vas deferens was removed during the vasectomy, a vasectomy reversal procedure was considered to be too complicated and was unlikely to be successful. Today, however, the development of new microsurgical techniques has provided a way to bypass an epididymal blockage and correct a shortened vas deferens. These new techniques have led to improved pregnancy rates following vasectomy reversal even in the most extreme cases.

7. Does health insurance cover vasectomy reversal?

It is important to check with your health insurance plan to identify what costs of vasectomy reversal may be covered.

The costs of vasectomy reversal will include: the surgeon's fee, the hospital's fee for the use of the operating room and ambulatory care facility, and the fee for anesthesia. These costs can range from approximately $5,000 to $15,000.

8. How have microsurgical techniques improved results of vasectomy reversal?

Most surgeons attribute the increased success following vasectomy reversal to the advent and skilled use of the operating microscope (microsurgery).

The advantage of using an operating microscope is that the ends vas deferens can be rejoined more accurately. The diameter of the vas

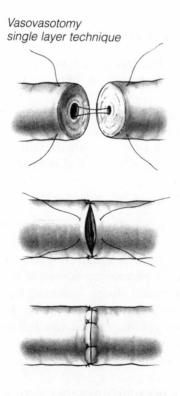

*Vasovasotomy
single layer technique*

Figure 16.7.

deferens is barely perceptible to the human eye (.3 to.5 mm in diameter). As a result the placement of sutures with the aid of optical magnification (10 to 40 times) is far more accurate.

Microsurgical techniques for the correction of epididymal obstruction (vasoepididymostomy) have also led to improved pregnancy rates following vasectomy reversal. A surgeon who has microsurgical expertise can move from a vasovasostomy to an more complicated vasoepididymostomy when the need arises. There are two microsurgical techniques available for vasovasostomy: A single layer approximation and a multi-layer approximation. In the single layer technique, the inner and outer layers of the vas deferens are joined with the same suture. Six to eight sutures are generally used. Gaps in the outer layer of the vas deferens may be present after the initial sutures are tied. In this case, additional sutures may be used to close these gaps. This is called a modified single layer approximation.

In the multi-layer technique, the inner and outer layers of the vas deferens are each connected separately. Microsurgery for vasoepididymostomy has made it possible to connect the vas deferens precisely to a single epididymal tubule with greater accuracy.

The inner layer of the vas deferens is precisely connected with sutures to a small opening in a single epididymal tubule. The outer layer of both the vas deferens and the epididymis are then connected to obtain the final result.

9. **Are the success rates for a multi-layer vasovasostomy different from a single layer vasovasostomy?**

Success rates for both single- and multi-layer vasovasostomy are similar as long as microsurgical techniques are employed by an experienced microsurgeon. In fact, according to a recent report, success rates after a modified single-layer closure was slightly better than a multi-layer closure (57 percent vs 51 percent pregnancy rates respectively). Many experienced physicians believe that potential drawbacks to the multi-layer vasovasostomy technique are the increased cost to the patient (more sutures are needed), increased operative time and longer anesthesia time.

10. **When would a surgeon perform a vasoepididymostomy rather than a vasovasostomy?**

While a vasovasostomy is the first choice of treatment for vasectomy reversal, vasoepididymostomy, the more complex procedure, is required in approximately one third of cases.

At the beginning of the reversal surgery, the surgeon isolates and excises the scarred ends of the vas deferens. As soon as this is done, the cut ends of the vas deferens closest to the testicles are examined for sperm content and vas fluid quality. Fluid is extracted from the vas deferens by syringe and inspected using a laboratory microscope. In general, if sperm is present in the vas fluid, a vasovasostomy is performed. If sperm is not present in the vas fluid, a vasoepididymostomy is performed. Lack of sperm in the vas fluid usually indicates rupture and blockage of the epididymal tubules induced by the back pressure which forms after vasectomy. A vasoepididymostomy merely connects the vas deferens to the epididymis at a site which will allow sperm to flow from the epididymis directly into the vas deferens thereby bypassing the site of the blockage.

Vas fluid quality, particularly clarity, is also important. Usually, when sperm are absent, the vas fluid has a cheesy, thick opaque appearance. When this occurs, a vasoepididymostomy is needed. In some rare instances, however, the vas fluid has a watery consistency and is clear in color. When this occurs, even if sperm is absent from the vas fluid, a vasovasostomy is performed. On average, two thirds of these surgeries result in sperm in the ejaculate and one third of couples will become pregnant.

11. How do I select a surgeon?

The skill and experience of the surgeon who performs your reversal surgery is one of the main determinants of your postoperative success.

It is a good idea to ask your potential surgeon whether he or she can perform a vasoepididymostomy using an operating microscope. During surgery, the surgeon needs to be experienced in assessing the vas fluid quality, evaluating signs of epididymal blockage, and determining the best location for a vasoepididymostomy if needed. A vasoepididymostomy is necessary in approximately one-third of cases, and the need for it can only be definitively determined during surgery.

12. My vasectomy was done years ago. How does that affect my chances for a successful reversal?

While the length of time from vasectomy to reversal surgery correlates with success, no interval is considered too long to perform reversal surgery.

Data from the largest research study on vasectomy reversal reveals progressively less favorable results as the time from vasectomy to reversal increases. These are the rates for 1,247 men studied who underwent vasovasostomy:

Table 16.1. Years between vasectomy and reversal

Years	Sperm Return	Pregnancy Rate
< 3	97%	76%
3 - 8	88%	53%
9 - 14	79%	44%
> 15	71%	30%

These data nevertheless indicate that despite long periods of time from vasectomy to reversal surgery (even greater than 15 years), vasectomy reversal can result in successful pregnancies.

One reason for lower success rates with longer intervals between vasectomy and reversal surgery is the increased rate of epididymal blockage as the time interval lengthens. Rupture and obstruction of the epididymal tubule is caused by increased pressure in the vas deferens and epididymis below the level of the vasectomy site. If the epididymis is blocked, vasoepididymostomy needs to be performed to accomplish the reversal.

13. Does the way my vasectomy was performed affect my chances for a successful reversal?

The site of the vasectomy is a factor in the outcome of reversal surgery. A vasectomy can be performed close to the testicle and epididymis or farther away. A disruption of the vas deferens farther away from the testicle will leave a long length of vas deferens (vas remnant) and increase the chance of a successful reversal. The shorter the vas remnant, the greater the chance of scarring and obstruction in the epididymis necessitating a more difficult vasoepididymostomy.

14. Can my doctor predict the outcome of my vasectomy reversal by examining me before surgery?

Your doctor will examine you before surgery by physically palpating your scrotum to determine the firmness and size of the testicles. If you have one or more shrunken testicles, this may indicate irreversible testicular failure; Therefore, surgery may not be able to restore fertility. If your doctor encounters an engorged and perhaps firm epididymis, this indicates that an epididymal blockage may be present. While not definitive, these findings may suggest that a vasoepididymostomy will need to be performed. On the other hand, if the epididymis is not engorged, a vasovasostomy is still not guaranteed.

Your doctor will also attempt to determine the length of the vas deferens that has remained after vasectomy (vas remnant) during the same scrotal examination. The longer the vas remnant, the better the chance for vasovasostomy and future success. The shorter the vas remnant, the greater the chance that the epididymis will have developed a blockage, necessitating a vasoepididymostomy.

In the rare event that a very long segment of the vas deferens is missing, it is more likely that extensive surgery will be necessary. On occasion, prior surgery such as hernia repair can cause damage to the vas deferens, resulting in a missing segment.

Lastly, disorders of the testicles such as varicoceles (an engorgement of the veins surrounding the testicles which cause damage) can be detected by your physician by examining your scrotal contents. These disorders may need to be corrected at a later date if vasectomy reversal surgery alone does not lead to pregnancy.

15. I've already had a vasectomy reversal with no success. Does it make sense to try it again?

A frequent cause of reversal surgery failure is that a vasovasostomy was performed when, on the basis of intraoperative findings, a vasoepididymostomy was indicated. Some other reasons for vasovasostomy failure are inaccurate approximation of the vas due to poor surgical technique, and blockage from scarring as a result of disruption of the blood supply. Success rates after repeat reversal surgery are slightly lower than success rates after first reversals, mainly because the duration of vas obstruction is longer for repeat reversal surgery.

Comparison of Overall Results in First and Repeat Reversals

Number of men with sperm in semen:

- First Reversal: 865 out of 1026 (86 percent)
- Second Reversal: 150 out of 199 (75 percent)

Number of couples that achieved a pregnancy:

- First Reversal: 421 out of 808 (52 percent)
- Second Reversal: 52 out of 120 (43 percent)

The large case study described above compared the results of first and repeat vasectomy reversals. This study reported that, following repeat reversals, sperm were present in the semen of three-fourths (150 out of 199) of men postoperatively and that pregnancy was reported in 52 out of 120 couples (43 percent) who were evaluated for pregnancy. These results are very similar to those of first reversals and many men feel that these results are high enough to try reoperation.

Chances of a successful reoperative reversal may be predicted by the sperm content of the intraoperative vas fluid sampled at the time of the first reversal. If sperm was present in the vas fluid during the initial vasovasostomy and the individual fails to produce sperm in the ejaculate, obstruction at the site of vas reapproximation may exist and the patient may need to repeat the vasovasostomy. If, on the other hand, sperm were absent in the vas fluid, the patient likely required a vasoepididymostomy during the first procedure and will likely require a vasoepididymostomy if the reversal surgery is repeated.

16. Is *in-vitro* fertilization (IVF) a better option for me than vasectomy reversal?

Recent medical and surgical advances have created many options for infertile couples. Choice of infertility treatments usually depends on weighing the likelihood of conceiving with a specific treatment versus other more complex and costly treatments. IVF is a relatively new technique that can help couples initiate a pregnancy who might not otherwise be able to conceive through natural methods. IVF involves incubation of human eggs and sperm in a culture dish. For fertilization to occur, the egg must have optimal maturity and the sperm must function normally. Once a fertilized egg develops into an embryo it is transferred back into the female.

Assisted fertilization techniques like IVF are appropriate for men with severe sperm function defects or for men in whom no cause of infertility can be found. Pregnancy rates, however, are very low with routine IVF and are usually coupled with gamete micromanipulation which requires special preparation of the egg and sperm. Intracytoplasmic sperm injection (ICSI) is the most useful micromanipulation technique developed so far to enhance IVF fertilization rates in patients with severe male factor infertility This procedure involves the direct injection of a single sperm into an egg.

For men who have undergone a vasectomy, sperm is obviously absent from the ejaculate. Therefore, since the IVF/ICSI procedure requires sperm, sperm must be retrieved from the testicle or epididymis through a minor surgical procedure. The procedure for obtaining sperm is less complicated than reversal surgery, but entails local anesthesia, and insertion of a needle into the scrotum (into the testicle or epididymis) to obtain sperm.

The cost of one cycle of IVF can range from $8,000 to $15,000 depending on the array of infertility factors involved and whether sperm retrieval procedures for the man is necessary. Currently, the national birth rate for IVF, as reported by The Society for Assisted Reproductive Technology, and its parent organization, the American Society for Reproductive Medicine, is only 18.3 percent per cycle.

Because of the expense, lower pregnancy rates, and potential side effects from hormonal therapy for the female partner, reversal surgery, and in most cases, repeat reversal surgery are options of first choice for vasectomized men. IVF is an option to consider if vasectomy reversal is unsuccessful, rather than as an alternative to surgery.

17. **We don't plan on trying to conceive right away. When would be the best time for me to have a vasectomy reversal?**

Even if you plan to postpone attempts to conceive, for most couples, it is probably best not to delay the reversal procedure.

Keep in mind that the average time interval from a vasectomy reversal until pregnancy is 12 months, and it takes 24 months postoperatively until the highest percentage of pregnancies is achieved.

Also, the longer the interval between vasectomy and reversal, the less the chance that pregnancy after reversal would occur. This should be understood in context. In other words, although many successful reversals are done several years after vasectomy, when you have the option, sooner is better.

18. **Do I need any tests before surgery?**

No special preoperative tests are needed before a vasectomy reversal other than the standard lab tests required by some hospitals, ambulatory surgery facilities or anesthesiologists. For men more than 40 years old, an EKG is usually required.

19. **Do tests for anti-sperm antibodies or follicle stimulating hormone levels help predict the success of my surgery?**

Measurement of serum antisperm antibodies appears to be of little prognostic value with regard to male fertility potential.

Anti-sperm antibodies are proteins that can inhibit the movement and function of sperm. Some research indicates that anti-sperm antibodies may decrease the chances for pregnancy after reversal surgery, however, studies have found little correlation between preoperative testing for anti-sperm antibodies and pregnancy.

The difficulty in testing for anti-sperm antibodies before reversal surgery is that only serum (blood) antibodies can be tested, which do not accurately predict the antibodies that may be found in the semen after the operation. Because of these difficulties, most surgeons do not find anti-sperm antibody testing to be useful.

Follicle-stimulating hormone (FSH) is not routinely assayed in men requesting vasectomy reversal.

FSH is a hormone produced in the pituitary gland that stimulates the testes to produce sperm. An elevated FSH level suggests reduced sperm production and testicular failure, and can indicate that there is less possibility of obtaining a good sperm count after surgery. Men who have a history of fertility prior to vasectomy rarely have an elevated FSH level. On the other hand, if serum FSH is low or normal, it does not necessarily mean sperm production is normal.

It is not unreasonable to measure serum FSH preoperatively in men who have never fathered a child, in men who have abnormally small testicles, or in men whose vasectomies were performed many years prior to reversal surgery.

20. **Should my wife undergo any tests before I have my vasectomy reversal?**

Your wife should undergo a gynecological exam to ensure adequate fertility potential. For older couples or those whose family history indicates, genetic counseling may also be helpful.

21. **Will I be able to go home the day of the surgery?**

The surgery may be performed either in an ambulatory surgery center or hospital, generally on a day-surgery basis. In most cases, the man arrives in the morning and leaves the hospital the same day.

22. **What type of anesthesia is used?**

Vasectomy reversal may be performed with local, regional or general anesthesia, depending on the preference of surgeon and patient. General anesthesia is commonly used because it affords maximum patient comfort considering the length and nature of the surgery.

23. **How long will the surgery take?**

Microsurgical vasovasostomy averages 2 to 3 hours, while vasoepididymostomy may take as long as 5 hours. The patient is then observed in the recovery room for an additional 3 more hours.

The length of surgery depends on the type of procedure, the amount of scarring present from prior surgery, the presence of and degree of inflammation, and the ease with which sperm can be identified in the vas deferens or epididymal tubule.

24. **Where are the incisions made?**

A vasectomy reversal is usually performed through incisions in the front of each side of the scrotum.

The incision is vertical (up and down) so that it can be extended if more length is needed. If there is difficulty in locating the site of the vasectomy, if the vasectomy was performed at a very high scrotal level, or if a long segment of the vas deferens was removed, it may be necessary to extend the scrotal incisions up to the lower inguinal (abdominal) region.

If a prior hernia procedure was performed, inadvertent blockage of the vas deferens may have occurred. If this is the case, an incision into the site of the prior hernia repair may be necessary.

25. **What are the complications that can occur?**

Normal signs and symptoms after surgery include: slight swelling, bruising or discoloration of the scrotal area. These generally do not require a doctor's attention. A sore throat, headache, nausea, constipation and general "body ache" due to the anesthesia and surgery may also be present. These symptoms usually resolve within a few days.

Severe complications that require additional surgery are rare. Postoperative complications that require prompt attention are wound infections and severe scrotal hematoma (black and blue bruised scrotum). A wound infection is present if you develop a fever or if your incision becomes warm, swollen, red, or painful. A hematoma is present if excessive bleeding under the skin occurs and is accompanied by a throbbing pain and a bulging of the incision site.

26. How much pain can I expect after surgery?

Discomfort after vasectomy reversal varies from patient to patient. In general, pain may be similar or slightly more severe than the pain experienced after the original vasectomy. Pain medication such as codeine is prescribed and is usually only necessary for one to two days after the surgery, after which acetaminophen (such as Tylenol) or ibuprofen (such as Motrin or Advil) is all that is needed. To decrease the pain and swelling after surgery, ice packs are recommended, which are placed on the scrotum for approximately ten minutes every half hour for the first post-operative day. A scrotal support is worn for four weeks after the surgery to decrease discomfort and lessen swelling. Normal strenuous activity can be resumed four weeks after the surgery if indicated by your physician.

27. How soon can I have sex after surgery?

It is generally best to wait three weeks after the surgery before resuming any type of sexual activity.

28. How long after the surgery will it take for sperm to reappear?

The first semen analysis is obtained one or two months after the surgery and again at two to three month intervals, either until sperm counts and motility are normal, or pregnancy occurs.

Three months after a vasovasostomy the semen analysis often reveals a good sperm count with poor motility. After 6 months the count is usually stable or slightly improved and the motility is significantly improved. After a vasoepididymostomy, sperm usually takes longer to appear in the ejaculate, and in most cases takes at least 4 to 6 months to appear.

29. Is there any chance that my sperm count will decline after an initially successful vasectomy reversal?

Studies have shown that, following initially successful reversal surgery, where good sperm counts and motility have been obtained, a significant number of men subsequently experience significant deterioration in sperm counts. Approximately 10 percent of men following successful vasovasostomy and approximately 20 percent of men following successful vasoepididymostomy will experience deterioration in sperm counts when followed for at least two years after surgery.

A decline in sperm counts after successful surgery can be caused by the formation of scar tissue which can occur from sperm leakage at the reversal site or from a disruption of the blood supply at the site of the surgery.

In light of the 10 to 20 percent of patients that deteriorate after successful surgery, sperm banking should be a consideration, particularly after a vasoepididymostomy.

30. How soon can I expect a pregnancy to occur after my vasectomy reversal?

The average time from reversal surgery to conception is 12 months. Studies indicate that pregnancies after reversal surgery can occur from one month to 82 months after reversal surgery. Most pregnancies occur within 24 months of reversal surgery.

31. What are my options if the surgery is unsuccessful?

About 14 percent of men with vasovasostomies and 40 percent with vasoepididymostomies have no sperm in their semen after surgery. After vasovasostomy, sperm is usually present in the semen after two months and should certainly be present within six months. After vasoepididymostomy, sperm usually appear in the semen during the first six months, although they may not appear for as long as 12 to 15 months. If sperm are not present in the semen by six months after vasovasostomy or by 12 to 18 months after vasoepididymostomy, then the reversal surgery is considered a failure.

If surgery is unsuccessful you can consider reoperation (see question #14) or assisted reproductive techniques such as in-vitro fertilization (IVF) with intracytoplasmic sperm injection (ICSI) (see question #15). For a man who has no sperm in the ejaculate after reversal surgery, sperm for IVF/ICSI can be obtained through a minor surgical procedure (sperm retrieval) which extracts sperm directly from the testicles and/or epididymis.

Glossary

Antisperm antibodies. Immunological substances that can inhibit sperm movement and function.

Epididymis. Tightly coiled, very small tubes covering the back and sides of the testis, where sperm collect after leaving the testis.

Follicle stimulating hormone (FSH). A pituitary hormone that stimulates the testes to make sperm.

ICSI Intracytoplasmic sperm injection. An in-vitro fertilization procedure that requires the direct injection of a single sperm into an egg.

IVF In-vitro fertilization. A fertility procedure where human eggs and a suspension of sperm are incubated together in a culture dish (test-tube). Once embryos are formed, they are placed back into the uterus of the female.

Microsurgery. Surgery using optical magnification provided by an operating microscope.

Prostate gland. Located below the bladder, the gland where the ejaculatory ducts, the two vas deferens and the urethra join.

Semen. The combination of sperm and glandular fluid released by the urethra when a man ejaculates.

Suture. The material (thread) used during vasectomy reversal surgery.

Scrotum. The sac that contains the testicles, epididymis and vas deferens.

Testes. Located in the scrotum, the male reproductive glands which produce sperm.

Urethra. The tube running from the bladder to the penis that carries urine and semen.

Vas deferens. The tubes that carry sperm from the testicle and epididymis to the urethra.

Vas remnant. The length of the vas deferens from the epididymis to the site of the vasectomy.

Vasectomy. A surgical procedure that provides infertility by blocking the transport of sperm from the epididymis to the urethra via the vas deferens.

Vasoepididymostomy. A surgical procedure to reverse the effects of vasectomy by connecting the vas deferens to the epididymis to bypass obstruction in the epididymis.

Vasovasostomy. A surgical procedure to restore fertility by reconnect the ends of vas deferens that were severed when vasectomy was performed.

References

Belker AM, Thomas AJ Jr, Fuchs EF, Konnak JW, Sharlip ID. Results of 1,469 microsurgical vasectomy reversals by the Vasovasostomy Study Group. J Urol 1991; 145:505-511.

Thomas AJ Jr, Pontes, JE, Rose NR, Segal S, Pierce JM Jr. Microsurgical vasovasostomy: immunologic consequences and subsequent fertility. Fertil Steril 1981;35:447-50.

Linnet L. Clinical immunology of vasectomy and vasovasostomy. Urology 1983;22:101-14. Silber SJ. Microscopic vasectomy reversal. Fertil Steril 1977;28:1191-1202.

Thomas AJ Jr. Vasoepididymostomy. Urol Clin North Am 1987;14:527:38. Bronson R. Cooper G, Rosenfeld D. Sperm antibodies: their role in infertility. Fertil Steril 1984;42:171-83.

The American Fertility Society Guideline for Practice: Vasectomy Reversal. The American Fertility Society 1992.

Goldstein M. Surgery of male infertility and other scrotal disorders. Campbell's Urology, 6th ed. Edited by PC Walsh, AB Retik, TA Stamey and ED Vaughan, Jr. Philadelphia: W.B. Saunders Co., vol. 3, chapt. 87, pp 3114-3149, 1992.

Jarow JP, Sigman M, Buch JP, Oates RD. Delayed appearance of sperm after end-to-side vasoepididymostomy. J Urol 1995; 153:1156.

Lee HY. A 20-year experience with epididymovasostomy for pathologic epididymal obstruction. Fertil Steril 1987;47:487.

Witt MA, Heron S, Lipshultz Li. The post vasectomy length of the testicular vasal remnant: a predictor of surgical outcome in microscopic vasectomy reversal. J Urof 1994; 151:892-894.

Matthews GJ, Schlegel PN, Goldstein M. Patency following microsurgical vasoepididymostomy and vasovasostomy: temporal considerations. J Urol 1995; 154: 2070-73.

Belker A. Repeating the Vasectomy Reversal. Contemporary Urology Sept 1993, 54-66.

Fisch H, Goluboff E. Simplified One-Layer Vasovasostomy. Current Surgical Techniques in Urology; Oisson CA, ed. Delaware, MPI, 1993.

Fuchs EF Restoring fertility through epididymovasostomy. Contemporary Urology, December 1991, 27-38.

Goldstein M. Surgery of Male Infertility. W.B. Saunders Co., 1995.

Gvakharia M, et al. Treating male-factor infertility with ICSI. Contemporary Urology, September, 1995, 58-67.

Lamb DJ, Stockton JD, Lipshultz LI. New roads to fertility. Contemporary Urology, January 1991, 32-41.

Neumann PJ, Gharib SD, Weinstein MC. The cost of a successful delivery with in-vitro fertilization. NEJM 1994: 239-43.

Sharlip ID. What is the best pregnancy rate that may be expected from vasectomy reversal? J Urol 1993: 1469-71.

Sigman M. A guide to assisted reproductive techniques. Contemporary Urology, March 1991, 31-39.

Part Four

Circumcision

Chapter 17

Medical Benefits of
Circumcision

Circumcision is the removal of a fold of loose skin (the foreskin) that covers the head (glans) of the unerect penis. The amount of this skin varies from virtually none, to a considerable amount that droops down from the end of the flaccid penis. The practice is common amongst many divergent human cultures. A variety of methods are, moreover, used and the amount of foreskin removed also varies.

Historically circumcision has been a topic of emotive and often irrational debate. At least part of the reason is that a sex organ is involved. (Compare, for example, ear piercing.) During the past two decades the medical profession in Australia have tended to advise parents not to circumcise their baby boys. In fact there have even been reports of harassment by medical professionals of new mothers, especially those belonging to religious groups that practice circumcision, in an attempt to stop them having this procedure carried out. Such attitudes are a far cry from the situation years ago when baby boys were circumcised routinely in Australia. But over the past 20 years the rate has declined to as low as 16-19 percent (55).

However, a reversal of this trend is starting to occur. In the light of an increasing volume of medical scientific evidence pointing to the benefits of neonatal circumcision, a new policy statement was formulated

©1997 Brian J. Morris, PhD DSc. Fax: 61-2-9351-2058, University Academic (in medical sciences) Email:brianm@physiol.usyd.edu.au. This review can be found on the world-wide web: (http://www.physiol.usyd.edu.au/brianm/ circumcision.htm). Last updated July 1997. The author freely grants permission for others to copy and distribute this review. Reprinted with acknowledgment.

by a working party of the Australian College of Paediatrics in August 1995 and adopted by the College in May 1996 (5). In this document medical practitioners are now urged to fully inform parents of the benefits of having their male children circumcised. Similar recommendations were made recently by the Canadian Paediatric Society who also conducted an evaluation of the literature, although concluded that the benefits and harms were very evenly balanced. The American College of Pediatrics has moved far closer to an advocacy position and many recognized authorities in the USA strongly advocate circumcision of all newborn boys. More details of their statements appear below.

In the present literature review I would like to focus principally on the protection afforded by circumcision against infection by micro-organisms, some of which can cause disease and even death, but will also touch on other aspects, including sexual benefits. I might add that I am a university academic who teaches medical and science students and who does medical research, including that involving genital cancer virology, as well as molecular biology and genetics. I am not Jewish, nor a medical practitioner or lawyer, so have no religious bias or medico-legal concerns that might impede a rational presentation of the information that has been published in reputable journals.

Why the Foreskin Increases Infection Risk

The increased risk of infection in the uncircumcised may be a consequence of the fact that the foreskin presents the penis with a larger surface area, the moist skin under it represents a thinner epidermal barrier than the drier, more cornified skin of the circumcised penis (the glans of which develops a thick stratum corneum layer), the presence of a prepuce is likely to result in greater microtrauma during sexual intercourse, thereby permitting an entry point into the bloodstream for infectious agents, and, as one might expect, the warm, moist mucosal environment under the foreskin favors growth of micro-organisms. The preputial sac has even been referred to by Dr Gerald Weiss, an American surgeon, as a "cesspool for infection," as its unfortunate anatomy draped around the end of the penis results in accumulation of secretions, excretions (urine), dead cells and growths of bacteria. Parents are told not to retract the foreskin of male infants which makes cleaning difficult. Even if optimal cleansing is performed there is no evidence that it confers protection (96, 97).

470

History

Circumcision has been practiced widely in Western countries this century. From at least the mid-1940s to mid-1970s over 90 percent of boys in the USA and Australia were circumcised soon after birth. The major benefits at that time were seen as improved lifetime genital hygiene, elimination of phimosis (inability to retract the foreskin) and prevention of penile cancer. The trend not to circumcise started in the mid to late 1970s, after the American Academy of Paediatrics Committee for the Newborn stated, in 1971, that there are "no valid medical indications for circumcision." In 1975 this was modified to "no absolute valid . . . ," which remained in the 1983 statement, but in 1989 it changed significantly to "New evidence has suggested possible medical benefits . . . "(31).

Dr Edgar Schoen, Chairman of the Task Force on Circumcision of the American Academy of Pediatrics, has stated that the benefits of routine circumcision of newborns as a preventive health measure far exceed the risks of the procedure. During the period 1985-92 there was an increase in the frequency of post-newborn circumcision and during that same time Schoen points out that the association of lack of circumcision and urinary tract infection has moved from "suggestive" to "conclusive." Moreover, it heralded the finding of associations with other infectious agents, including HIV. In fact he goes on to say that "Current newborn circumcision may be considered a preventive health measure *analogous to immunization* in that side effects and complications are immediate and usually minor, but benefits accrue for a lifetime." Benefits included: a decrease in physical problems such as phimosis reduction in balanitis (inflammation of the glans, the head of the penis (24), reduced urinary tract infections, problems with erections at puberty, decrease in certain sexually transmitted diseases (STDs) such as HIV, and, in older men, elimination of penile cancer and a decrease in urological problems and infections [reviewed in (2, 5, 25, 47, 73, 76)]. Therefore, the benefits are different at different ages.

Different Specialists See Different Things

Neonatologists only see the problems of the operation itself. Moreover such problems occur in only a minor proportion of boys, and generally because of poor technique by an inexperienced operator. However, urologists who see and have to treat the problems of uncircumcised men cannot understand why all newborns are not circumcised [76, 77]. Other health care workers in hospitals and aged care homes also have adverse comments about the uncircumcised penises

471

they see. The demand for circumcision later in childhood has increased, but, with age, problems, such as anaesthetic risk, are higher. Thus Schoen states "Current evidence concerning the life-time medical benefit of newborn circumcision favors an affirmative choice"(77).

Anti-Circumcision Lobby Groups

In a letter written by Dr Schoen to Dr Terry Russell in Brisbane in 1994 Schoen derides an organization known as "NOCIRC" for their use of "distortions, anecdotes and testimonials to try to influence professional and legislative bodies and the public, stating that in the past few years they have become increasingly desperate and outrageous as the medical literature has documented the benefits. For example they have compared circumcision with female genital mutilation, which is equivalent to cutting off the penis. In 1993 the rate of circumcision had risen to 80 percent in the USA and Schoen suggests that "Perhaps NOCIRC has decided to export their 'message' to Australia since their efforts are proving increasingly futile in the US." One only has to do a search on the World Wide Web to read the statements from this group and others like it and any intelligent person can quickly make up their own mind about the quality of their material and the message they are trying to promulgate. Some of these people mean well and some are intelligent, but lack a broad perspective. Dr Schoen also noted that when Chairman of the Task Force his committee was bombarded with inaccurate and misleading communications from this group. They even publish their own journals, e.g., "*Circumcision.*" Another of these groups is "UNCIRC," which promotes procedures to reverse circumcision, by, for example, stretching the loose skin on the shaft of the retracted penis or the use of surgery. This has led to genital mutilation (88). Claimed benefits of "increased sensitivity" in reality appear to be a result of the friction of the foreskin, whether intact or newly created, on the moist or sweaty glans and undersurface of the prepuce in the unaroused state and would obviously in the "re-uncircumcised" penis have nothing to do with an increase in touch receptors. Indeed, nerves do not regenerate. Moreover, the sensitivity during sexual intercourse is in fact identical, according to men circumcised as adults.

Benefits Outweigh the Risks

Dr Tom Wiswell, a respected authority in the USA was a strong opponent, but then switched camps as a result of his own research findings and the findings of others. This is what he has to say: "As a pediatrician and neonatologist, I am a child advocate and try to do what is best for children. For many years I was an outspoken opponent of circumcision . . . I have gradually changed my opinion" (93, 94). This ability to keep an open mind on the issue and to make a sound judgement on the balance of all available information is to his credit; he did change his mind.

Wiswell looked at the complication rates of having or not having it performed in a study of 136,000 boys born in US army hospitals between 1980 and 1985, 100,000 were circumcised and 193 (0.19 percent) had complications, with no deaths, but of the 36,000 who were not circumcised the complication rate was 0.24 percent and there were 2 deaths (98). A study by others found that of the 11,000 circumcisions performed at New York's Sloane Hospital in 1989, only 6 led to complications, none of which were fatal (73).

A retrospective study of boys aged 4 months to 12 years found significantly greater frequency of penile problems (14 percent vs 6 percent; $P<0.001$) and medical visits for penile problems (10 percent vs 5 percent; $P<0.05$) among those who were uncircumcised, compared with those who were circumcised (36).

Pain and Memory

No adverse psychological aftermath has been demonstrated (75). It must be recognized that there are many painful experiences encountered by the child before, during and after birth (54). Circumcision, if performed without anaesthetic is just one of these. Cortisol levels have registered an increase during and shortly after the procedure, indicating that the baby is not unaware of having had something done in its unanesthetized state and one has to weigh up the need to inflict this short term pain in the context of a lifetime of gain from prevention or reduction of subsequent problems. Anaesthetic creams and other means appear to be at least partially effective in reducing trauma and some babies show no signs of distress at all when the procedure is performed without anaesthetic. Many, however, do, and this may be contributed by the restraining procedure, as well as the surgery itself.

Penile Hygiene

The proponents of not circumcising nevertheless stress that lifelong penile hygiene is required. This acknowledges that something harmful or unpleasant is happening under the prepuce. Moreover, a study of British schoolboys found that penile hygiene does not exist (73). Furthermore, Dr Terry Russell, an Australian medical practitioner states "What man after a night of passion is going to perform penile hygiene before rolling over and snoring the night away (with pathogenic organisms multiplying in the warm moist environment under the prepuce)"(73). The bacteria start multiplying again immediately after washing and explain the whitish film, termed "smegma," that is found under the foreskin. Bacteria give off an offensive odor, necessitating several showers a day by uncircumcised men, some of whom, together with their partners, find the stench so unpleasant that this smell has caused these men to seek a circumcision on this basis alone. For mothers and fathers, it is far easier to maintain cleanliness of their son's penis if it is circumcised. If their son isn't the messages are confusing: "leave it alone," "clean under it," "pull it back sometimes," "irrigate occasionally!"

What Motivates Parents to Get Their Baby Boy Circumcised and the Rates

The reasons for circumcision, at least in a survey carried out as part of a study at Sydney Hospital, were: 3 percent for religious reasons, 1-2 percent for medical, with the remainder suggested by the researchers as "to be like dad" or a preference of one or both parents for whatever reason (22). The main reason may have more to do with hygiene and appearance, as will be discussed later in the section on socio-sexual aspects. The actual proportion of men who were circumcised when examined at this clinic was 62 percent. Of those studied, 95 percent were Caucasian, with younger men just as likely to be circumcised as older men. In Adelaide, South Australia, a similar proportion has been noted, with 55 percent of younger men being circumcised. In Britain, however, the rate is only 7-10 percent, much like Europe. Rates in Africa, Asia and India vary according to religion and culture, with higher rates amongst Muslims and certain tribes and low rates amongst other groups and nations. In the USA, as indicated above, the rate of circumcision has always been high, although differs in different regions: the rates for 1991, 1992, 1993 and 1994 in the northeast region were 62 percent, 68 percent, 65 percent and 70 percent, in each respective year; for the Midwest they were 78 percent, 78 percent, 74 percent and 80 percent, respectively; for the southern region: 64 percent, 63 percent, 61 percent and 65 percent; and for the western region: 41 percent, 38 percent, 36 percent and 34 percent (58). The actual rates are higher than indicated by this data, as they represent only the numbers reported, whereas not all are. In Canada the rate varies markedly between different regions. Even in the same province, Ontario, for example, the rate between different districts ranges from 2 percent to 70 percent, with a mean of around 50 percent.

Physical Problems

Phimosis (inability to retract the foreskin) affects 2-10 percent of uncircumcised males, and can lead to urinary retention, vesica-ureteral reflux and hypertension. *Paraphimosis* (where the retracted foreskin cannot be brought back again over the glans) is a very painful problem, relieved by circumcision or slitting the dorsal surface of the foreskin. To paediatric surgeons, the most obvious medical reasons for circumcision are balanitis (inflammation of the glans) and posthitis (inflammation of the foreskin), which are very painful conditions virtually limited to uncircumcised males. In babies, balanitis is caused by soiled diapers, playing and sitting in dirty areas, antibiotic therapy, as well as yeast and other micro-organisms. Balanoposthitis (inflammation of the foreskin and glans) is common in uncircumcised diabetic men owing to a weakened, shrunken penis (24), and such men also have more problems associated with intercourse. Diabetes is common and inherited, so a family history of this disease may add to considerations in favor of circumcision at birth. Uncircumcised boys may entrap their foreskin in zippers, resulting in pain, trauma, swelling and scarring of this appendage.

In elderly men, infections and pain from balanoposthitis, phimosis and paraphimosis are seen and carers report problems in achieving optimal hygiene in uncircumcised men. The need for an appliance for urinary drainage in quadriplegics and in senile men is facilitated if they are circumcised. Boys and men who are not circumcised can be a source of irritation if they do not retract the foreskin when they urinate, as "splatter" will occur. Although not a medical problem, it is a source of annoyance for other people (such as a parent or partner) if it is they that have the job of cleaning the bathroom. Foreskin problems also mean intercourse is painful.

Neonatal Urinary Tract Infections

In 1982 it was reported that 95 percent of urinary tract infections (UTIs) in boys aged 5 days to 8 months were in uncircumcised infants

(32). This was confirmed by Wiswell (100) and a few years later Wiswell and colleagues found that in 5261 infants born at one US Army hospital, 4 percent of UTI cases were in uncircumcised males, but only 0.2 percent in those who were circumcised (101). Wiswell then went on to examine the records for 427,698 infants (219,755 boys) born in US Armed Forces hospitals from 1975-79 and found that the uncircumcised had an 11-fold higher incidence of UTIs (98). During this decade the frequency of circumcision in the USA decreased from 84 percent to 74 percent and this decrease was associated with an increase in rate of UTI (102). Reviews by others in the mid-80s concluded there was a lower incidence in circumcised boys (50, 71). The rate in girls was stable during the period it was increasing in boys, in whom circumcision was in a decline. In a 1993 study by Wiswell of 209,399 infants born between 1985 and 1990 in US Army hospitals world-wide, 1046 (496 boys) got UTI in their first year of life (99). The number was equal for boys and girls, but was 10-times higher for uncircumcised boys. Among the uncircumcised boys younger than 3 months, 23 percent had bacteremia, caused by the same organism responsible for the UTI. It should be noted that these studies gave figures for infants admitted to hospital for UTI, so that the actual rate would undoubtedly have been higher. The infection can travel up the urinary tract to affect the kidney and a higher rate of problems such as pye lonephritis and renal scarring (seen in 7.5 percent (92) is reported in uncircumcised children (72, 82). These and other reports (e.g., 29, 35, 72, 82) all point to the benefits of circumcision in reducing UTI.

Indeed, Wiswell performed a meta-analysis of all 9 studies that had been published up until 1992 and observed that every one had found an increase in UTI in the uncircumcised (99). The average was 12-fold higher and the range was 5 to 89-fold, with 95 percent confidence intervals of 11-14 (99). Meta-analyses by others have reached similar conclusions. There have been other studies since then that have added further support. One of these was in Sydney and involved boys under 5 years of age (mean 6 months). It found that 6 percent of uncircumcised boys got a UTI, but only 1 percent of circumcised (16).

The benefit appears to extend beyond childhood and into adult life. In a study of men aged, on average, 30 years, and matched for race, age and sexual activity, the circumcised had a lower rate of UTI (81).

The fact that fimbriated strains of the bacterium *Escherichia coli* which are pathogenic to the urinary tract and pyelonephritogenic, have been shown to be capable of adhering to the foreskin, satisfies one of the criteria for causality (27, 30, 40, 41, 82, 102, 103). Thus, in infancy and childhood the prepuce becomes colonized with bacteria.

Fimbriated strains of *Proteus mirabilis*, non-fimbriated *Pseudomonas*, as well as species of *Klebsiella* and *Serratia* also bind closely to the mucosal surface of the foreskin within the first few days of life (27, 30, 103). Circumcision prevents such colonization and subsequent ascending infection of the urinary tract (71).

Since the absolute risk of UTI in uncircumcised boys is approx. 1 in 25 (0.05) and in circumcised boys is 1 in 500 (0.002), the absolute risk reduction is 0.048. Thus, 20 baby boys need to be circumcised to prevent one UTI. However, the potential seriousness and pain of UTI, which can in rare cases even lead to death, should weigh heavily on the minds of parents. The complications of UTI that can lead to death are: kidney failure, meningitis and infection of bone marrow. The data thus show that much suffering has resulted from leaving the foreskin intact. Lifelong genital hygiene in an attempt to reduce such infections is also part of the price that would have to be paid if the foreskin were to be retained. However, given the difficulty in keeping bacteria at bay in this part of the body (63, 77), not performing circumcision would appear to be far less effective than having it done in the first instance (77).

Sexually-Transmitted Diseases

In 1947 a study of 1,300 consecutive patients in a Canadian Army unit showed that being uncircumcised was associated with a 9-fold higher risk of syphilis and 3-times more gonorrhea (91). Work in the mid-70s showed higher chancroid, syphilis, papillomavirus and herpes in uncircumcised men (85). At the University of Western Australia a 1983 study showed twice as much herpes and gonorrhea, 5-times more candidiasis and 5-fold greater incidence of syphilis (64). Others have reported higher rates of non-gonococcal urethritis in uncircumcised men (80). In South Australia a study in 1992 showed that uncircumcised men had more chlamydia (odds ratio 1.3) and gonococcal infections (odds ratio 2.1). Similarly in 1988 a study in Seattle of 2,800 heterosexual men reported higher syphilis and gonorrhea in uncircumcised men, but no difference in herpes, chlamydia and non-specific urethritis (NSU). Like this report, a study in 1994 in the USA, found higher gonorrhea and syphilis, but no difference in other common STDs (15). In the same year Dr Basil Donovan and associates reported the results of a study of 300 consecutive heterosexual male patients attending Sydney STD Centre at Sydney Hospital (22). They found no difference in genital herpes, NSU, seropositivity for HSV-2 and genital warts (i.e., the benign, so-called "low-risk" human papillomavirus types 6 and 11, which are visible on physical examination, unlike the "high-risk" types 16 and 18, which are not). As mentioned above, 62 percent were circumcised and the two groups had a similar age, number of partners and education. Gonorrhea, syphilis and hepatitis B were too uncommon in this Sydney study for them to conclude anything about these other STDs. Similar findings were obtained in the National Health and Social Life Survey in the USA, which asked about gonorrhea, syphilis, chlamydia, non-gonococcal urethritis, herpes and HIV (which is more often acquired intravenously) (48), although some under-reporting by uncircumcised men was likely as they tended to be less educated. Also, circumcision at birth was assumed, so that the number who sought circumcision later in life for problems, such as STDs and/or other infections, and therefore had switched group, was not taken into account. Design aspects of a number of the studies have in fact been criticized. As a result there is still no overwhelming agreement. Nevertheless, on the bulk of evidence it would seem that at least some STDs could be more common in the uncircumcised, but this conclusion is by no means absolute in Western settings, and the incidence may be influenced by factors such as the degree of genital hygiene, availability of running water and socioeconomic group being studied. In some more recent studies in developed nations, in which hygiene is good, no difference was apparent.

Cancer of the Penis

The incidence of penile cancer in the USA is 1 per 100,000 men per year (i.e., 750-1000 cases annually) and mortality rate is 25-33 percent (44, 51). It represents approximately 1 percent of all malignancies in men in the USA. This data has to be viewed, moreover, in the context of the high proportion of circumcised men in the USA, especially in older age groups, and the age group affected, where older men represent only a portion of the total male population. Thus 1 in 100,000 per year of life translates to 75 in 100,000 during each man's lifetime, but since it occurs almost entirely in uncircumcised men, if we assume that these represent 30 percent of males in the USA, the chance an uncircumcised man will get it would be 75 per 30,000 = 1 in 400. In a study in Melbourne in 1990, although 60 percent of affected men were over 60 years of age, 40 percent were under 60 (74). In 5 major series in the USA since 1932 (104), not one man with penile cancer had been circumcised neonatally (51), i.e., this disease is almost completely confined to uncircumcised men and, less commonly, in those circumcised after the newborn period. The finite residual risk in those circumcised later is the major contributing factor to estimates of lifetime risk in the total population of circumcised men of 1 in 50,000 to 1 in 12,000,000 (96, 97). The predicted life-time risk for an uncircumcised man has been estimated as 1 in 600 in the USA and 1 in 900 in Denmark (44). In underdeveloped countries the incidence is higher: approx. 3-6 cases per 100,000 per year (44) and in Uganda it is the most common malignancy in males, leading to calls for greater circumcision in that country (21). In Australia, the most recent figures of the New South Wales Cancer Council (for 1993) show 28 cases per year (including one in a child), with 5 deaths, which is similar to the 1 in 100,000 figure above and applies to a population in which the majority of the older men are circumcised. The rate is set to escalate, however, as more of the males who were not circumcised during the period after the mid 1970s reach the ages when this cancer generally begins to appear.

The so-called "high-risk" papillomavirus types 16 and 18 (HPV 16/18) are found in a large proportion of cases and there is good reason to suspect that they are involved in the causation of penile cancer (53), as is true for most, if not all, cases of cervical cancer (see below). HPV 16 and 18 are, moreover, more common in uncircumcised males (60). These types of HPV produce flat warts that are normally only visible by application of dilute acetic acid (vinegar) to the penis and the data on high-risk HPVs should not be confused with the incidence figures for genital warts, which although large and readily visible, are caused by the relatively benign HPV types 6 and 11 (42). Other factors, such as smoking, poor hygiene and other STDs have been suspected as contributing to penile cancer as well (11, 51), but it would seem lack of circumcision is the primary prerequisite, with such other factors adding to the risk in the uncircumcised man. Financial considerations are, moreover, not inconsiderable. In the USA it was estimated that the cost for treatment and lost earnings in a man of 50 with cancer in 1980 was $103,000 (34). The amount today is higher.

In Australia between 1960 and 1966 there were 78 deaths from cancer of the penis and 2 from circumcision. (Circumcision fatalities today are virtually unknown.) At the Peter McCallum Cancer Institute 102 cases of penile cancer were seen between 1954 and 1984, with twice as many in the latter decade compared with the first. Moreover, several authors have linked the rising incidence of penile cancer to a decrease in the number of neonatal circumcisions (17, 74). It would thus seem that "prevention by circumcision in infancy is the best policy." Indeed it would be an unusual parent who did not want to ensure their child was completely protected by this simple procedure.

There is also some data to suggest that circumcised males may have half the incidence of prostate cancer, which is very common (27 percent of new cancers in males and 7 percent of all deaths (59).

Cervical Cancer in Female Partners of Uncircumcised Men

A number of studies have documented higher rates of cervical cancer in women who have had one or more male sexual partners who were uncircumcised. These studies have to be looked at critically, however, to see to what extent cultural and other influences might be contributing in groups with different circumcision practices. In a study of 5,000 cervical and 300 penile cancer cases in Madras between 1982 and 1990 the incidence was low amongst Muslim women, when compared with Hindu and Christian, and was not seen at all in Muslim men (31). In a case-control study of 1107 Indian women with cervical cancer, sex with uncircumcised men or those circumcised after the age of 1 year was reported in 1993 to be associated with a 4-fold higher risk of cervical cancer, after controlling for factors such as age, age of first intercourse and education (1).

Another study published in 1993 concerning various types of cancer in the Valley of Kashmir concluded that universal male circumcision in the majority community was responsible for the low rate of cervical cancer compared with the rest of India (18). In Israel, a 1994 report of 4 groups of women aged 17-60 found that gynaecologically healthy Moshav residents had no HPV 16/18, whereas healthy Kibbutz residents had a 1.8 percent incidence (38). Amongst those with gynecological complaints HPV 16/18 was found in 9 percent of Jewish and 12 percent of non-Jewish women. So-called "high-risk" HPV types 16, 18 and some rarer forms are responsible for virtually every case of cervical cancer (87). These same high-risk HPVs also cause penile intraepithelial neoplasia (PIN). In a study published in the *New England Journal of Medicine* in 1987 it was found that women with cervical cancer were more likely to have partners with PIN, the male equivalent of cervical intraepithelial neoplasia (CIN) (9). CIN may lead to cancer or, more often, it goes away. Thus co-factors are suspected. Interestingly, smegma (the film of bacteria, secretions and other material under the foreskin), obtained from human and horse has been shown to be capable of producing cervical cancer in mice in one study (67), but not in another (70). Thus the epidemic of cervical cancer in Australia, and indeed most countries in the world, would appear to be contributed, at least in part, by the uncircumcised male and would therefore be expected to get even worse as the large proportion of men that were born in the past 10-20 years and not circumcised reach sexual maturity.

AIDS Virus

In the USA the estimated risk of HIV per heterosexual exposure is 1 in 10,000 to 1 in 100,000. If one partner is HIV positive and otherwise healthy then a single act of unprotected vaginal sex carries a 1 in 300 risk for a woman and as low as a 1 in 1,000 risk for a man (12). (The rates are very much higher for unprotected anal sex and intravenous injection). In Africa, however, the rate of HIV infection is up to 10 percent in some cities. (A possible reason for this big difference will be discussed later.) In Nairobi it was first noticed that among 340 men being treated for STDs they were 3-times as likely to be HIV positive if they had genital ulcers or were uncircumcised (11 percent of these men had HIV) (79). Subsequently another report showed that amongst 409 African ethnic groups spread over 37 countries the geographical distribution of circumcision practices indicated a correlation of lack of circumcision and high incidence of AIDS (10). In 1990 Moses in the *International Journal of Epidemiology* reported that amongst 700 African societies involving 140 locations and 41 countries there was a considerably lower incidence of HIV in those localities where circumcision was practiced (56, 57). Truck drivers, who generally exhibit more frequent prostitute contact, have shown a higher rate of HIV if uncircumcised. Interestingly, in a West African setting, men who were circumcised but had residual foreskin were more likely to be HIV-2 positive than those in whom circumcision was complete (65).

Of 33 cross-sectional studies, 22 have reported statistically significant association (e.g., 20, 37, 39, 68, 88), by univariate and multivariate analysis, between the presence of the foreskin and HIV infection (4 of these were from the USA). Five reported a trend (including 1 U.S. study). The 6 that saw no difference were 4 from Rwanda and 2 from Tanzania. In addition there have been 5 prospective studies and 2 from Kenya and 1 from Tanzania reported statistically significant association. The increased risk in the significant studies ranged from 1.5 to 9.6. The findings have, moreover, led various workers such as Moses and Caldwell to propose that circumcision be used as an important intervention strategy in order to reduce AIDS (12, 26, 37, 43, 52, 56, 57). Such advice has been taken up, with newspaper advertisements from clinics in Tanzania offering this service to protect against AIDS.

Perhaps the most interesting study of the risk of HIV infection imposed by having a foreskin is that by Cameron, Plummer and associates published as a large article in *Lancet* in 1989 (13). It was conducted in Nairobi. Rather than look at the existing infection rate in each group, these workers followed HIV negative men until they became infected. The men were visiting prostitutes, numbering approx. 1000, amongst whom there had been an explosive increase in the incidence of HIV from 4 percent in 1981 to 85 percent in 1986. These men were thus at high risk of exposure to HIV, as well as other STDs. From March to December 1987, 422 men were enrolled into the study. Of these, 51 percent had presented with genital ulcer disease (89 percent chancroid, 4 percent syphilis, 5 percent herpes) and the other 49 percent with urethritis (68 percent being gonorrhea). Twelve percent were initially positive for HIV-1. Amongst the whole group, 27 percent were not circumcised. They were followed up each 2 weeks for 3 months and then monthly until March 1988. During this time 8 percent of 293 men seroconverted (i.e., 24 men), the mean time being 8 weeks. These displayed greater prostitute contact per month (risk ratio = 3), more presented with genital ulcers (risk ratio = 8; $P<0.001$) and more were uncircumcised (risk ratio = 10; $P<0.001$). Logistic regression analysis indicated that the risk of seroconversion was independently associated with being uncircumcised (risk ratio = 8.2; $P<0.0001$), genital ulcers (risk ratio = 4.7; $P=0.02$) and regular prostitute contact (risk ratio = 3.2; $P= 0.02$). The cumulative frequency of seroconversion was 18 percent and was only 2 percent for men with no risk factors, compared to 53 percent for men with both risk factors. Only one circumcised man with no ulcer seroconverted. Thus, 98 percent of seroconversion was associated with either or both cofactors. In 65 percent there appeared to be additive synergy, because ulcers increase infectivity for HIV. This involves increased viral shedding in the female genital tract of women with ulcers, where HIV-1 has been isolated from surface ulcers in the genital tract of HIV-1 infected women.

It has been suggested that the foreskin could physically trap HIV-infected vaginal secretions and provide a more hospitable environment for the infectious inoculum. Also, the increased surface area, traumatic physical disruption during intercourse and inflammation of the glans penis (balanitis) could aid in recruitment of target cells for HIV-1. The port of entry could potentially be the glans, subprepuce and/or urethra. In a circumcised penis the drier, cornified skin may prevent entry and account for the findings.

In this African study the rate of transmission of HIV following a single exposure was 13 percent (i.e., very much higher than in the

USA). It was suggested that concomitant STDs, particularly chancroid (12), may be a big risk factor, but there could be other explanations as well. Studies in the USA have not been as conclusive. Some studies have shown a higher incidence in uncircumcised men. But in one in New York City, for example, no significant correlation was found, although the patients were mainly intravenous drug users and homosexuals, so that any existing effect may have been obscured. A study in Miami, however, of heterosexual couples did find a higher incidence in men who were uncircumcised, and, in Seattle homosexual men were twice as likely to be HIV positive if they were uncircumcised (45).

In an editorial review in 1994 of 26 studies it was pointed out that more work was needed in order to reduce potential biases in some of the previous data (19). At least one study since then has controlled for such potential confounding factors, confirming a significantly lower HIV prevalence among circumcised men (86).

The reason for the big difference in apparent rate of transmission of HIV in Africa and Asia, where heterosexual exposure has led to a rapid spread through these populations and is the main method of transmission, compared with the very slow rate of penetration into the heterosexual community in the USA and Australia, now appears to be related at least in part to a difference in the type of HIV-1 itself (46). In 1995 an article in *Nature Medicine* discussed findings concerning marked differences in the properties of different HIV-1 subtypes in different geographical locations (62). A class of HIV-1 termed "clade E" is prevalent in Asia and differs from the "clade B" found in developed countries in being highly capable of infecting Langerhans cells found in the foreskin, so accounting for its ready transmission across mucosal membranes. The Langerhans cells are part of the immune system and in turn carry the HIV to the T-cells, whose numbers are severely depleted as a key feature of AIDS. The arrival of the Asian strain in Australia was reported in Nov 1995 and has the potential to utilize the uncircumcised male as a vehicle for rapid spread through the heterosexual community of this country in a similar manner as it has done in Asia. It could thus be a time-bomb about to go off and should be a major concern for health officials.

Sexual transmission of HIV and other STDs would be reduced by use of barrier protection such as condoms. Despite the campaigns, passion will over-ride compliance on occasions in the most sexually promiscuous, at-risk group, who are at an age when risk-taking behavior is prevalent (cf. smoking in young people vis-a-vis the anti-smoking campaign), with tragic consequences. Thus education is only part of the answer and where an additional simple procedure is available to reduce the risk, then logic dictates that it should be used. The result will be many lives saved.

Socio-Sexual Aspects

In the setting of Australia, a survey of circumcised vs uncircumcised men and their partners that was conducted by Sydney scientist James Badger (7, 8) (who regards himself as neutral on the issue of circumcision) found that:

- 18 percent of uncircumcised males underwent circumcision later in life anyway.

- 21 percent of uncircumcised men who didn't, nevertheless wished they were circumcised. (There were also almost as many men who wished they hadn't been circumcised and it could be that at least some men of either category may have been seeking a scapegoat for their sexual or other problems. In addition, this would no doubt be yet another thing children could blame their parents for, whatever their decision was when the child was born.)

- No difference in sexual performance (consistent with Masters & Johnson).

- Slightly higher sexual activity in circumcised men.

- No difference in frequency of sexual intercourse for older uncircumcised vs. circumcised men.

- Men circumcised as adults were very pleased with the result. The local pain when they awoke from the anaesthetic was quickly relieved by pain killers (needed only for one day), and all had returned to normal sexual relations within 2 weeks, with *no decrease in sensitivity* of the penis and claims of "better sex." (Badger's findings are, moreover, consistent with every discussion the author has ever had with men circumcised as adults, as well as email received from a number of such men. The only cases to the contrary were a testimonial in a letter I received from a member of UNCIRC and a very brief email message that didn't say why.)

- Women with circumcised lovers were more likely to reach a simultaneous climax.

- Women with uncircumcised lovers were 3 times as likely to fail to reach orgasm. (These data could, however, possibly reflect behaviors of uncircumcised males that might belong to lower socio-economic classes and/or ethnic groups whose attitudes concerning sex and women may differ from the better educated groups in whom circumcision is more common.)

- Circumcision was favored by women for appearance and hygiene. (Furthermore, some women were nauseated by the smell of the uncircumcised penis, where, as mentioned above bacteria and other micro-organisms proliferate under the foreskin.)

- The uncircumcised penis was found by women to be easier to elicit orgasm by hand.

- The circumcised penis was favored by women for oral sex (fellatio).

These findings are consistent with other studies. In a survey of new mothers, hygiene and appearance were the two major reasons for choosing to have their newborn son circumcised (90). There was a strong correlation between their son's circumcision status and the woman's ideal male partner's circumcision status for intercourse. Thus by being circumcised they thought that their sons would likewise be more attractive to a future sexual partner (with the implication that they would be at an advantage in passing on their, and therefore the mother's, genes to the subsequent generation). Their own preference thus affected their choice for their sons. Ninety-two percent said the circumcised penis was cleaner, 90 percent said it looked "sexier," 85 percent it felt nicer to touch and 55 percent smelled more pleasant. Even women who had only ever had uncircumcised partners preferred the look of the circumcised penis. Only 2 percent preferred an uncircumcised penis for fellatio, with 82 percent preferring the circumcised variety. Preference for intercourse for circ vs uncirc was 71 percent vs 6 percent, respectively; manual stimulation, 75 percent vs 5 percent; visual appeal, 76 percent vs 4 percent. What then is sexier about a circumcised penis? Quite likely it is that the glans is exposed in both the erect and unerect state. American producers of erotic films and publishers of photographic works choose circumcised men, or at least uncircumcised men whose foreskin is smooth and free from loose, wrinkled skin, as the latter lacks visual appeal, especially to those who are not used to seeing an uncircumcised penis.

As far as sex is concerned, the National Health and Social Life Survey in the USA found that uncircumcised men were more likely to experience sexual dysfunctions (48); this was slight at younger ages, but became quite significant later in life and included finding it twice as difficult in achieving or maintaining an erection. It was also discovered that circumcised men engaged in a more elaborate set of sexual practices. Not surprisingly, in view of the findings above, circumcised men received more fellatio. However, they also masturbated more, a finding that, ironically, contradicts the wisdom in Victorian times that circumcision would reduce the urge to masturbate. As noted in other studies, circumcision rates were greatest among whites and those who were better-educated, reflecting their exposure to and ability to evaluate and respond to scientific information about circumcision. There was little difference between different religious groups.

In Britain a class distinction is associated with circumcision, with the Royal Family and the upper classes being circumcised and the lower classes generally not. Some ancient cultures and some even today practice infibulation (drawing a ring or similar device through the prepuce or otherwise occluding it for the principle purpose of making coition impossible) (78). This is the opposite of circumcision. It was, moreover, espoused in Europe and Britain in previous centuries as a way of reducing population growth amongst the poor and to prevent masturbation (78).

Consistent with the accounts above of men circumcised as adults, clinical and neurological testing has not detected any difference in penile sensitivity between men of each category (102, 103). Sexual pleasure also appears to be the same.

The Procedure Itself

Circumcision of the neonate: There is no evidence of any long-term psychological harm arising from circumcision. The risk of damage to the penis is extremely rare and avoidable by using a competent, experienced doctor. Unfortunately, because it is such a simple, low-risk procedure, it had been the practice to assign this job to junior medical staff and nurses, with occasional devastating results. Parents or patients need to have some re-assurance about the competence of the operator. Also the teaching of circumcision to medical students and practitioners should be given greater attention because it is so commonly performed and needs to be done well. Surgical methods often use a procedure that protects the penis during excision of the foreskin. The most commonly used devices are the GOMCO clamp, MOGEN clamp and PlastiBell. The latter clamps the foreskin, which then falls off after a few days, and so eliminates the need to actually cut the foreskin off (28).

However, some of these more elaborate methods take up to 15-30 min to perform and therefore expose the baby to a greater period of discomfort. Circumcision can be completed in 15-30 seconds by a competent practitioner using more traditional approaches. Rather than tightly strapping the baby down, swaddling and a pacifier has been suggested (95-97). Dr Tom Wiswell strongly advocates the neonatal period as being the best time to perform circumcision, pointing out that the child will not need ligatures or general anaesthesia, nor additional hospitalization (95-97).

Without an anaesthetic the child experiences pain and pain is also present for from a few up to a maximum of 12-24 hours afterwards. The child does not, however, have any long term memory of having been circumcised. A greater responsiveness to subsequent injection for routine immunization may, however, suggest the baby could remember for a short time (84). Complication rate is very low (0.2 percent), as is cost (less than $100).

In the past no anaesthetic was used. However, several anaesthetic procedures are available today. These include dorsal penile nerve block, which works well, with no serious complications. There are also anaesthetic creams. One that has been advocated for newborns and infants recently by various experts is Emla cream (5 percent lidocaine/prilocaine; Astra) (84, 95-97), with hard evidence of its effectiveness, not only for circumcision [83, 84], but also for relieving the pain of antecubital venepuncture in newborn babies (69). A sugar-coated pacifier can also help. General anaesthetic and alcohol are too dangerous. For some circumcisions, cultural or religious beliefs dictate the method.

Children: For children aged 4 months to 15 years a general anaesthetic is generally used and this carries a small risk. Also, ligatures are usually needed. Recently, excellent cosmetic results were reported for all of 346 patients aged 14 to 38 months using electrosurgery, which presents a bloodless operative field (66). Metal of any kind (such as the Gomco clamp) have to of course be avoided in this procedure. Circumcision later obviously requires a separate (often overnight) visit to hospital. Rate of complications is also greater, but still low (1.7 percent). Pain lasts for days afterwards and those older than 1-2 years may remember. Cost is also much greater.

Adults: In adults it may be even more expensive, but can be performed on an outpatient basis, sometimes with local anaesthetic, and pain can last for a week or so, during which time absence from work is required.

In relation to cost, on average the amount per circumcision across all ages versus mean lifetime medical costs in those not circumcised works out about the same (49). In this analysis it was stated that if the rate of surgical complications from circumcision was less than 0.6 percent or if risk of penile problems in uncircumcised males exceeded 17 percent (cf. current baseline of 14 percent) then circumcision would be preferred on a cost and lifespan basis (49).

Thus, when considering when is the best time, it would appear that circumcision in the newborn period is safer, cheaper and technically easier than later in life.

Whose Responsibility?

It is argued by opponents of circumcision that the male himself should be allowed to make the decision about whether he does or does not want to be circumcised. However, there are problems with this argument, not the least of which is the fact that the greatest benefits occur the earlier in life the procedure is performed. If left till later ages the individual has already been exposed to the risk of urinary tract infections, the physical problems and carries a residual risk of penile cancer. Moreover, it would take a very street-wise, outgoing, adolescent male to make this decision and under-take the process of ensuring that is was done. Most males in the late teens and 20s, not to mention many men of any age, are reti-cent to confront such issues, even if they hold private convictions and preferences about their penis. Moreover, despite having prob-lems with this part of their anatomy, many will suffer in silence rather than seek medical advice or treatment. Really though pa-rental responsibility must over-ride arguments based on "the rights of the child." Think what would happen if we allowed children to reach the age of legal consent in relation to, for example, immuni-zation, whether they should or should not be educated, etc, etc. A period of great benefit would have been lost, to the potential det-riment of the person concerned. Parents have the legal right to authorize surgical procedures in the best interests of their children (3, 23). For them to make this decision medical practitioners are obliged to disclose to them fully and objectively all information relating to circumcision. This includes benefits and risks, progno-sis and alternative methods.

Risks

Having described the benefits, let's look at the risks. These are (95-97):

Excessive bleeding: Occurs in 1 in 1000—treated with pressure or locally-acting agents, but 1 in 4000 may require a ligature and 1 in 20,000 need a blood transfusion because they have a previously unrecognized bleeding disorder. Hemophilia in the family is of course a contra-indication for circumcision.

Infection: Local infections occur in 1 in 100-1000 and are easily treated with local antibiotics. Systemic infections may appear in 1 in 4000 and require intravenous or intramuscular injection of antibiotics.

Subsequent surgery: Needed for 1 in 1000 because of skin bridges, or removal of too much or too little foreskin. Repair of injury to penis or glans required for 1 in 15,000. Loss of entire penis: 1 in 1,000,0000, and is avoidable by ensuring the practitioner performing the procedure is competent.

Local anaesthetic: The only risk is when the type of anaesthetic used is a dorsal penile nerve block, with 1 in 4 having a small bruise at the injection site. This will disappear.

Death: The records show that between 1954 and 1989, during which time 50,000,000 circumcisions were performed in the USA there were only 3 deaths. (But there were 11,000 from penile cancer, a disease essentially confined to the uncircumcised (96).

Why Are Human Males Born with a Foreskin?

The foreskin probably protected the head of the penis from long grass, shrubbery, etc when humans wore no clothes, where evolutionarily our basic physiology and psychology are little different from our cave-dwelling ancestors. However, Dr Guy Cox from The University of Sydney has recently supplemented this suggestion with a novel idea, namely that the foreskin could be the male equivalent of the hymen, and served as an impediment to sexual intercourse during adolescence before humans became civilized (15). The physical difficulties may explain why the word for uncircumcised in Hebrew means "obstruction" or "to impede," so explaining the Biblical term "uncircumcised heart" when referring to obstructionism.

What Caused Many Cultures to Ritually Remove it?

According to Cox, the ritual removal of the foreskin in diverse human traditional cultures, ranging from Muslims to Aboriginal Australians could be a sign of civilization in that human society acquired the ability to control, through education and religion, the age at which sexual intercourse could begin. Food for thought and discussion!

Another compelling explanation involves the ritualization of circumcision's prophylactic effects, especially as many different human groups and cultures that live in desert or other hot environments have adopted it as part of their customs. Infections, initiated by the aggravation of dirt and sand, are not uncommon under such conditions and have even crippled whole armies, where it is difficult to achieve sanitation during prolonged battle. Historically it was not uncommon for soldiers to be circumcised in preparation for active service.

The Judeo-Muslim practice of circumcision quite likely had its origin in Egyptian civilization, where illustrations of the operation itself, as well as of circumcised Pharaohs, date back to 3000 BC. One possible reason the Egyptians could have circumcised themselves and their slaves might have been to prevent schistosomal infection. Urinary tract obstruction and hematuria are common in localities such as the Nile Valley that are inhabited by the blood fluke, *Schistosoma haematobium*, and the foreskin would undoubtedly possess the adverse ability of being able to hold water infected with the cercaria stage of the life cycle of this parasite and so facilitate its entry into the body. The perpetuation of the procedure by the Jews may have subsequently been driven by a desire to maintain cleanliness in an arid, sandy desert environment. Such considerations could also explain why it is practiced in multiple other cultures that live in such conditions. In each instance, the original practical reason became lost as the ritual persisted as a religious rite in many of the various cultures of the world.

In the Muslim religion circumcision occurs near the time of puberty. In other cultures it is associated with preparation for marriage and as a sign of entry into manhood.

Interestingly, in Japan, which, like most of Asia, is traditionally a non-circumcising nation, circumcision has recently started to become a fashion amongst young men. The procedure is currently being promoted by way of articles and advertisements in the vast array of "girlie,"sex magazines read by young males. The message is that it improves hygiene and attractiveness to women.

To Summarize

Lack of Circumcision

- Is responsible for a 12-fold higher risk of urinary tract infections. Risk = 1 in 20.

- Carries a higher risk of death in the first year of life (from complications of urinary tract infections: viz. kidney failure, meningitis and infection of bone marrow).

- One in ~400-900 uncircumcised men will get cancer of the penis. A quarter of these will die of it and the rest will require at least partial penile amputation as a result. (In contrast, penile cancer *never or rarely* occurs in men circumcised at birth). (Data from studies in the USA, Denmark and Australia, which are not to be confused with the often quoted, but misleading, annual incidence figures of 1 in 100,000).

- Is associated with balanitis (inflammation of the glans), posthitis (inflammation of the foreskin), phimosis (inability to retract the foreskin) and paraphimosis (constriction of the penis by a tight foreskin). Up to 18 percent of uncircumcised boys will develop one of these by 8 years of age, whereas all are unknown in the circumcised. Risk of balanoposthitis = 1 in 6. Obstruction to urine flow = 1 in 10-50.

- Means problems that may result in a need for circumcision later in life: complication risk = 1 in 100 (compared with 1 in 1000 in the newborn). Also, the cost can be 10 times higher for an adult.

- Is the biggest risk factor for heterosexually-acquired AIDS virus infection in men. 8-times higher risk by itself, and even higher when lesions from STDs are added in. Risk per exposure = 1 in 300.

- Is associated with higher incidence of cervical cancer in the female partners of uncircumcised men.

Conclusion

The information that appears in this review should prove informative to medical practitioners and health workers and thereby enhance the quality of information that is conveyed to parents of male children and to adult men. It should also prove to have educational value to others. It is hoped that as a result the choice that has to be made concerning circumcision, especially of male infants, is much more informed. Although there are benefits to be had at any age, they are greater the younger the child. Issues of "informed consent" may be analogous to those parents have to consider for other medical procedures, such as whether or not to immunize their child. The question to be answered is "do the benefits outweigh the risks." When considering each factor in isolation there could be some difficulty in choosing. However, when viewed as a whole, in my opinion the answer to whether to circumcise a male baby is "yes." Nevertheless, everybody needs to weigh up all of the pros and cons for themselves and make their own best decision. I trust that the information I have provided in this article will help in the decision-making process.

Brian J. Morris, PhD DSc

Fax: 61-2-9351-2058
University Academic (in medical sciences)
Email: brianm@physiol.usyd.edu.au

This review can be found on the world-wide web: (http://www.physiol.usyd.edu.au/brianm/circumcision.htm)

The author freely grants permission for others to copy and distribute this review.

References

1. Agarwal SS, Sehgal A, Sardana S, Kumar A, Luthra UK. Role of male behavior in cervical carcinogenesis among women with one lifetime sexual partner. *Cancer* 1993; 72: 1666-9.

2. American Academy of Pediatrics. Task Force on Circumcision. Report of the Task Force on Circumcision. *Pediatrics* 1989; 84: 388-91

3. American Academy of Pediatrics Committee on Bioethics. Informed consent, parental permission, and assent in pediatric practice. *Pediatrics* 1995; 95 (5 pt 1): 314-7

4. Apt A. Circumcision and prostatic cancer. *Acta Med Scand* 1965; 178: 493-504

5. Australian College of Paediatrics. Policy statement on neonatal male circumcision. 1995

6. Aynaud O, Ionesco M, Barrasso R. Penile intraepithelial neoplasia - specific clinical features correlate with histologic and virologic findings. *Cancer* 1994; 74: 1762-7

7. Badger J. Circumcision. What you think. *Australian Forum* 1989; 2 (11): 10-29

8. Badger J. The great circumcision report part 2. *Australian Forum* 1989; 2 (12): 4-13

9. Barrasso R, De Brux J, Croissant O, Orth G. High prevalence of papillomavirus associated penile intraepithelial neoplasia in sexual partners of women with cervical intraepithelial neoplasia. *N Engl J Med* 1987; 317: 916-23

10. Bongaarts J, Peining P, Way P, Conont F. The relationship between male circumcision and HIV infection in African populations. *AIDS* 1989; 3: 373-7

11. Brinton LA, Li JY, Rung SD, Huang S, Xiao BS, Shi BG, Zhu ZJ, Schiffman MH, Dawsay S. Risk factors for penile cancer: results from a case-control study in China. *Int J Cancer* 1991; 47: 504-9

12. Caldwell JC, Caldwell P. The African AIDS epidemic. *Sci Am* 1996; 274: 40-46

13. Cameron BE, Simonsen JN, D'Costa LJ, Ronald AR, Maitha GM, Gakinya MN, Cheang M, Ndinya-Achola JO, Piot P, Brunham RC, Plummer FA. Female to male transmission of human immunodeficiency virus type 1: risk factors for seroconversion in men. *Lancet* 1989; ii: 403-7

14. Cook LS, Kovtsky LA, Holmes Circumcision and sexually transmitted diseases. *Am J Publ Health* 1994; 84: 197-201

15. Cox G. De virginibus Puerisque: The function of the human foreskin considered from an evolutionary perspective. *Med Hypoth* 1995; 45: 617-621

16. Craig JC, Knight JF, Sureshkumar P, Mantz E, Roy LP. Effect of circumcision on incidence of urinary tract infection in preschool boys. *J Pediatr* 1996; 128: 23-7

17. Dagher R, Selzer ML, Lapides J. Carcinoma of the penis and the anti-circumcision crusade. *J Urol* 1973; 110: 79-80

18. Dahr GM, Sah GN, Nahees B, Hafiza. Epidemiological trend in the distribution of cancer in Kashmir Valley. *J Epidemiol Comm Hlth* 1993; 47: 290-2

19. De Vincenzi I, Mertens T. Male circumcision a role in HIV prevention? (editorial) *AIDS* 1994; 8: 153-60

20. Diallo MO, Ackah AN, Lafontaine MF, Doorly R, Roux R, Kanga JM, Heroin P, De Cock KM. HIV-1 and HIV-2 infections in men attending sexually transmitted disease clinics in Abidjan, Cote d'Ivoire. *AIDS* 1992; 6: 581-5

21. Dodge OG, Linsell CA. Carcinoma of the penis in Uganda and Kenya Africans. *Cancer* 1963; 18: 1255-63

22. Donovan B, Basset I, Bodsworth NJ. Male circumcision and common sexually transmissible diseases in a developed nation setting. *Genitourin Med* 1994; 70: 317-20

23. Etchells E, Sharpe G, Walsh P. Consent for circumcision. *Can Med Assoc J* 1997; 156: 18

24. Fakjian N, Hunter S, Cole GW, et al. An argument for circumcision. Prevention of balanitis in the adult. *Arch Dermatol* 1990; 126: 1046-7

25. Fetus and Newborn Committee, Canadian Paediatric Society. Neonatal circumcision revisited. *Can Med Ass J* 1996; 154: 769-780

26. Fink AJ. Newborn circumcision: a long-term strategy for AIDS prevention. *J Roy Soc Med* 1990; 83: 673

27. Fussell EN, Kaak BM, Cherry R, et al. Adherence of bacteria to human foreskin. *J Urol* 1988; 140: 997-1001

28. Gee WF, Ansell JS. Neonatal circumcision: A ten-year overview, with comparison of the Gomco clamp and the Plastibell device. *Pediatrics* 1976; 58: 824-7

29. Ginsburg CM, McCracken GH. Urinary tract infections in young children. 1982; 69: 409-12

30. Glennon J, Ryan PI, Keane CT, Rees JPR. Circumcision and periurethral carriage of *Proteus mirabilis* in boys. *Arch Dis Child* 1988; 63: 556-7

31. Galalakshmi CK, Shanta V. Association between cervical and penile cancers in Madras, India. *Acta Oncol* 1993; 32: 617-20

32. Ginsburg CM, McCracken GH Jr. Urinary tract infections in young infants. *Pediatrics* 1982; 69: 409-12

33. Glennon J, Ryan PJ, Keane CT, et al. Circumcision and peri-urethral carriage of Proteus mirabilis in boys. *Arch Dis Child* 1988; 63: 556-7

34. Harturian NS, Smart CN, Thompson MS. The incidence and economic costs of cancer, motor vehicle injuries, coronary heart disease and stroke: a comparative analysis. *Am J Public Health* 1980; 70: 1249-60

35. Herzog LW. Urinary tract infections and circumcision: a case-control study. *Am J Dis Child* 1989; 143: 348-50

36. Herzog LW, Alvarez SR. The frequency of foreskin problems in uncircumcised children. *Am J Dis Child* 1986; 140: 254-6

37. Hunter DJ. AIDS in sub-Saharan Africa: the epidemiology of heterosexual transmission and the prospects of prevention (Review). *Epidemiology* 1993; 4: 63-72

38. Isacsohn M, Dolberg L, Sabag SL, Mitrani-Rosenbaum S, Nubani N, Diamant YZ, Goldsmidt R. The inter-relationship of herpes virus, papilloma 16/18 virus infection and Pap smear pathology in Israeli women. *Israel J Med Sci* 1994; 30: 383-7

39. Jessamine PG, Plummer FA, Ndinya Achola JO, Wainberg MA, Wamolo I, D'Costa JL, Cameron DW, Simonsen JN, Plouroe P, Ronald AR. Human immunodeficiency virus, genital ulcers and the male foreskin: synergism in HIV-1 transmission. *Scand J Infect Dis* 1990 (suppl 69): 181-6

40. Kallenius G, Moillby R, Svenson SB, Helin I, Hultberg H, Cedergren B, Winberg J. Occurrence of P-fimbriated *Escherichia coli* in urinary tract infections. *Lancet* 1981; ii: 1369-72

41. Kallenius G, Svenson S, Mollby R, et al. Structure of carbohydrate part of receptor on human uroepithelial cells for pyelonephritogenic *Escherichia coli. Lancet* 1981; ii: 604-6

42. Katelaris PM, Cossart YE, Rose BR, Thompson CH, Sorich E, Nightingale B, Dallas PB, Morris BJ. Human papillomavirus: the untreated male reservoir. *J Urol* 1988; 140: 300-5

43. Kirby PK, Munyao T, Kreiss J, Holmes KK. The challenge of limiting the spread of human immunodeficiency virus by controlling other STDs. *Arch Dermatol* 1991; 127: 237-42

44. Kochen M, McCurdy S. Circumcision and risk of cancer of the penis. A life-table analysis. *Am J Dis Child* 1980; 134: 484-6

45. Kreiss JK, Hopkins SG. The association between circumcision status and human immunodeficiency virus infection among homosexual men. *J Infect Dis* 1993; 168: 1404-8

46. Kunanusont C, Foy HM, Kreiss JK, Rerky-Ngaram S, Phanuphak P, Raktham S, Pau CP, Young NL. HIV-1 subtypes and male-to-female transmission in Thailand. *Lancet* 1995; 34 5: 1078-83

47. Lafferty PM, MacGregor FB, Scobie WG. Management of fore-skin problems. *Arch Dis Childhood* 1991; 66: 696-7

48. Laumann EO, Maal CM, Zuckerman EW. Circumcision in the United States. Prevalence, prophylactic effects, and sexual practice. *J Am Med Assoc* 1997; 277: 1052-7

49. Lawler FH, Bisonni RS, Holtgrave DR. Circumcision: a cost deci-sion analysis of its medical value. *Fam Med* 1991; 23: 587-93

50. Lohr JA. The foreskin and urinary tract infections. *J Pediatr* 1989; 114: 502-4

51. Maden C, Sherman KJ, Beckmann AM, Huslop TK, Heh OZ, Ashley RL, Daling JR. History of circumcision, medical condi-tions, and sexual activity and risk of penile cancer. *J Nat Canc Inst* 1993; 85: 19-24

52. Marx JL. Circumcision may protect against the AIDS virus. *Science* 1989; 245: 470-1

53. McCance DJ, Kalache A, Ashdown K, et al. Human papilloma-virus types 16 and 18 in carcinoma of the penis from Brazil. *J Cancer* 1986; 37: 55-9

54. McIntosh N. Pain in the newborn, a possible new starting point. *Eur J Pediatr* 1997; 156: 173-7

55. Medicare Estimates and Statistics Section, Australia, Feb 1994

56. Moses S, Bradley JE, Nagelkerke NJ, Ronald AR, Ndinya Achola JO, Plummer FA. Geographical patterns of male cir-cumcision practices in Africa: association with HIV seroprevalance. *Int J Epidemiol* 1990; 19: 693-7

57. Moses S, Plummer FA, Bradley JF, Ndinya-Achola JO, Nagelkerke NJ, Ronald AR. The association between lack of male circumcision and risk for HIV infection: a review of the epidemiological data. *Sexually Transm Dis* 1994; 21: 201-9

58. National Center for Health Statistics of the Department of Health and Human Services. 1991-1994

59. New South Wales Cancer Council. *Cancer in New South Wales. Incidence and Mortality 1993.*

60. Niku SD, stock JA, Kaplan GW. Neonatal circumcision (review). *Urol Clin N Am* 1995; 22: 57-65

61. Ohjimi H, Ogata K, Ohjimi T. A new method for the relief of adult phimosis. *J Urol* 1995; 153: 1607-9

62. Osborne JE: HIV: The more things change, the more they stay the same. *Nature Med* 1995; 1: 991-3

63. Oster J. Further fate of the foreskin: incidence of preputial adhesions, phimosis and smegma among Danish schoolboys. *Arch Dis Child* 1968; 43: 200-3

64. Parker SW, Stewart AJ, Wren MN, et al. Circumcision and sexually transmissible diseases. *Med J Aust* 1983; 2: 288-90

65. Pepin J, Quigby M, Todd J, Gage I, Jenneh M, Van Dyck E, Rot P, Whittle H. Association between HIV-2 infection and genital ulcer disease among male sexually transmitted disease patients in The Gambia. *AIDS* 1992; 6: 489-93

66. Peters KM, Kass EJ. Electrosurgery for routine pediatric penile procedures. *J Urol* 1997; 157: 1453-5.

67. Plaut A, Kohn-Speyer AC. The carcinogenic action of smegma. *Science* 1947; 105: 391-2.

68. Prual A, Chacko S, Koch-Weser D. Sexual behaviour, AIDS and poverty in Sub-Saharan Africa. *Int J STD AIDS* 1991; 2: 1-9

69. Ramet J, Benatar A, Diltoer M, Spapen H, Huyghens L. Neonatal circumcision. *Lancet* 1997; 349: 1257

70. Reddy DG, Baruah IK. Carcinogenic action of human smegma. *Arch Pathol* 1963; 75: 414

71. Roberts JA. Does circumcision prevent urinary tract infections? *J Urol* 1986; 135: 991-2

72. Rushton HG, Majd M. Pyelonephritis in male infants: how important is the foreskin? *J Urol* 1992; 148: 733-6

73. Russell T. The case for circumcision. *Med Observer* 1993 (1 Oct issue)

74. Sandeman TF. Carcinoma of the penis. *Australasian Radiol* 1990; 34: 12-6

75. Schlosberger NM, Turner RA, Irwin CE Jr. Early adolescent knowledge and attitudes about circumcision: methods and implications for research. *J Adolescent Hlth* 1992; 13: 293-7

76. Schoen EJ. The status of circumcision of newborns. *N Engl J Med* 1990; 332: 1308-12

77. Schoen EJ. Circumcision updated-implicated? *Pediatrics* 1993; 92: 860-1

78. Schwarz GS. Infibulation, population control, and the medical profession. *Bull NY Acad Med* 1970; 46: 964-80

79. Simonsen JNM, Cameron DW, Gakinya MN, Ndinya-Achola JO, D'Costa LJ, Karasira P. HIV infection among men with STDs. *N Engl J Med* 1988; 319: 274-8

80. Smith GL, Greenup R, Takafuji ET. Circumcision as a risk factor for urethritis in racial groups. *Am J Publ Health* 1987; 77: 452-4

81. Spach DH, Stapleton AE, Stamm WE. Lack of circumcision increases the risk of urinary tract infections in young men. *J Am Med Assoc* 1992; 267: 679-81

82. Stull TL, LiPuma JJ: Epidemiology and natural history of urinary tract infections in children (Review). *Med Clin N Am* 1991; 75: 287-97

83. Taddio A, Katz J, Herisch AL, Koren G. Effect of neonatal circumcision on pain response during subsequent routine vaccination. *Lancet* 1997; 349: 599-603

84. Taddio A, Stevens B, Craig K, Rastogi P, Bendavid S, Shennan A, Mulligan P, Koren G. Efficacy and safety of lidocaine-prilocaine cream for pain during circumcision. *N Engl J Med* 1997; 336: 1197-1201

85. Taylor PK, Rodin P. Herpes genitalis and circumcision. *Br J Ven Dis* 1975; 51: 274-7

86. Urassa M, Todd J, Boerma JT, Hayes R, Islingo R. Male circumcision and susceptibility to HIV infection among men in Tanzania. *AIDS* 1997; 11: 73-80

87. Walboomers JMM, Meijer CJL. Do HPV-negative cervical carcinomas exist? (editorial) *J Path* 1997; 181: 253-4

88. Walter G, Streimer J. Genital self-mutilation: attempted foreskin reconstruction. *Brit J Psychiat* 1990; 156: 125-7

89. Whittington WL, et al. HIV-1 in patients with genital lesions attending a North American STD clinic: Assessment of risk factors. *Int Conf AIDS* 1989; 5: 409

90. Williamson ML, Williamson PS. Women's preferences for penile circumcision in sexual partners. *J Sex Educ Hlth* 1988; 14: 8-12

91. Wilson RA. Circumcision and venereal disease. *Can Med Ass J* 1947; 56: 54-6

92. Winberg J, Bollgren I, Gothefors L, et al. The prepuce: a mistake of nature? *Lancet* 1989; I: 598-9

93. Wiswell TE. Do you favor routine neonatal circumcision? Yes. *Postgrad Med* 1988; 84: 98-104

94. Wiswell TE. Circumcision—an update. *Curr Problems Pediat* 1992; 10: 424-31

95. Wiswell TE. Neonatal circumcision: a current appraisal. *Focus & Opinion Pediat* 1995; 1: 93-9

96. Wiswell TE. Circumcision circumspection. *N Engl Med J* 1997; 336: 1244-5

97. Wiswell TE. Neonatal circumcision: a current appraisal. 1997; http://www.geocities.com/HotSprings/ 2754/

98. Wiswell TE, Geschke DW. Risks from circumcision during the first month of life compared with those for uncircumcised boys. *Pediatrics* 1989; 83: 1011-5

99. Wiswell TE, Hachey WE. Urinary tract infections and the circumcision state: an update. *Clin Pediat* 1993; 32: 130-4

100. Wiswell TE, Roscelli JD. Corroborative evidence for the decreased incidence of urinary tract infections in circumcised male infants. *Pediatrics* 1982; 69: 96-9

101. Wiswell TE, Smith FR, Bass JW. Decreased incidence of urinary tract infections in circumcised male infants. *Pediatrics* 1985; 75: 901-3

102. Wiswell TE, Enzenauer RW, Holton ME, et al. Declining frequency of circumcision: implications for changes in the absolute incidence and male to female sex ratio of urinary tract infections in early infancy. *Pediatrics* 1987; 79: 338-41

103. Wiswell TE, Miller GM, Gelston HM Jr, Jones SK. Effects of circumcision status on periurethral bacterial flora during the first year of life. *J Paediat* 1988; 113: 442-6

104. Wolbarst AL. Circumcision and penile cancer. *Lancet* 1932; i: 150-3.

Chapter 18

Frequently Asked Questions about Foreskin Restoration

I've received literally hundreds of e-mail messages from around the globe from men considering or who are currently undertaking non-surgical foreskin restoration. While I have stated many times that I am not a doctor, nor do I consider myself a particular "expert" on restoration, I have attempted to answer as many of the more common questions as possible, and this FAQ reflects that effort.

NOTE: This FAQ is a general one for people thinking or wondering about foreskin restoration. We also have a t-tape and strap FAQ, that addresses questions about the t-tape and strap restoration method, for those already undertaking foreskin restoration available on the Derrick Townsend website (http://www.foreskin.denver.co.us./).

I consider this FAQ a work-in-progress, and as such, you should check it occasionally for new additions, corrections, etc. So with that, and in no particular order, here is the FAQ:

What exactly is non-surgical foreskin restoration?

Non-surgical foreskin restoration refers to any number of techniques for restoring a prepuce or "foreskin" on a circumcised male without involving the use of plastic surgery to get the job done. All the various techniques use the application of tension to the penile shaft skin (i.e., pulling the skin) and leaving the tension applied for

---

©1995 Derrick Townsend, (http://www.tde.com/~derrick/restore~faq.html). Reprinted with permission.

extended periods. Most employ medical tape (to hold the skin) and weights (or equivalents) to provide the tension.

Is this permanent? Won't the stretching eventually return to normal?

Yes, it is permanent, and no, it will not return to normal. Also, this is not stretching! Non-surgical foreskin restoration is often referred to as "stretching, but it's a complete misnomer. The tension that results from the process causes the body to generate completely new skin cells, essentially growing new skin at the site of the tension. A more appropriate term is skin expansion."

Is "skin expansion" medically proven, or is all this a modern version of snake oil?

Yes, the principle is medically proven; plastic surgeons use it to grow skin for skin grafts in some cases (like separating conjoined [i.e., Siamese] twins). In their method, they implant a balloon under the skin and over time (days, weeks) inflate it. The principle is the same, only the method varies. In any event, the elasticity of your skin will provide a difference almost immediately after starting, as a result of true stretching alone, and that much will "snap back" after you stop. But don't confuse this with the permanent results that take time and will not go away when you stop!

Does it hurt?

No, not if you do it correctly. Pain comes from putting on tape too tight, using too much tension, and so on. If it hurts, then you've not exercised due care in applying or using the method you've chosen. You may well feel tension on the skin, and that's normal. Pain is not normal. If it hurts, stop.

What's all this talk about tape?

The various methods (and there are many) for non-surgical foreskin restoration almost all employ the use of tape (usually medical or first aid tape) to pull what skin you have now up over the glans (head) of your penis as far as possible. You can use straps side to side over the glans: o-tapes or tape rings that go around the circumference of the penis after pulling the skin forward; t-tapes that use an elastic leg or other strap to provide tension; a foam cone over the glans then pull the skin up onto it and tape it in place; metal weights of some sort (again, pull the skin up and tape in place onto the weight), and so on. Most people start with the tape straps (across the glans in an X), graduate to the tape rings, then use some other system. Personally, I think the t-tape and leg strap approach from beginning to end is best. The *Joy* book (described in the resource list has more details.)

How long does it take?

It varies. Some people get where they want after a year of dedicated taping. Some get there in a couple of years. Some more. It depends on several things: how much skin you have to start with; how much you want to add, how dedicated you are to the process (i.e., how often do you tape up and how long do you keep it that way), and so forth. The more you stay taped, the sooner it will happen. It is not a fast process. It requires great dedication to the effort, and a very great deal of patience. If you want instant gratification, non-surgical foreskin restoration is not for you.

I have heard from two different sources that the t-tape and strap method is capable of adding 1/16th square inches of new skin daily. This assumes 24 hour a day use, with "ideal" tension. And this is square inches, i.e., surface area, not overall length of foreskin. If you measure the circumference of your penis and do the math, you can probably get a round figure for how long you can expect it to take under ideal circumstances.

Can't you do anything to speed it up?

Not really. Using an effective restoration method is the best way to ensure results, and the one described on the Foreskin Restoration Site (in the how to section) is one of the most popular and fastest working. Otherwise, patience is key here, and there's nothing you can do to speed-up nature's work.

Am I too young to restore?

I strongly recommend that non-adult males (those younger than 18) worry about their sexual function and penile appearance later in life when they've had more experience with which to assess their relative pleasure or displeasure with things as they are. When I was under 18, I never liked being told I was "too young" to do something, but in this case, I'm telling you you're too young. To begin with, your body has not stopped developing, and anything that would or could interfere with nature's own processes is not something you should entertain now. Frankly, I wouldn't do anything at all with regard to restoration until you're at least 21, as I don't believe anyone younger will have enough experience to judge with. If you feel strongly that you want to do this, at least discuss it with your doctor. And if you're too embarrassed to talk to your doctor about it, then you're probably not emotionally ready to proceed with it, SO DON'T!

Am I too old to restore?

No. Some men with comparative data have indicated that restoration takes longer in older men, and this may make some sense considering that the properties of skin change with age. However, a great many men have successfully begun and completed to their satisfaction the restoration process. Age should not discourage you from proceeding. As always, if you're concerned, seek the assistance of a competent health care professional.

How will my penis look when I'm done? Does it look like an intact penis?

For all practical purposes, nobody will be able to distinguish a penis with a restored foreskin from a penis with an intact foreskin. The structural differences (you cannot restore a frenulum, which is described in the anatomy section of the Foreskin Restoration Site) are not apparent to anyone, unless someone knows what an intact foreskin looks like and how it functions, and they perform a manual, physical examination of your penis. Externally, there is simply not a way to tell. I've heard several reports of even doctors not being able to tell from looking.

Do I have to see a doctor about this like you suggest?

You should. Some people have medical conditions that make non-surgical foreskin restoration by conventional means dangerous. (Read more about it on our cautions and warnings page.) Persons who are prone to bleeding or who have any problems related blood circulation; persons with diabetes, hypoglycemia, or peyronies; persons who are "keloid formers"; those whose immune systems are diminished or are otherwise prone to chronic infections of any type; and those who have allergic reactions to adhesive chemicals in tape products should not begin restoration without a doctor's specific approval, recommendation, and supervision!

504

If you are in good health, have no known circulatory or other health problems, are not prone to contracting infections, and have no known allergies, you can probably proceed safely. You are still strongly encouraged to visit your doctor.

Not all general practice (or other) physicians are familiar with non-surgical restoration techniques; many are not even aware that it's possible. If your regular physician is unable to assist you, see your urologist, or ask for a referral to one or another appropriate specialist. Some doctors are, in fact, quite well informed about restoration, and have access to information and resources to help you. If you are in doubt for any reason, search for and locate an informed and understanding physician who can help ensure your safety and productivity with your restoration program.

Why would anyone somebody want to do this? Seems like a lot of trouble, and I've never had any problem with being circumcised.

If you don't have a problem with being "cut" or circumcised, then by all means enjoy your penis as-is. Many men do. Many men, however, feel a sense of victimization over the fact that their penis was mutilated by a doctor without their consent after birth. Many men simply like the appearance of an "uncut" penis better. The reasons truly vary, but virtually everyone who has restored even some of their foreskin report greatly enhanced sexual sensitivity and function. Think about it; the glans (head) of a cut penis rubs against clothing, sheets, or whatever it's in contact with all the time. This constant rubbing "numbs" it to some degree. (In some men, to such a degree that there is a severe loss of sexual function.) Nature intended the glans to be an internal organ, covered constantly by the foreskin. By restoring, you can bring that back, and restore the incredible sensitivity of the glans, and hence, increase sexual pleasure.

Isn't it just a bunch of queers doing this restoration stuff? Seems that way.

There may be a lot of interest in foreskin restoration among gay men due to the increased attention paid to the male sexual organ, but foreskin restoration is not a "queer" activity; it's the activity of circumcised male who is less than pleased with the physical and/or emotional result of their circumcision. Men of all sexual orientations, backgrounds, religions, and so on investigate foreskin restoration, many of them choose to proceed, and there's not really much more to it than that. I've personally spoken with hundreds of men, gay and straight, who are pleased to have discovered foreskin restoration, and are happier with themselves for it. Afterall, it's what you need and you want for yourself and your penis that matters here not what everyone else is doing or thinking.

My girlfriend/boyfriend/wife/husband/sex partner doesn't like uncircumcised men.

Bully for them. It's your penis. If you want to restore, restore. If I were you, I'd spend some time questioning the nature and depth of your relationship if this is such a big issue. Should it be a discussion point? Absolutely. But remember whose body it is and whose sexual function it is that we're concerned about there (namely yours).

Don't uncut men smell? Doesn't an uncut penis get all cheesy?

This propaganda is disseminated by pro-circumcision folks as one of the reasons for circumcising men in the first place. "It's so much easier to keep clean." Yes, well, your armpit probably wouldn't get smelly if you cut your arm off, either. This is ridiculous. The answer is yes, any part of your body that is moist and enclosed, whether an armpit, rectum, or foreskin, can develop an odor. This is the primary reason behind an invention called a "shower." Washing yourself (and generally clear water is all that's needed for your foreskin) is the solution. If you don't wash it, it gets cheesy and smelly. Even when you do keep clean, the natural moisture under your foreskin has its own unique aroma that is quite natural, and, to most people, not objectionable.

How do you know a restored foreskin is so superior?

Foreskin restoration isn't new. Most who have completed it, and many who've even started it and kept with it for very long, report the benefits. It's true that some men don't seem to notice (or won't admit) the differences. In any case, they are far outnumbered by the hundreds of men I've personally heard from in the two years I've known about foreskin restoration who make remarks like, "It's the best decision I ever made." "I can't believe the difference!" And so forth. Certainly a cut man who never starts has no way of knowing what he's lost. An uncut man who never gets circumcised doesn't know what he has. That's actually a unique advantage we have as men who've been cut and have restored; we know both sides of the fence personally!

What about surgical restoration?

Some have undergone surgical restoration, but it's problematic. Like all plastic surgery, foreskin restoration involves the use of skin grafts—skin that is removed from one area of the body, and essentially "transplanted" to another area. The problem with skin grafts is that skin color, concentration of hair, and skin thickness varies all over our bodies. It's extemely difficult to graft skin onto the penis shaft and have it look even remotely natural in terms of hair, color, and thickness.

Then, there are the problems with the surgery itself. Skin grafts are not always successful, and when they fail, you'll end-up with less skin on your penis than you started with, not to mention a very unsightly result. Surgical restoration is a very risky procedure! It's also complicated, very expensive, and difficult to have done. But if you want to learn more, the *Joy* book I mention in the resources section has some information about it.

What is a surgical touch-up?

Once you have used non-surgical restoration to fully restore your foreskin, it is possible to have very minor plastic surgery performed to help make the visual appearance of the result more natural. Intact men have a frenulum which keeps the skin forward over the glans (if you don't know these terms, refer to the anatomy section). Circumcised males who have restored don't have one. The purpose of the touch-up surgery is to make the restored skin taper over the tip in a more natural-looking fashion. The *Joy* book mentioned in the resources section has details.

Can you surgically restore a frenulum after non-surgically restoring the foreskin?

Not to the best of my knowledge (if someone has credible information to the contrary, let me know). The frenulum has a rather unique purpose, and a rather unique structure. It cannot be non-surgically restored, and it's doubtful that a surgical restoration of it is possible either (since the skin structure itself is the only one of its type on the body).

Will my penis get longer from all the stretching?

Some have claimed that non-surgical foreskin restoration lengthens the penis. Medical sources I trust have indicated to me that supposed penis lengthening as a result of restoration efforts is, simply, totally false. I have, however, had men tell me that they are convinced some lengthening has occurred. First, don't expect penis lengthening, as it is unlikely. Secondly, even if your restoration efforts do lengthen your penis, most men wouldn't find that particularly bothersome, so don't lose sleep over it. But as I said, don't start the process thinking this is going to be a side-effect, because it probably isn't going to turn out that way.

Are there creams or ointments I can use to speed things up?

Not that I'm aware of. The restoration process and the principle behind it is not something that occurs at the surface of your skin where some sort of cream could possibly have any effect. The entire thickness of the skin tissue comes into play here. Creams or ointments may make the skin feel better as you "rest" things between tapings, but they're not likely to actually speed the process along.

When overweight people lose weight, their skin snaps back. Why doesn't this?

Nobody believes me when I say this is permanent. In any case, a doctor could probably give a more scientifically correct response, but essentially it's like this: When people are overweight, the actual tension on the skin tissue is not all that significant. Unless a person is grossly obese, it's very unlikely that the tension is high enough to result in the addition of significant new skin cells to the tissue. When weight is lost, skin elasticity will cause it to return to its normal state, especially if one is only modestly overweight.

With foreskin restoration efforts, the actual tension presented to the skin tissue is fairly significant, often well over a pound of weight directly focused on just a few specific inches of skin surface area. It is this high amount of tension that prompts the skin to actually grow.

In fact, lack of significant tension is why some men fail to achieve desired results in their restoration efforts. Applying some light tension is not enough to do anything on a permanent basis.

Terminology Guide

Here is a guide to the terminology used herein, and some additional important terms as well:

Circumcision scar. The scar left after the healing fusion of shaft skin and inner foreskin. It may differ in pigmentation and/or texture from the surrounding skin.

Corona. The rounded ridge of the glans.

Foreskin. A retractable covering of skin that partially or completely covers the glans in an uncircumcised male. A more technical term is the prepuce. During infant circumcision, most or all of the outer foreskin and much of the inner foreskin is removed. In adult circumcisions, larger portions of the inner and outer foreskin may remain.

Frenar band. Elastic tissue at the tip of the foreskin (between the inner and outer foreskin) that helps contract the tip of the foreskin allow it to remain positioned over the glans.

Frenulum. An elastic band of tissue under the glans that conects to the foreskin and helps contract the foreskin over the glans. It is often partially or totally removed during circumcision.

Glans (or glans penis). The head or tip of the penis.

Overhang. The portion of the foreskin that extends beyond the tip of the glans.

Shaft skin. A part of the penile sheath that covers the shaft up to the foreskin or circumcision scar. During restoration, stimulation of this skin along with remnants of the inner foreskin generates new skin which creates the restored foreskin.

Sulcus. The grooved connection between the glans and the shaft of the penis.

Urethra. The tube through the penis in which urine and semen flow.

Urinary meatus. Opening at the tip of the penis where urine and semen exit the body.

Resources Online

Restoration chat channel. On the EFnet IRC network, you'll find the #restore channel. A bot or two, and some regular users, normally are parked in the channel (if not, hang out awhile and you'll typically run across some chatty and helpful guys). I regularly participate in the channel. Use your own IRC client, or if you have one that's configured to support it, try clicking #restore and see if that works. (Details on using IRC links on the

web can be found at http://www.mirc.co.uk/mirclink.html.)
Make sure you are using EFnet IRC servers. (If you don't know
what EFnet is, ask your ISP, or a friend experienced with IRC
chat systems.)

Circumcision Information Resource Centre. This site, located
in Montréal, is available in French and English. The main page
is http://www.infocirc.org/ (which is in French, just click the link
near the top of the page to visit the English version of the site).
A great deal of information is available here about a wide range
of circumcision and restoration related issues.

The "original" foreskin restoration web resource. I have a
lot of information here, but I strongly suggest you also visit the
original web resource for restoration information. The site has
information as well as pictures showing some of the other restoration techniques we don't cover here, so you can see what this
all looks like. It's all at http://www.eskimo.com/~gburlin/restore/

Foreskin restoration mailing list. There is not currently a
newsgroup available for restoration, but the next best thing (a
mailing list) is. An information sheet about it can be read by
opening http://www.eskimo.com/~gburlin/restore/rest.html.
PLEASE NOTE: THIS IS NOT MY MAILING LIST! I DO NOT
HOST IT, SO DO NOT SEND QUESTIONS ABOUT THE LIST
TO MY ATTENTION. THANKS!

**Geoffrey Falk's Circumcision Information and Resource
Pages (CIRP).** Another web site with a variety of information
about circumcision, as well as foreskin restoration. Located at
http://www.cirp.org/CIRP/.

**American Bodycrafters manufactures the P.U.D. (penis
uncircumcising device).** A combination weight and penis extension that you can use for restoration efforts. Their home
page is at http://www.tfa2.com/abi. I've never used one, but I've
heard many reports of great satisfaction with this device.

Offline Resources

**The book: *The Joy of Uncircumcising, Restore Your Birth-
right and Maximize Sexual Pleasure.*** If you're interested in

foreskin restoration, or about circumcision and its history in general, the Bible for us is a book you may be interested in, entitled *The Joy of Uncircumcising, Restore Your Birthright and Maximize Sexual Pleasure.* It's written by Jim Bigelow, Ph.D., and is published by Hourglass Book Publishing, P. O. Box 171, Aptos, CA, 95001. Its ISBN (handy for ordering it from your local bookseller) is 0-9630482-1-X. If you click that link, you'll be swept off to the web site of Book Stacks Unlimited, an online bookstore where you can order a copy conveniently. You can also find it at many bookstores. This book covers a great deal of territory, including the history and methodology of the circumcision practice, and all the various popular methods of restoration. A real "must have" resource for anyone considering or undertaking foreskin restoration.

Finding other offline sources. There are other "offline" resources available, but I'll leave it to some of the web sites mentioned above for details. In particular, the restoration section of the CIRP site has some contact places to write for information on support groups and the like. In addition, the resource section in the back of the *Joy* book has a lot of information too (another reason to buy a copy).

Part Five

Sleep Disorders

Chapter 19

Sleep Apnea

What is sleep apnea?

Sleep apnea is a serious, potentially life-threatening condition that is far more common than generally understood. First described in 1965, sleep apnea is a breathing disorder characterized by brief interruptions of breathing during sleep. It owes its name to a Greek word, *apnea*, meaning "want of breath." There are two types of sleep apnea: central and obstructive. Central sleep apnea, which is less common, occurs when the brain fails to send the appropriate signals to the breathing muscles to initiate respirations. Obstructive sleep apnea is far more common and occurs when air cannot flow into or out of the person's nose or mouth although efforts to breathe continue.

In a given night, the number of involuntary breathing pauses or "apneic events" may be as high as 20 to 30 or more per hour. These breathing pauses are almost always accompanied by snoring between apnea episodes, although not everyone who snores has this condition. Sleep apnea can also be characterized by choking sensations. The frequent interruptions of deep, restorative sleep often lead to early morning headaches and excessive daytime sleepiness.

Early recognition and treatment of sleep apnea is important because it may be associated with irregular heartbeat, high blood pressure, heart attack, and stroke.

NIH Publication No. 95-3798. September 1995.

515

Who gets sleep apnea?

Sleep apnea occurs in all age groups and both sexes but is more common in men (it may be under-diagnosed in women) and possibly young African Americans. It has been estimated that as many as 18 million Americans have sleep apnea. Four percent of middle-aged men and 2 percent of middle-aged women have sleep apnea along with excessive daytime sleepiness. People most likely to have or develop sleep apnea include those who snore loudly and also are overweight, or have high blood pressure, or have some physical abnormality in the nose, throat, or other parts of the upper airway. Sleep apnea seems to run in some families, suggesting a possible genetic basis.

What causes sleep apnea?

Certain mechanical and structural problems in the airway cause the interruptions in breathing during sleep. In some people, apnea occurs when the throat muscles and tongue relax during sleep and partially block the opening of the airway. When the muscles of the soft palate at the base of the tongue and the uvula (the small fleshy tissue hanging from the center of the back of the throat) relax and sag, the airway becomes blocked, making breathing labored and noisy and even stopping it altogether. Sleep apnea also can occur in obese people when an excess amount of tissue in the airway causes it to be narrowed. With a narrowed airway, the person continues his or her efforts to breathe, but air cannot easily flow into or out of the nose or mouth. Unknown to the person, this results in heavy snoring, periods of no breathing, and frequent arousals (causing abrupt changes from deep sleep to light sleep). Ingestion of alcohol and sleeping pills increases the frequency and duration of breathing pauses in people with sleep apnea.

How is normal breathing restored during sleep?

During the apneic event, the person is unable to breathe in oxygen and to exhale carbon dioxide, resulting in low levels of oxygen and increased levels of carbon dioxide in the blood. The reduction in oxygen and increase in carbon dioxide alert the brain to resume breathing and cause an arousal. With each arousal, a signal is sent from the brain to the upper airway muscles to open the airway; breathing is resumed, often with a loud snort or gasp. Frequent arousals, although necessary for breathing to restart, prevent the patient from getting enough restorative, deep sleep.

What are the effects of sleep apnea?

Because of the serious disturbances in their normal sleep patterns, people with sleep apnea often feel very sleepy during the day and their concentration and daytime performance suffer. The consequences of sleep apnea range from annoying to life-threatening. They include depression, irritability, sexual dysfunction, learning and memory difficulties, and falling asleep while at work, on the phone, or driving. It has been estimated that up to 50 percent of sleep apnea patients have high blood pressure. Although it is not known with certainty if there is a cause and effect relationship, it appears that sleep apnea contributes to high blood pressure. Risk for heart attack and stroke may also increase in those with sleep apnea. In addition, sleep apnea is sometimes implicated in sudden infant death syndrome.

When should sleep apnea be suspected?

For many sleep apnea patients, their spouses are the first ones to suspect that something is wrong, usually from their heavy snoring and apparent struggle to breathe. Coworkers or friends of the sleep apnea victim may notice that the individual falls asleep during the day at inappropriate times (such as while driving a car, working, or talking). The patient often does not know that he or she has a problem and may not believe it when told. It is important that the person see a doctor for evaluation of the sleep problem.

How is sleep apnea diagnosed?

In addition to the primary care physician, pulmonologists, neurologists, or other physicians with specialty training in sleep disorders may be involved in making a definitive diagnosis and initiating treatment. Diagnosis of sleep apnea is not simple because there can be many different reasons for disturbed sleep. Several tests are available for evaluating a person for sleep apnea.

Polysomnography. Polysomnography is a test that records a variety of body functions during sleep, such as the electrical activity of the brain, eye movement, muscle activity, heart rate, respiratory effort, air flow, and blood oxygen levels. These tests are used both to diagnose sleep apnea and to determine its severity.

The Multiple Sleep Latency Test (MSLT). The Multiple Sleep Latency Test (MSLT) measures the speed of falling asleep. In this test, patients are given several opportunities to fall asleep during the course of a day when they would normally be awake. For each opportunity, time to fall asleep is measured. People without sleep problems usually take an average of 10 to 20 minutes to fall asleep. Individuals who fall asleep in less than 5 minutes are likely to require some treatment for sleep disorders. The MSLT may be useful to measure the degree of excessive daytime sleepiness and to rule out other types of sleep disorders.

Diagnostic tests usually are performed in a sleep center, but new technology may allow some sleep studies to be conducted in the patient's home.

How is sleep apnea treated?

The specific therapy for sleep apnea is tailored to the individual patient based on medical history, physical examination, and the results of polysomnography. Medications are generally not effective in the treatment of sleep apnea. Oxygen administration may safely benefit certain patients but does not eliminate sleep apnea or prevent daytime sleepiness. Thus, the role of oxygen in the treatment of sleep apnea is controversial, and it is difficult to predict which patients will respond well. It is important that the effectiveness of the selected treatment be verified; this is usually accomplished by polysomnography.

Behavioral Therapy

Behavioral changes are an important part of the treatment program, and in mild cases behavioral therapy may be all that is needed. The individual should avoid the use of alcohol, tobacco, and sleeping pills, which make the airway more likely to collapse during sleep and prolong the apneic periods. Overweight persons can benefit from losing weight. Even a 10 percent weight loss can reduce the number of apneic events for most patients. In some patients with mild sleep apnea, breathing pauses occur only when they sleep on their backs. In such cases, using pillows and other devices that help them sleep in a side position is often helpful

Physical or Mechanical Therapy

Nasal continuous positive airway pressure (CPAP). Nasal continuous positive airway pressure (CPAP) is the most common effective treatment for sleep apnea. In this procedure, the patient wears a mask over the nose during sleep, and pressure from an air blower forces air through the nasal passages. The air pressure is adjusted so that it is just enough to prevent the throat from collapsing during sleep. The pressure is constant and continuous. Nasal CPAP prevents airway closure while in use, but apnea episodes return when CPAP is stopped or used improperly.

Variations of the CPAP device attempt to minimize side effects that sometimes occur, such as nasal irritation and drying, facial skin irritation, abdominal bloating, mask leaks, sore eyes, and headaches. Some versions of CPAP vary the pressure to coincide with the person's breathing pattern, and others start with low pressure, slowly increasing it to allow the person to fall asleep before the full prescribed pressure is applied.

Dental appliances. Dental appliances that reposition the lower jaw and the tongue have been helpful to some patients with mild sleep apnea or who snore but do not have apnea. Possible side effects include damage to teeth, soft tissues, and the jaw joint. A dentist or orthodontist is often the one to fit the patient with such a device.

Surgery

Some patients with sleep apnea may need surgery. Although several surgical procedures are used to increase the size of the airway, none of them is completely successful or without risks. More than one procedure may need to be tried before the patient realizes any benefits

Some of the more common procedures include removal of adenoids and tonsils (especially in children), nasal polyps or other growths, or other tissue in the airway and correction of structural deformities. Younger patients seem to benefit from these surgical procedures more than older patients.

Uvulopalatopharyngoplasty (UPPP). Uvulopalatopharyngoplasty (UPPP) is a procedure used to remove excess tissue at the back of the throat (tonsils, uvula, and part of the soft palate). The success of this technique may range from 30 to 50 percent. The long-term side effects and benefits are not known, and it is difficult to predict which patients will do well with this procedure.

Laser-assisted uvulopalatoplasty (LAUP). Laser-assisted uvulopalatoplasty (LAUP) is done to eliminate snoring but has not been shown to be effective in treating sleep apnea. This procedure involves using a laser device to eliminate tissue in the back of the throat. Like UPPP, LAUP may decrease or eliminate snoring but not sleep apnea itself. Elimination of snoring, the primary symptom of sleep apnea, without influencing the condition may carry the risk of delaying the diagnosis and possible treatment of sleep apnea in patients who elect LAUP. To identify possible underlying sleep apnea, sleep studies are usually required before LAUP is performed.

Tracheostomy. Tracheostomy is used in persons with severe, life-threatening sleep apnea. In this procedure, a small hole is made in the windpipe and a tube is inserted into the opening. This tube stays closed during waking hours, and the person breathes and speaks normally. It is opened for sleep so that air flows directly into the lungs, bypassing any upper airway obstruction. Although this procedure is highly effective, it is an extreme measure that is poorly tolerated by patients and rarely used.

Other procedures. Patients in whom sleep apnea is due to deformities of the lower jaw may benefit from surgical reconstruction. Finally, surgical procedures to treat obesity are sometimes recommended for sleep apnea patients who are morbidly obese.

For More Information

Information about sleep disorders research can be obtained from the NCSDR. In addition, the NHLBI Information Center can provide you with sleep education materials as well as other publications relating to heart, lung, and blood diseases.

National Center on Sleep Disorders Research.
Two Rockledge Center, Suite 7024
6701 Rockledge Drive
MSC 7920
Bethesda, MD 20892-7920
(301)435-0199
(301)480-3451 (fax)

NHLBI
PO Box 30105
Bethesda, MD 20824-0105
(301)251-1222
(301)251-1223 (fax)

Chapter 20

Snoring

Chapter Contents

Section 20.1

Snoring May Be Hazardous to Your Health

NCRR Reporter, September/October 1993.

Intermittent snoring, interrupted by silent pauses and then gasping breaths, has driven many sleeping partners to desperation. Studies have shown that snoring accompanied by disturbed breathing during sleep is not only a bedroom nuisance, it also may have debilitating medical consequences. It has been unclear, however, how many people actually have serious sleep-breathing disorders. A new study of men and women in the general working population has now shown that the problem is more prevalent than previously thought.

Researchers at the University of Wisconsin General Clinical Research Center (GCRC) and the department of preventive medicine in Madison estimate that 2 percent of women and 4 percent of men between 30 and 60 years of age suffer from sleep apnea syndrome. This disorder is characterized by snoring, cessation of breathing during sleep, and excessive daytime sleepiness. Sleep apnea, which is often undiagnosed, represents a significant health problem because it may contribute to hypertension, heart disease, and stroke. Persons with sleep apnea may also have memory lapses, mood swings, and depression, which can make it difficult for them to maintain regular employment. An editorial in the *New England Journal of Medicine* calls sleep apnea a major public health problem and states that "The study by Young et al. should lay to rest any misconceptions about the high prevalence of obstructive sleep apnea."

During sleep the upper airways, which include the passages around the back of the mouth, tend to narrow and may completely close in susceptible persons. The flow of air through the constricted passages causes snoring. If the airways close, breathing—and snoring—stops for 15 to 90 seconds and then resumes when the sleeping person briefly wakes and gasps for air.

In the largest study of its kind, Dr. Terry Young, associate professor of preventive medicine at the University of Wisconsin, and her colleagues analyzed the sleep patterns of 602 men and women during an overnight stay at the GCRC. The subjects were selected from a random sample of Wisconsin state employees. The scientists used a technique known as polysomnography to measure and record data on nasal and oral airflow, throat noises, abdominal and chest respiratory effort, heart rate, eye movement, and other physiologic parameters.

The researchers identified a number of risk factors for sleep-breathing disorders, among them loud snoring, male gender, and obesity. Habitual snorers were most likely to have a more severe form of sleep apnea. Regardless of severity or age group, men were approximately three times as likely as women to have breathing disorders during sleep.

The most common method for estimating the severity of sleep-disordered breathing is to measure the number of episodes per hour of sleep when breathing either stops completely (apnea) or partially (hypopnea), according to Dr. Young. She and her colleagues found that habitual snorers and people with sleep-disordered breathing (five or more episodes of apnea or hypopnea per hour of sleep) are likely to be excessively sleepy during the day.

Although most people in the study had very few periods of apnea or hypopnea during sleep, some had as many as 89 abnormal breathing events per hour. Sleepers who have 15 or more episodes of apnea per hour have a more severe form of the syndrome and often require treatment at a sleep disorder clinic.

The researchers found that about one-quarter of the men and 10 percent of the women studied had undiagnosed sleep-breathing disorders that ranged from mild to severe. Of these patients, approximately 23 percent of women and 16 percent of men also reported excessive daytime drowsiness, which placed them in the category of having sleep apnea syndrome. "The undiagnosed disorders included more than just the very mild or preclinical physiological levels of sleep apnea. A portion of the patients we studied had undiagnosed sleep apnea that was as severe as might be encountered in a sleep disorder clinic," says Dr. Young.

Because study participants were culled from the work force, they are likely to be more healthy than the general public overall, says Dr. Young. Therefore, the prevalence of breathing disorders during sleep may be even higher in the general population than this study indicates.

Dr. Young and her colleagues are now collecting follow-up data, bringing all the study participants back to the GCRC for another overnight analysis. It will take 4 years to study the entire cohort, which now numbers more then 950 volunteers, in the two-bed laboratory.

In the follow-up studies the researchers will investigate whether persons who now have mild apnea or hypopnea can be expected to have full-blown sleep apnea 5 years from now. They also hope to determine why obesity is associated with breathing disorders during sleep. These studies would help them to pinpoint the most appropriate types of intervention.

According to Dr. Young, a promising line of research is the relationship between apnea and blood pressure fluctuations. Her group plans to monitor volunteers' blood pressure every 20 minutes over a 24-hour period. The scientists already have learned that blood pressure fluctuations at night are different for people with sleep apnea than for those who do not have this syndrome.

Since sleep-breathing disorders have been described as a syndrome only within the last 15 years, several basic questions still await answers. "It is very important to determine what level of abnormality is clinically significant. For example, do patients with 10 apneas per hour of sleep require treatment? At what point should we consider this a disease?" says Dr. Young. "Whether to treat or not is an important issue, especially with scarce medical resources."

Additional Reading

Young, T., Palta, M., Dempsey, J., et al. The occurrence of sleep-disordered breathing among middle-aged adults. *New England Journal of Medicine* 328: 1230-1235, 1993.

Phillipson, E. A., Sleep Apnea—a major public health problem. *New England Journal of Medicine* 328:1271-1273,1993.

Ancoli-Israel S., Epidemiology of sleep disorders. *Clinics in Geriatric Medicine* 5:347-361.

This study was supported by the General Clinical Research Centers Program of the National Center for Research Resources and by the National Heart, Lung, and Blood Institute.

—John S. Makulowich

Section 20.2

Doctor, Can You Cure My Snoring?

Snoring, Not Funny, Not Hopeless

Forty-five percent of normal adults snore at least occasionally, and 25 percent are habitual snorers. Problem snoring is more frequent in males and overweight persons, and it usually grows worse with age.

More than 300 devices are registered in the U.S. Patent and Trademark Office as cures for snoring. Some are variations on the old idea of sewing a sock that holds a tennis ball on the pajama back to force the snorer to sleep on his side. (Snoring is often worse when the person sleeps on his back.) Some devices reposition the lower jaw forward; some open nasal air passages; a few others have been designed to condition a person not to snore by producing unpleasant stimuli when snoring occurs. But if you snore, the truth is that it is not under your control whatsoever; if anti-snoring devices work, that is probably because they keep you awake.

What causes snoring?

The noisy sounds of snoring occur when there is an obstruction to the free flow of air through the passages at the back of the mouth and nose. This area is the collapsible part of the airway (see Figure 20.1) where the tongue and upper throat meet the uvula. When these structures strike each other and vibrate during breathing, that is snoring.

Persons Who Snore May Suffer From:

- **poor muscle tone in the tongue and throat.** When muscles are too relaxed, either from alcohol or from drugs that cause sleepiness, the tongue falls backwards into the airway or the

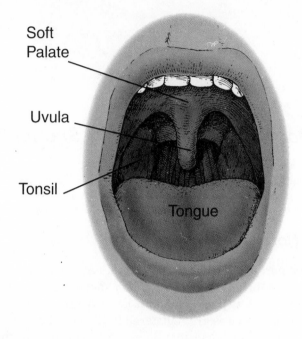

Soft Palate

Uvula

Tonsil

Tongue

Figure 20.1.

throat muscles draw in from the sides into the airway. This can also happen in deep sleep.

- **excessive bulkiness of throat tissue.** Children with large tonsils and adenoids, often snore. Overweight persons have bulky neck tissue, too. Cysts or tumors could also cause bulk, but they are rare.

- **long soft palate and/or uvula.** A long palate narrows the opening from the nose into the throat. As it dangles, it acts as a noisy flutter valve during relaxed breathing. A long uvula makes matters even worse.

- **obstructed nasal airways.** A stuffy or blocked nose requires extra effort to pull air through it. This creates an exaggerated

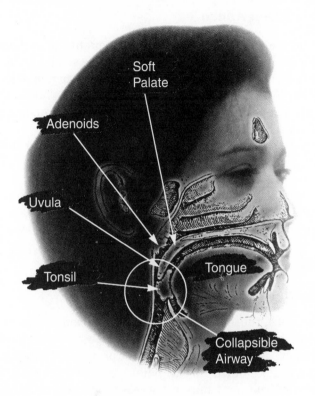

Figure 20.2.

vacuum in the throat, pulls together the floppy tissues of the throat, and snoring results. So, snoring often occurs only during the hay fever season or with a cold or sinus infection.

Also, deformities of the nose or nasal septum, such as a deviated septum (a deformity of the wall that separates one nostril from the other), can cause such an obstruction.

Is snoring serious?

Socially—yes. It can be, when it makes the snorer an object of ridicule and causes others sleepless nights and resentfulness.

Medically—yes. It disturbs the sleeping pattern and deprives the snorer of appropriate rest. When snoring is severe (see below), it can cause serious long-term health problems.

Obstructive Sleep Apnea

When loud snoring is interrupted by frequent episodes of totally obstructed breathing, it is known as obstructive sleep apnea. Serious episodes last more than 10 seconds each and occur more than seven times per hour. Apnea patients may experience 30 to 300 such events per night. These episodes can reduce blood oxygen levels, causing the heart to pump harder.

The immediate effect of sleep apnea is that the snorer is forced to sleep lightly and keep his muscles tense in order to keep airflow to the lungs. Because the snorer does not get a good rest, he may be sleepy during the day, which impairs job performance and makes him a hazardous driver or equipment operator. After many years with the disorder, high blood pressure and heart enlargement may occur.

Diagnosis, Prognosis, and Treatment

Can heavy snoring be cured?

Heavy snorers, those who snore in any position or are disruptive to the family, should seek medical advice to ensure that sleep apnea is not a problem. An otolaryngologist will provide a thorough examination of the nose, mouth, throat, palate, and neck. A sleep study in a laboratory environment may be necessary to determine how serious the snoring is and what effect(s) it has on the snorer's health.

Treatment

Treatment depends on the diagnosis. An examination will reveal if the snoring is caused by nasal allergy, infection, deformity, or tonsils and adenoids. Snoring/sleep apnea may respond best to surgery on the throat and palate that tightens flabby tissues and expands air passages, an operation known as uvulopalatopharyngoplasty (UPPP). If surgery is too risky or unwanted, the patient may sleep every night with a nasal mask that delivers air pressure into the throat (CPAP).

A chronically snoring child should be examined for problems with his or her tonsils and adenoids. A tonsillectomy and adenoidectomy may be required to return the child to full health.

Self-help for the Light Snorer

Adults who suffer from mild or occasional snoring should try the following self-help remedies:

1. Adopt a healthy and athletic lifestyle to develop good muscle tone and to lose weight.

2. Avoid tranquilizers, sleeping pills, and antihistamines before bedtime.

3. Avoid alcohol for at least 4 hours and heavy meals or snacks for 3 hours before retiring.

4. Establish regular sleeping patterns.

5. Sleep on your side rather than back.

6. Tilt the head of your bed upwards 4 inches.

Remember, snoring means obstructed breathing, and obstruction can be serious. It's not funny and not hopeless.

What is Otolaryngology—Head and Neck Surgery (Ear, Nose, and Throat Specialist)?

An otolaryngologist is a physician concerned with the medical and surgical treatment of the ears, nose, throat, and related structures of the head and neck.

The American Academy of Otolaryngology—Head and Neck Surgery, Inc. represents more than 7,500 ear, nose, and throat specialists. For more information or a list of otolaryngologists practicing in your area, please contact the Academy.

Part Six

Diet, Nutrition, and Fitness

Chapter 21

Hair Loss and Its Treatment

Chapter Contents

Section 21.1

Male Pattern Hair Loss

Dating as far back as history will take us, baldness has been a part of the aging process that many men fear the most. Before Rogaine, hair transplants and hair additions, men coped in various ways from magic ointments to the styling of their hair. Julius Caesar grew his hair long in the back and combed it all forward. Napoleon did the same thing. Somehow we often disregard history and the fact that this has been an age-old condition. We can't imagine or accept the fact that there is not a cure.

Understanding the cause of male pattern hair loss may better indicate exactly why it presently has no cure.

Androgenetic Alopecia

Androgenetic Alopecia. The modern medical term for either male or female pattern hair loss can be broken down in two parts:

1. Androgenetic,

    -   consisting of ANDROGEN (any of the various hormones that control the appearance and development of masculine characteristics such as testosterone), and

    -   GENETIC—the inheritance of genes from either the mother or the father's side of the family.

    -   Add AGE, which when coupled with genetics, represents a time clock that will signal the hair follicle to produce an enzyme named 5 alpha reductase. When the testosterone present in the follicle combines with the enzyme 5 alpha reductase, it produces dihydrotestosterone (DHT). Hair follicle receptors are sensitive to DHT and thereby start the process of male or female pattern hair loss.

2. Alopecia meaning hair loss, of which there are many types.

Put simply, scientists are working against aging, hormones and genetics. This is no easy task. Add the fact that male or female pattern hair loss is not life threatening, and it is easy to see why many physicians do not view hair loss as a priority in scientific research.

What is working for you in terms of research is that large pharmaceutical firms now know that a cure for hair loss could mean a fortune in revenue for their companies and stockholders. This is fuel enough and the race HAS begun.

Although we may not see a cure in our lifetime, it is possible. Science is closer to understanding hair loss due to many recent advancements. To say the cure is around the corner would only be speculation but hope certainly is alive.

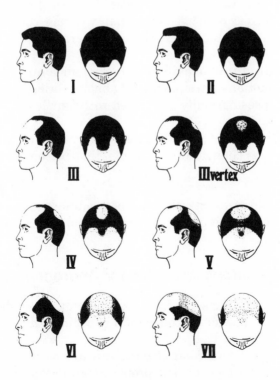

Figure 21.1. The Norwood Classifications of Hair Loss

Until then, since there are other causes of hair loss, it is advisable to consult with a dermatologist who is competent and experienced with diagnosing hair loss. Confirming the type of hair loss you have will make it possible for you to know which treatment options may be best for you.

Other Causes

Alopecia areata: Generally thought to be an autoimmune disorder. Causes "patchy" hair loss, often in small circular areas in different areas of the scalp.

Alopecia totalis: Total hair loss of the scalp, (an advanced form of alopecia areata).

Alopecia universalis: Hair loss of the entire body, (also an advanced form of alopecia areata).

Traction alopecia: Hair loss caused by physical stress and tension on the hair such as prolonged use of hair weaving, corn rows etc. Done too tightly on weak hair these can cause permanent hair loss.

Telogen effluvium: (usually temporary hair loss) CAUSES: Physical stress, emotional stress, thyroid abnormalities, medications and hormonal causes normally associated with females.

Anagen effluvium: Generally due to internally administered medications, such as chemotherapy agents, that poison the growing hair follicle.

All of these represent only a few of the different types of hair loss. Androgenetic alopecia represents close to 95 percent of all hair loss however.

Treatment Options Available for Androgenetic Alopecia

- **Learning to live with hair loss.** Often the assistance of a professional counselor can be helpful in coping with hair loss.

- **Hair styling and cosmetic techniques** such as permanent waves and hair colors. The proper haircut alone can make a vast difference in diffusing hair.

- **Rogaine**, the only FDA approved topical treatment for male or female pattern hair loss. Although Rogaine is not effective in stimulating new hair growth in many males, it appears to be more effective in retarding hair loss in a substantial number of both males and females.

- **Hair additions** have made many advances in both simulation of natural appearance and more secure attachment methods.

- **Hair replacement surgery** has also made many advances towards more natural appearing results. Modern surgical techniques have made transplantation for females a viable treatment option providing they are qualified candidates and have realistic expectations.

- A **combination** of Hair Additions with Hair Replacement Surgery.

To find out more about these options contact the American Hair Loss Council for consumer's guidelines to finding qualified specialists.

Myths Related to Hair Loss

- Frequent shampooing contributes to hair loss.
- Hats and wigs cause hair loss.
- 100 strokes of the hair brush daily will create healthier hair.
- Permanent hair loss is caused by perms, colors and other cosmetic treatments.
- Shaving one's head will cause the hair to grow back thicker.
- Standing on one's head will cause increased circulation and thereby stimulate hair growth.
- Dandruff causes permanent hair loss.
- There are cosmetic products that will cause the hair to grow thicker and faster.
- Stress causes permanent hair loss.
- Hair loss does not occur in the late teens or early twenties.
- Hair loss affects only intellectuals.
- There is a cure for Androgenetic Alopecia.

These are only a few of the common myths heard by physicians and other hair loss specialists on a daily basis. The AHLC suggests that you first have your hair loss diagnosed by a competent dermatologist who sees hair loss patients on a regular basis. Once you know the diagnosis, you will have a better understanding of exactly which treatment option may be best for you.

The American Hair Loss Council is a nonprofit organization and does not endorse individual physicians or business firms. It is advisable to consult with several specialists in order to be a well informed patient/consumer.

Section 21.2

Hair Replacement: What Works, What Doesn't

FDA Consumer, April 1997.

When the advertising slogan "Be Like Mike" caught America's fancy, it wasn't because every man decided to go for the Michael Jordan look by reaching for a razor and shaving his head.

Sure, men like Jordan, Charles Barkley, and "Star Trek's" Patrick Stewart are part of a small minority who are proud of their baldness. But combating and covering up hair loss hasn't turned into an estimated $1 billion-a-year industry because Americans like the idea of hair collecting in the shower drain.

"It probably represents aging," says Ken Washenik, M.D., director of dermatopharmacology at New York University Medical Center. "I think our concept of a bald person is of an older person. I think anything that reminds us in the mirror every day of the inevitability of aging is less than optimal."

When you talk about restoring hair, you're essentially looking at three different approaches. The first is to medicate, using a 2 percent solution of minoxidil found in Rogaine (and other brands since Pharmacia & Upjohn's patent expired in February 1996). Minoxidil is the only drug approved by the Food and Drug Administration for regrowing hair.

That doesn't mean minoxidil is by any means the panacea that men have been searching for since at least 1150 B.C., when Egyptians covered their baldness with a mixture of fats from ibex (a mountain goat), lion, crocodile, serpent, goose, and hippopotamus.

Surgical procedures, including hair transplantation and scalp reduction, are another modern-day approach. And, finally, there's the solution that Julius Caesar, according to legend, used in ancient days—cover it up. The most powerful man in the Roman Empire is said to have turned to the ceremonial wreath of laurel leaves to hide his ever-emerging scalp. The modern alternative is the hairpiece.

Uncovering Baldness

When discussing baldness, which affects an estimated 40 million men and 20 million women in the United States, the topic is generally about a hereditary condition called androgenetic alopecia. Ninety-five percent of hair loss is of this variety.

Male-pattern baldness refers to the upward retreat of the hairline from the forehead, as well as an expanding area of fallout from the crown of the head. In the end, all that might be left is a horseshoe-shaped fringe around the sides and back of the head. Female-pattern baldness, which recently has received more attention since Pharmacia & Upjohn began packaging and marketing Rogaine separately for women, refers to a diffuse pattern of hair loss throughout the scalp.

Research continues in search of ways to treat androgenetic alopecia and allow hair to sprout in barren scalps. But, at this time, all you can do, if you're a man, is to look at your father's head and your mother's father's head to see how they fared, because chances are you'll wind up with a similar fate. In addition, female-pattern baldness can be passed down from mother to daughter.

"I think it's just the luck of the draw what your genetics are," says Allan Kayne, M.D., a dermatologist and assistant clinical professor of medicine at the University of Washington Medical Center in Seattle.

In male- and female-pattern baldness, the culprit is something called dihydrotestosterone, or DHT, which is derived from androgen, a male hormone. Circulating through the bloodstream, androgen is converted to DHT by the enzyme 5-alpha reductase. Those with greater enzyme activity have more DHT binding to hair-follicle receptors. If flooded by DHT, the follicles sprout thinner and thinner hairs until nothing regrows, and the follicles eventually wither away.

Minoxidil

Currently, if you want to regrow hair, topical minoxidil is the only approved way to go. As Washenik explains, no one is quite certain how minoxidil, an oral medication originally approved to treat high blood pressure, works to grow hair.

To be effective, minoxidil must be used twice a day. It works better on those who are younger and whose hair loss is recent, according to clinical studies by Pharmacia & Upjohn.

Those studies show that 26 percent of men between 18 and 49 reported moderate to dense hair regrowth after four months of Rogaine treatment. An additional 33 percent had minimal hair regrowth. Almost 20 percent of women between 18 and 45 had moderate regrowth, while an additional 40 percent showed minimal regrowth.

A company spokesman said the research accounted for the fully pigmented hair fibers normally seen on the scalp and not vellus hair, which is more like peach fuzz. Many doctors, however, say the number of their patients who have as much success is much lower, and some find that only vellus hair appears.

"I have not been that impressed that it helps regrow hair," Kayne says. "I think that occurs in a very small minority."

One plus that Denise Cook, M.D., medical officer in FDA's division of dermatologic and dental drug products, points out is that patients report a decrease in shedding due to minoxidil use, though whether that perception is the result of fewer hairs being lost or more hairs being produced is unknown. Normally, you should lose only about 100 hairs a day.

One possible side effect of minoxidil is an itchy scalp. Another drawback is that it must be used for life or any regrown hair will fall out. Also, only those people losing hair on the crown, not in front, are candidates for regrowth.

Researchers are optimistic that more products to boost hair regrowth will be coming down the pike. For example, Proscar (finasteride), now used to treat enlarged prostate glands, has anti-androgen properties that may make it marketable as a hair-loss prescription, Washenik says. Theoretically, he says, if a drug can be targeted to halt the conversion of testosterone to DHT in the scalp region only, it could stop hair from falling out. He foresees combinations of medications as the wave of the future.

Surgery

Twenty years ago, many people felt they risked looking like a Cabbage Patch doll if they chose surgery to eliminate baldness. Now, says Carlos Puig, D.O., director of Puig Medical Group, which is headquartered in Houston, better surgical techniques—used by increasingly skilled surgeons—are getting more eye-pleasing results.

"When I started in 1973 . . . it was like the Stone Age," the cosmetic surgeon says, referring to the equipment and techniques in use. Now, he says, surgeons have learned to create a much more natural-looking hair line, using scalpels to cut either small slits or holes in the scalp to receive transplanted hair.

While there are numerous types of surgery, they can be sifted into two main categories: transplantation and scalp reduction.

Transplantation involves moving hair from densely covered sites on the sides or back of the head to bald areas of the scalp.

The key to success, explains Anthony Santangelo, president of the American Hair Loss Council, is to have good sites on the sides or back of the head from which to move hairs. Otherwise, patients can't expect ample coverage. Because their hair loss is diffuse, women generally lack good donor sites, making transplantation impractical for them.

The biggest improvement in transplants is with "micro" or "mini" grafts. "You're looking at one to two hairs shot into the head with a needle," Santangelo says. "It achieves a very, very fine, natural-looking hair line. The significant difference there is you need a lot of hair to do that."

Surgeons also use larger round plugs of seven to 10 hairs. Line grafts, the shifting of strips of nine to 12 hairs, are common, too.

One thing to keep in mind is that prosthetic hair fibers for transplantation are banned by FDA. Implanting them, according to Stephen Rhodes, acting chief of FDA's plastic and reconstructive surgery devices branch, caused a high incidence of adverse reactions, including infection.

If male-pattern baldness has left you with too much balding area to cover, you may benefit from scalp reduction: the surgical removal of large sections of a bald scalp. Extenders and expanders, elastic devices placed under the skin to stretch the hair-bearing scalp regions on the side of the head, have been used as a complement to reduction surgery.

Another surgical method is the flap technique, which rotates hair-bearing scalp areas from the sides or moves those areas from the back forward. The flap technique has the highest complication rate, though, Puig says. Bleeding, scarring and infection can occur from surgery. But advances, such as knowing what size flap to use and how to enhance blood supply to the region, have cut down on the visibility of scars.

Hairpieces

Finally, if you prefer to dodge the pain, time and cost of surgery, there's always the old, reliable hairpiece.

Obviously, all toupees and wigs are not created equal. Just as the transplant is only as good as the surgeon, the hairpiece is only as good as the person creating it and the materials used.

There are a variety of ways of affixing the hairpiece, which consists of human or synthetic hair implanted one hair at a time into a nylon netting. No method is permanent.

The hair weave involves sewing a wig into existing hair.

Also there are more traditional methods: You can use bonding (a type of glue), metal clips, or simple tape to attach the hairpiece to the scalp. Unlike the weaves, these give you the option to take the hairpiece on or off with ease. Many companies advertise "hair systems" or "hair clubs," which, according to Santangelo, offer check-ups to clean, color and tighten the hairpiece.

Lark Lambert, consumer complaint coordinator for FDA's Office of Cosmetics and Colors, notes that in addition to maintaining the cleanliness of hairpieces and wigs, it is important not to neglect the scalp under the wig. Keeping it clean and healthy avoids skin irritation and disease, he says. Also, as a precautionary safety measure, first-time users of hairpiece adhesives and solvents should test a patch of skin for 48 hours to determine possible skin sensitization to these products.

Health-Related Hair Loss

While hair loss is more harmful to the psyche than anything else, some of the causes of baldness may represent serious health problems. That's why it's important to talk about hair loss with a physician.

One problem, says FDA's Cook, could be a condition called alopecia areata. It's an autoimmune disease of unknown cause in which inflammatory cells attack the bulbs of the follicles under the scalp, leaving hairless patches. In more serious cases, hair may fall out from the entire head—eyebrows and beard included—and the entire body. Many times, though, the hair returns spontaneously.

Childbirth, severe malnutrition, chemotherapy, thyroid problems, and a form of lupus can also cause hair loss.

Something as simple as pigtails or cornrows, if worn too long, can cause hair loss, too, because of the stress they cause to the hair shaft.

The medical opinion concerning the role of emotional stress in balding is mixed. If stress does play a role, however, it's only at times of extreme emotional trauma, according to Kayne at the University of Washington Medical Center.

Mythical Treatments

The mythology of hair loss is a book unto itself. Wearing hats won't cause it, doctors say. Nor will standing on your head to increase blood flow cure it. Massaging your scalp and brushing your hair won't save you. Toweling off your head lightly rather than vigorously will only postpone the inevitable for a few days.

Perhaps the biggest myth is that cleaning your scalp of sebum (the semifluid secretion of glands attached to the follicle) will unclog those follicles and allow hair to grow. Surgeons will tell you that when they're performing transplants, there's no trapped hair to be found.

In 1989, FDA banned all nonprescription hair creams, lotions, or other external products claiming to grow hair or prevent baldness. And it has taken action against companies that continue to sell such products. In 1996, the agency sent a warning letter to Daniel Rogers Laboratories Inc., of Paramus, N.J., the manufacturer of "Natural Hairs," for claiming its product could promote hair growth and prevent hair loss. Two years earlier, after an FDA investigation, a U.S. district court judge enjoined the marketing of "Solution 109 Herbal Shampoo" because of claims that the product warded off hair loss.

Advertisements for "hair farming" products and others that hint they can regrow hair are still plentiful. But if you're desperate, keep one thing in mind:

"There will be never be a secret [ingredient] that works for hair loss," NYU's Washenik says. And, if they were to find it, he says: "It will be on the cover of the New York Times. It will be on the nightly news . . . . When this happens, it's going to be wildness. You're not going to need an expert to tell you the name of the drug."

The Thick and Thin of Hair Cosmetics

While Rogaine and other minoxidil-based products are giving consumers hopes of regrowing hair, another part of the hair-care industry has been jumping into the fray.

Drugstore chains, beauty shops, and salons are offering a number of products claiming to make hair appear thicker or fuller. While they won't solve baldness, such products can help women in particular by giving the appearance of more hair—if, and only if, the products are used regularly.

"The reality is," says Anthony Santangelo, president of the American Hair Loss Council, "[the products] just build hair for the day."

A quick walk down the store aisle shows a multitude of shampoos, conditioners, gels, mousses, and volumizers competing for your dollars. Many labeling claims target people with thinning hair, while others hint they can regrow hair, creating controversy about whether such a claim constitutes going too far. Any product claiming to regrow hair would have to file a new drug application. The Food and Drug Administration has approved only one product, the drug minoxidil, for regrowing hair.

"It's marketing; it's puffery," Santangelo says. "They'll take it as close as they possibly can without crossing the line, and they'll run with it."

Many of these products seem to thicken hair by coating it with chemicals called polymers. Hair has a negative charge, and the polymers' positive charge causes the polymers to adhere to the hair shaft, says Charles Fox, a Fair Lawn, N.J., consultant to the cosmetics industry. That results in better hair manageability and shine, he says. The hair also retains moisture, causing the shaft to swell and its diameter to expand slightly.

Also, says Stanley Milstein, Ph.D., special assistant to the director of FDA's Office of Cosmetics and Colors, some products coat the hair with various oils, waxes and silicone, claiming to restore moisture balance as they thicken hair.

Clarence Robbins, vice president of advanced technology for Colgate-Palmolive Co. and author of Chemical and Physical Behavior of Human Hair, says that if the products work, it's because they keep hair shafts from sliding past each other (think of the fly-away hair you get after blow-drying on a winter day.) In that way, hair volume appears greater.

If you're one to use bleach (peroxide) occasionally, he says, the bleach can achieve that sliding effect. Perms also make your hair wavier and fuller looking.

Many promoters of these products say their pro-vitamin B5 (panthenol) formulas can lead to fuller hair. Experts say don't bet on it, and according to the agency, the claim has never been proved.

By the way, there are products that simply color your scalp to create the appearance of hair. "But get any closer than 20 feet from an individual, they're gonna see your head's been spray-painted or covered with powder," Santangelo says.

—Larry Hanover

Larry Hanover is a writer in Mount Laurel, N.J.

Chapter 22

Diet and Nutrition

Chapter Contents

Section 22.1

Understanding Adult Obesity

NIH Publication No. 94-3680. National Institute of Diabetes &
Digestive & Kidney Diseases (NIDDK).

Many Americans are at increased health risk because they are
obese. The U.S. Surgeon General, in a 1988 report on nutrition and
health, estimated that one-fourth of adult Americans are overweight.
Obesity is a known risk factor for chronic diseases including heart disease, diabetes, high blood pressure, stroke, and some forms of cancer.

This section provides basic information about obesity: what it is,
what causes it, how to measure it. NIDDK published companion fact
sheets provide more in-depth information about some aspects addressed briefly here, such as health risks of obesity and treatment
options for the condition.

How Is Obesity Measured?

Everyone needs a certain amount of body fat for stored energy, heat
insulation, shock absorption, and other functions. As a rule, women
have more fat than men. Doctors generally agree that men with more
than 25 percent body fat and women with more than 30 percent body
fat are obese. Precisely measuring a person's body fat, however, is not
easy. The most accurate method is to weigh a person underwater—a
procedure limited to laboratories with sophisticated equipment.

There are two simpler methods for estimating body fat, but they can
yield inaccurate results if done by an inexperienced person or if done on
someone with severe obesity. One is to measure skinfold thickness in
several parts of the body. The second involves sending a harmless amount
of electric current through a person's body (bioelectric impedance analysis). Both methods are commonly used in health clubs and in commercial weight-loss programs, but results should be viewed skeptically.

Because measuring a person's body fat is tricky, doctors often rely
on other means to diagnose obesity. Two widely used measurements

548

are weight-for-height tables and body mass index. While both measurements have their limitations, they are reliable indicators that someone may have a weight problem. They are easy to calculate and require no special equipment.

Weight-for-Height Tables

Most people are familiar with weight-for-height tables. Doctors have used these tables for decades to determine whether a person is overweight. The tables usually have a range of acceptable weights for a person of a given height.

Table 22.1. Suggested Weights for Adults

SUGGESTED WEIGHTS FOR ADULTS	Height[1]	Weight in pounds[2]	
		19 to 34 years	35 years and over
[1]Without shoes.	5'0"	97-128	108-138
[2]Without clothes.	5'1"	101-132	111-143
[3]The higher weights in	5'2"	104-137	115-148
the ranges generally	5'3"	107-141	119-152
apply to men, who tend	5'4"	111-146	122-157
to have more muscle	5'5"	114-150	126-162
and bone; the lower	5'6"	118-155	130-167
weights more often	5'7"	121-160	134-172
apply to women,	5'8"	125-164	138-178
who have less muscle	5'9"	129-169	142-183
and bone.	5'10"	132-174	146-188
	5'11"	136-179	151-194
	6'0"	140-184	155-199
	6'1"	144-189	159-205
	6'2"	148-195	164-210
	6'3"	152-200	168-216
	6'4"	156-205	173-222
	6'5"	160-211	177-228
	6'6"	164-216	182-234

One problem with using weight-for-height tables is that doctors disagree over which is the best table to use. Many versions are available, all with different weight ranges. Some tables take a person's frame size, age, and sex into account; others do not. A limitation of all weight-for-height tables is that they do not distinguish excess fat from muscle. A very muscular person may appear obese, according to the tables, when he or she is not. Still, weight-for-height tables can be used as general guidelines.

Table 22.2. Body weights in pounds according to height and body mass index* *Each entry gives the body weight in pounds (lb.) for a person of a given height and body mass index. Pounds have been rounded off. To use the table, find the appropriate height in the left-hand column. Move across the row to a given weight. The number at the top of the column is the body mass index for the height and weight. Adapted with permission from Bray C.A.. Gray. D.S. Obesity. Part 1. Pathogenesis. West J Med 1988: 149: 429-41.

Body Mass Index (kg/m²)

Height (in.)	19	20	21	22	23	24	25	26	27	28	29	30	35	40
	Body Weight (lb.)													
58	91	96	100	105	110	115	119	124	129	134	138	143	167	191
59	94	99	104	109	114	119	124	128	133	138	143	148	173	198
60	97	102	107	112	118	123	128	133	138	143	148	153	179	204
61	100	106	111	116	122	127	132	137	143	148	153	158	185	211
62	104	109	115	120	126	131	136	142	147	153	158	164	191	218
63	107	113	118	124	130	135	141	146	152	158	163	169	197	225
64	110	116	122	128	134	140	145	151	157	163	169	174	204	232
65	114	120	126	132	138	144	150	156	162	168	174	180	210	240
66	118	124	130	136	142	148	155	161	167	173	179	186	216	247
67	121	127	134	140	146	153	159	166	172	178	185	191	223	255
68	125	131	138	144	151	158	164	171	177	184	190	197	230	262
69	128	135	142	149	155	162	169	176	182	189	196	203	236	270
70	132	139	146	153	160	167	174	181	188	195	202	207	243	278
71	136	143	150	157	165	172	179	186	193	200	208	215	250	286
72	140	147	154	162	169	177	184	191	199	206	213	221	258	294
73	144	151	159	166	174	182	189	197	204	212	219	227	265	302
74	148	155	163	171	179	186	194	202	210	218	225	233	272	311
75	152	160	168	176	184	192	200	208	216	224	232	240	279	319
76	156	164	172	180	189	197	205	213	221	230	238	246	287	328

The table printed here is from the 1990 edition of Dietary Guidelines for Americans, a pamphlet printed jointly by the U.S. Departments of Agriculture and Health and Human Services. This table has a wide range for what the pamphlet calls "healthy" or "suggested" weights.

In this table, the higher weights generally apply to men, who tend to have more muscle and bone. The lower weights more often apply to women, who have less muscle and bone. The table also shows higher weights for people age 35 and older, which some experts question.

Body Mass Index (BMI). Body mass index, or BMI, is a new term to most people. However, it is the measurement of choice for many physicians and researchers studying obesity. BMI uses a mathematical formula that takes into account both a person's height and weight. BMI equals a person's weight in kilograms divided by height in meters squared. ($BMI = kg/m^2$). The table printed here has already done the math and metric conversions. To use the table, find the appropriate height in the left-hand column. Move across the row to the given weight. The number at the top of the column is the BMI for that height and weight.

In general, a person age 35 or older is obese if he or she has a BMI of 27 or more. For people age 34 or younger, a BMI of 25 or more indicates obesity. A BMI of more than 30 usually is considered a sign of moderate to severe obesity.

The BMI measurement poses some of the same problems as the weight-for-height tables. Doctors don't agree on the cutoff points for "healthy" versus "unhealthy" BMI ranges. BMI also does not provide information on a person's percentage of body fat. However, like the weight-for-height table, BMI is a useful general guideline.

Body Fat Distribution: "Pears" vs. "Apples"

Doctors are concerned with not only how much fat a person has but where the fat is on the body.

Women typically collect fat in their hips and buttocks, giving their figures a "pear" shape. Men, on the other hand, usually build up fat around their bellies, giving them more of an "apple" shape. This is not a hard and fast rule, though. Some men are pear-shaped and some women become apple-shaped, especially after menopause.

People whose fat is concentrated mostly in the abdomen are more likely to develop many of the health problems associated with obesity.

Doctors have developed a simple way to measure whether someone is an apple or a pear. The measurement is called waist-to-hip ratio.

Waist-to-Hip Ratio. To find out someone's waist-to-hip ratio, measure the waist at its narrowest point, then measure the hips at the widest point. Divide the waist measurement by the hip measurement. A woman with a 35-inch waist and 46-inch hips would do the following calculation:

$$35 \div 46 = 0.76$$

Women with waist-to-hip ratios of more than 0.8 or men with waist-to-hip ratios of more than 1.0 are "apples." They are at increased health risk because of their fat distribution.

What causes obesity?

In scientific terms, obesity occurs when a person's calorie intake exceeds the amount of energy he or she burns. What causes this imbalance between consuming and burning calories is unclear. Evidence suggests that obesity often has more than one cause. Genetic, environmental, psychological, and other factors all may play a part.

Genetic Factors. Obesity tends to run in families, suggesting that it may have a genetic cause. However, family members share not only genes but also diet and lifestyle habits that may contribute to obesity. Separating these lifestyle factors from genetic ones is often difficult. Still, growing evidence points to heredity as a strong determining factor of obesity. In one study of adults who were adopted as children, researchers found that the subjects' adult weights were closer to their biological parents' weights than their adoptive parents'. The environment provided by the adoptive family apparently had less influence on the development of obesity than the person's genetic makeup.

Nevertheless, people who feel that their genes have doomed them to a lifetime of obesity should take heart. As discussed in the next section, many people genetically predisposed to obesity do not become obese or manage to lose weight and keep it off.

Environmental Factors. Although genes are an important factor in many cases of obesity, a person's environment also plays a significant part. Environment includes lifestyle behaviors such as what a person eats and how active he or she is.

Americans tend to have high-fat diets, often putting taste and convenience ahead of nutritional content when choosing meals. Most Americans also don't get enough exercise.

People can't change their genetic makeup, of course, but they can change what they eat and how active they are. Some people have been able to lose weight and keep it off by:

- Learning how to choose more nutritious meals that are lower in fat.

- Learning to recognize environmental cues (such as enticing smells) that may make them want to eat when they are not hungry.

- Becoming more physically active.

Psychological Factors. Psychological factors also may influence eating habits. Many people eat in response to negative emotions such as boredom, sadness, or anger.

While most overweight people have no more psychological disturbance than normal-weight people, about 30 percent of the people who seek treatment for serious weight problems have difficulties with binge eating. During a binge eating episode, people eat large amounts of food while feeling they can't control how much they are eating. Those with the most severe binge eating problems are considered to have binge eating disorder. These people may have more difficulty losing weight and keeping the weight off than people without binge eating problems. Some will need special help, such as counseling or medication, to control their binge eating before they can successfully manage their weight.

Other Causes of Obesity. Some rare illnesses can cause obesity. These include hypothyroidism, Cushing's syndrome, depression, and certain neurologic problems that can lead to overeating. Certain drugs, such as steroids and some antidepressants, may cause excessive weight gain. A doctor can determine if a patient has any of these conditions, which are believed to be responsible for only about 1 percent of all cases of obesity.

What are the consequences of obesity?

Health Risks. Obesity is not just a cosmetic problem. It's a health hazard. Someone who is 40 percent overweight is twice as likely to die prematurely as an average-weight person. (This effect is seen after 10 to 30 years of being obese.)

Obesity has been linked to several serious medical conditions, including diabetes, heart disease, high blood pressure, and stroke. It is also associated with higher rates of certain types of cancer. Obese men are more likely than non-obese men to die of cancer of the colon, rectum, and prostate. Obese women are more likely than non-obese women to die of cancer of the gallbladder, breast, uterus, cervix, and ovaries.

Other diseases and health problems linked to obesity include:

- Gallbladder disease and gallstones.
- Osteoarthritis, a disease in which the joints deteriorate, possibly as a result of excess weight on the joints.
- Gout, another disease affecting the joints.
- Pulmonary (breathing) problems, including sleep apnea, in which a person can stop breathing for a short time during sleep.

Doctors generally agree that the more obese a person is, the more likely he or she is to have health problems.

Psychological and Social Effects. One of the most painful aspects of obesity may be the emotional suffering it causes. American society places great emphasis on physical appearance, often equating attractiveness with slimness, especially in women. The messages, intended or not, make overweight people feel unattractive. Many people assume that obese people are gluttonous, lazy, or both. However, more and more evidence contradicts this assumption.

Obese people often face prejudice or discrimination at work, at school, while looking for a job, and in social situations. Feelings of rejection, shame, or depression are common.

Who should lose weight?

Doctors generally agree that people who are 20 percent or more overweight, especially the severely obese person, can gain significant health benefits from weight loss.

Many obesity experts believe that people who are less than 20 percent above their healthy weight should try to lose weight if they have any of the following risk factors.

Risk Factors

- **Family history of certain chronic diseases.** People with close relatives who have had heart disease or diabetes are more likely to develop these problems if they are obese.

- **Pre-existing medical conditions.** High blood pressure, high cholesterol levels, or high blood sugar levels are all warning signs of some obesity-associated diseases.

- **"Apple" shape.** People whose weight is concentrated around their abdomens may be at greater risk of heart disease, diabetes, or cancer than people of the same weight who are pear-shaped.

Fortunately, even a modest weight loss of 10 to 20 pounds can bring significant health improvements, such as lowering one's blood pressure and cholesterol levels.

How is obesity treated?

Treatment options for obesity are explored in depth in other fact sheets. The method of treatment will depend on how obese a person is. Factors such as an individual's overall health and motivation to lose weight are also important considerations. Treatment may include a combination of diet, exercise, and behavior modification. In some cases of severe obesity, gastrointestinal surgery may be recommended.

Research on Obesity

The National Institute of Diabetes and Digestive and Kidney Diseases (NIDDK) is the part of the National Institutes of Health chiefly responsible for obesity research. NIDDK supports the study of obesity in its own labs and clinics and at universities, hospitals, and research centers across the United States. NIDDK-funded research has helped scientists learn more about the role of genes and metabolism in obesity. Other NIDDK-supported studies have examined the relationship between obesity and various medical conditions. Ongoing NIDDK research efforts include better ways to define and treat the various types of obesity and understanding how the body stores and uses fat.

NIDDK also oversees the National Task Force on Prevention and Treatment of Obesity. The task force comprises leading obesity and nutrition experts who gather and assess the latest information on obesity treatment and prevention. The task force also helps guide basic and clinical research on obesity. Scientific papers and general-interest brochures and pamphlets approved by the task force are available from the NIDDK's Obesity Resource Information Center.

In addition to NIDDK, other sections of the NIH sponsor obesity research. They include:

- the National Heart, Lung, and Blood Institute (NHLBI)
- the National Center for Research Resources (NCRR)
- the National Institute of Child Health and Human Development (NICHD)
- the National Institute on Mental Health (NIMH)
- the National Cancer Institute (NCI)
- the National Institute on Aging (NIA)
- the National Institute of Nursing Research (NINR)
- the National Institute of Arthritis and Musculoskeletal and Skin Diseases (NIAMS)
- the National Institute of Neurological Diseases and Stroke (NINDS)
- the National Institute of Environmental and Health Sciences (NIEHS).

Additional Reading on Obesity

"Are You Eating Right?" *Consumer Reports*, October 1992. This article summarizes advice from 68 nutrition experts, including a discussion on weight control and health risks of obesity. Available in public libraries.

Bray, G.A. "Pathophysiology of Obesity." *American Journal of Clinical Nutrition*. 1992; Supplement to Vol. 55 (2): 488S-494S. This article comes from the proceedings of an NIH Consensus Development Conference on Gastrointestinal Surgery for Severe Obesity. Written for health professionals in technical language. Available in medical libraries.

"Dietary Guidelines for Americans." Third Edition, 1990. Home and Garden Bulletin No. 232. This pamphlet, issued by the U.S. Agriculture and Health and Human Services Departments, contains information about maintaining a healthy weight, as well as dietary and nutrition recommendations. Available through the Government Printing Office, Publication No. 1990-273-930 and reprinted in this Sourcebook.

"Exercise and Weight Control." The President's Council on Physical Fitness and Sports, Department of Health and Human Services. This brochure discusses the difference between being "overweight" and "overeat" and the role diet and exercise can play in a weight loss program. Copies can be obtained from the President's Council on Physical Fitness and Sports, Dept. No. 176, 701 Pennsylvania Ave. NW, Washington, D.C. 20004.

"The Facts About Weight Loss Products and Programs." This brochure, produced by the Federal Trade Commission in conjunction with the Food and Drug Administration and the National Association of Attorneys General, has tips on evaluating diet claims and weight loss programs. Copies can be obtained from the FTC, Public Affairs Branch, Room 130, Sixth St. and Pennsylvania Ave. NW, Washington, D.C. 20580

"Getting Slim." *U.S. News & World Report*, May 14, 1990. This article, written for the general public, discusses definitions of obesity, the role of genes, body mass index, and apple/pear weight distribution patterns. Available in public libraries.

Long, P. "The Great Weight Debate." *Health*. February/March 1992, pp. 42-47. This article, written for the general public, discusses the controversy over which weight-for-height table is best to use. It also provides some simple guidelines for determining whether someone needs to lose weight. Available in public libraries.

"Methods for Voluntary Weight Loss and Control." *National Institutes of Health Technology Assessment Conference Statement*, March 30-April 1, 1992. This publication, written for health professionals, summarizes findings of a conference discussing success rates of various methods of weight loss, short-term and long-term effects of losing weight, and related topics. Copies are available from the Office of Medical Applications Research, National Institutes of Health, Federal Building, Room 618, Bethesda, MD 20892.

Yanovski, S.Z. "A Practical Approach to Treatment of the Obese Patient." *Archives of Family Medicine*. 1993; Vol. 2, No. 3, pp 309-316. Written for health professionals, this article provides guidance on evaluating overweight patients and developing plans for treatment.

Section 22.2

Facts about Overweight and Obesity

Extracted from NIH Publication No. 96-4158 July 1996.
NIDDK Web Document, (http://www.niddk.nih.gov/nutritiondocs.html).
This e-pub is not copyrighted. NIDDK and WIN encourage unlimited
duplication and distribution of this etext.

One in three or 58 million American adults aged 20 through 74 are overweight. According to data from the Third National Health and Nutrition Examination Survey (NHANES III), the number of overweight Americans increased from 25 to 33 percent between 1980 and 1991. The survey also shows that minority populations, specifically minority women, are disproportionately affected: approximately 50 percent of African American and Mexican American women are overweight. By a similar definition, more than one in five children and adolescents aged 6 through 17 are also overweight. Even using a more rigorous definition recommended for youths, 11 percent of children and adolescents are overweight, up from approximately 5 percent in the 1960s and 70s. Overweight and obesity is a known risk factor for diabetes, heart disease, high blood pressure, gallbladder disease, arthritis, breathing problems, and some forms of cancer.

What Is Overweight and Obesity?

Overweight is the excess amount of body weight that includes muscle, bone, fat, and water. Obesity is the excess accumulation of body fat. One can be overweight without being obese: a body builder who has a lot of muscle, for example. However, for practical purposes, most people who are overweight are also obese.

The Prevalence of Overweight in the United States

Total number of overweight adults: (20 through 74 years old) approximately one-third or 58 million Americans.[2] (numbers derived from NHANES III, 1988-91, which defines overweight as a BMI value of 27.3 percent or more for women and 27.8 percent or more for men)

Overweight adult females (20-74 years old): 32 million (1990)[2]

Overweight adult males (20-74 years old): 26 million (1990)[2]

Total number of overweight youths: 6 through 17 years old approximately 11 percent or 4.7 million children in this age group.[3] (numbers derived from NHES II and III, which defines overweight by the 95th percentile of BMI)

Other Overweight/Obesity-Related Statistics

- The percentage of dietary fat American adults eat:[4] 34

- The percentage of saturated fat American adults eat:[4] 12

- The number of extra calories a person must eat to gain a pound or burn to lose a pound:[5] 3,500

- Percentage of adult American women trying to lose weight at any given time:[6] 33 to 40 percent

- The percentage of adult American men trying to lose weight at any given time:[6] 20 to 24 percent

- The average number of calories a person burns eating:[7] .023 kcal per minute/per kilogram of body weight

- The annual number of deaths attributable to poor diet and inactivity:[8] 300,000 deaths

Economic Costs of Chronic Conditions Linked to Overweight/Obesity

Noninsulin-Dependent Diabetes Mellitus (NIDDM)

Nearly 80 percent of patients with NIDDM are obese.[9] Much of the estimated $11.3 billion dollars spent each year to diagnose, treat, and manage NIDDM, including treatment for diabetic ketoacidosis, diabetic coma, diabetic eye disease, and diabetic kidney disease, stems from obesity.[9]

Gallbladder Disease

The incidence of symptomatic gallstones soars as a person's body mass index (BMI) goes beyond 29.[10] Nearly $2.4 billion dollars or 30 percent of the total amount spent annually on gallbladder disease and gallbladder surgery are related to obesity.[10]

Heart Disease

Nearly 70 percent of the diagnosed cases of cardiovascular disease are related to obesity.

Obesity

Obesity accounts for $22.2 billion, or 19 percent, of the total cost of heart disease.[10]

High Blood Pressure

Obesity more than doubles one's chances of developing high blood pressure, which affects approximately 26 percent of obese American men and women. The annual cost of obesity-related high blood pressure is close to $1.5 billion dollars.[10]

Breast and Colon Cancer

Almost half of breast cancer cases are diagnosed among obese women; an estimated 42 percent of colon cancer cases are diagnosed among obese individuals. Obesity-related breast cancer and colon cancer account for 2.5 percent of the total costs of cancer, or $1.9 billion dollars, annually.[10]

Indirect Costs

Americans spend an additional $33 billion dollars annually on weight-reduction products and services, including diet foods, products, and programs.[10]

Sources

1. *Weighing the Options: Criteria for Evaluating Weight-Management Programs.* Institute of Medicine, National Academy of Sciences. 1995; 50-51.

2. Kuczmarski, R.J., Johnson, C.L., Flegal, K.M., Campbell, S.M. Increasing prevalence of overweight among US adults. *Journal of the American Medical Association.* 1994; 272: 205-211.

3. Troiano, R.P., Kuczmarski, R.J., Johnson, C.L., Flegal, K.M., Campbell, S.M. Overweight prevalence and trends for children and adolescents: The National Health and Nutrition Examination Surveys, 1963 to 1991. *Archives of Pediatrics and Adolescent Medicine.* 1995; 149:1085-1091.

4. Daily dietary fat and total food-energy intakes: Third National Health and Nutrition Examination Survey, Phase I, 1988-1991. *MMWR Morbidity and Mortality Weekly Report.* 1994; 43:116-117, 123-125.

5. Weight control: What works and why. *Medical Essay.* Mayo Foundation for Medical Education and Research, 1994.

6. *Methods of Voluntary Weight loss and Control.* National Institutes of Health Technology Assessment Conference Statement, March 30-April 1, 1992. Copies are available from the Office of Medical Applications Research, National Institutes of Health, Federal Building, Room 618, Bethesda, MD 20892.

7. McArdle, W.D., Katch, F.I. & Katch, V.L. *Exercise Physiology: Energy, Nutrition & Human Performance.* Philadelphia, Pa: Lea & Febiger; 1991.

8. McGinnis, J.M. & Foege, W.H. Actual causes of death in the United States. *Journal of the American Medical Association.* 1993; 270:2207-2212.

9. *Diabetes in America, 2nd Edition,* The National Institutes of Diabetes and Digestive and Kidney Diseases, 1995, NIH publication number 95-1468.

10. Colditz, G.A. Economic costs of obesity. *American Journal of Clinical Nutrition,* 1992; 55:503-507s.

Research on Obesity

The National Institute of Diabetes and Digestive and Kidney Diseases (NIDDK) is the part of the National Institutes of Health (NIH) primarily responsible for obesity and nutrition-related research. NIDDK supports the study of obesity in its own labs and clinics and at universities, hospitals, and research centers across the United States. NIDDK-funded research has helped scientists learn more about the role of genes and metabolism in obesity. Other NIDDK-supported studies have examined the relationship between obesity and other medical conditions such as breast cancer. Ongoing NIDDK research efforts include better ways to define and manage obesity and to understand how the body stores and uses fat.

Section 22.3

Physical Activity and Weight Control

NIH Publication No. 96-4031. NIDDK Web Document, (http://www.niddk.nih.gov/nutritiondocs.html). This e-pub is not copyrighted. WIN encourages unlimited duplication and distribution of this e-text. April 1996.

Regular physical activity is an important part of effective weight loss and weight maintenance. It also can help prevent several diseases and improve your overall health. It does not matter what type of physical activity you perform—sports, planned exercise, household chores, yard work, or work-related tasks—all are beneficial. Studies show that even the most inactive people can gain significant health benefits if they accumulate 30 minutes or more of physical activity per day. Based on these findings, the U.S. Public Health Service has identified increased physical activity as a priority in Healthy People 2000, our national objectives to improve the health of Americans by the year 2000.

Research consistently shows that regular physical activity, combined with healthy eating habits, is the most efficient and healthful way to control your weight. Whether you are trying to lose weight or maintain it, you should understand the important role of physical activity and include it in your lifestyle.

How can physical activity help control my weight?

Physical activity helps to control your weight by using excess calories that otherwise would be stored as fat. Your body weight is regulated by the number of calories you eat and use each day. Everything you eat contains calories, and everything you do uses calories, including sleeping, breathing, and digesting food. Any physical activity in addition to what you normally do will use extra calories.

Balancing the calories you use through physical activity with the calories you eat will help you achieve your desired weight. When you eat more calories than you need to perform your day's activities, your body stores the extra calories and you gain weight. When you eat fewer calories than you use, your body uses the stored calories and you lose weight. When you eat the same amount of calories as your body uses, your weight stays the same.

Any type of physical activity you choose to do—strenuous activities such as running or aerobic dancing or moderate-intensity activities such as walking or household work—will increase the number of calories your body uses. The key to successful weight control and improved overall health is making physical activity a part of your daily routine.

What are the health benefits of physical activity?

In addition to helping to control your weight, research shows that regular physical activity can reduce your risk for several diseases and conditions and improve your overall quality of life. Regular physical activity can help protect you from the following health problems.

- **Heart Disease and Stroke.** Daily physical activity can help prevent heart disease and stroke by strengthening your heart muscle, lowering your blood pressure, raising your high-density lipoprotein (HDL) levels (good cholesterol) and lowering low-density lipoprotein (LDL) levels (bad cholesterol), improving blood flow, and increasing your heart's working capacity.

- **High Blood Pressure.** Regular physical activity can reduce blood pressure in those with high blood pressure levels. Physical activity also reduces body fatness, which is associated with high blood pressure.

- **Noninsulin-Dependent Diabetes.** By reducing body fatness, physical activity can help to prevent and control this type of diabetes.

- **Obesity.** Physical activity helps to reduce body fat by building or preserving muscle mass and improving the body's ability to use calories. When physical activity is combined with proper nutrition, it can help control weight and prevent obesity, a major risk factor for many diseases.

- **Back Pain.** By increasing muscle strength and endurance and improving flexibility and posture, regular exercise helps to prevent back pain.

- **Osteoporosis.** Regular weight-bearing exercise promotes bone formation and may prevent many forms of bone loss associated with aging.

Studies on the psychological effects of exercise have found that regular physical activity can improve your mood and the way you feel about yourself. Researchers also have found that exercise is likely to reduce depression and anxiety and help you to better manage stress.

Keep these health benefits in mind when deciding whether or not to exercise. And remember, any amount of physical activity you do is better than none at all.

How Much Should I Exercise?

For the greatest overall health benefits, experts recommend that you do 20 to 30 minutes of aerobic activity three or more times a week and some type of muscle strengthening activity and stretching at least twice a week. However, if you are unable to do this level of activity, you can gain substantial health benefits by accumulating 30 minutes or more of moderate-intensity physical activity a day, at least five times a week.

If you have been inactive for a while, you may want to start with less strenuous activities such as walking or swimming at a comfortable pace. Beginning at a slow pace will allow you to become physically fit without straining your body. Once you are in better shape, you can gradually do more strenuous activity.

Moderate-intensity Activity

Moderate-intensity activities include some of the things you may already be doing during a day or week, such as gardening and housework. These activities can be done in short spurts—10 minutes here, 8 minutes there. Alone, each action does not have a great effect on your health, but regularly accumulating 30 minutes of activity over the course of the day can result in substantial health benefits.

To become more active throughout your day, take advantage of any chance to get up and move around. Here are some examples:

- Take a short walk around the block
- Rake leaves
- Play actively with the kids
- Walk up the stairs instead of taking the elevator
- Mow the lawn
- Take an activity break—get up and stretch or walk around
- Park your car a little farther away from your destination and walk the extra distance

The point is not to make physical activity an unwelcome chore, but to make the most of the opportunities you have to be active.

Aerobic Activity

Aerobic activity is an important addition to moderate-intensity exercise. Aerobic exercise is any extended activity that makes you breathe hard while using the large muscle groups at a regular, even pace. Aerobic activities help make your heart stronger and more efficient. They also use more calories than other activities. Some examples of aerobic activities include:

- Brisk walking
- Jogging
- Bicycling
- Swimming
- Aerobic dancing
- Racket sports
- Rowing
- Ice or roller skating
- Cross-country or downhill skiing
- Using aerobic equipment (i.e., treadmill, stationary bike)

To get the most health benefits from aerobic activity, you should exercise at a level strenuous enough to raise your heart rate to your target zone. Your target heart rate zone is 50 to 75 percent of your maximum heart rate (the fastest your heart can beat). To find your target zone, look for the category closest to your age in the chart below and read across the line. For example, if you are 35 years old, your target heart rate zone is 93-138 beats per minute.

To see if you are exercising within your target heart rate zone, count the number of pulse beats at your wrist or neck for 15 seconds, then multiply by four to get the beats per minute. Your heart should be beating within your target heart rate zone. If your heart is beating faster than your target heart rate, you are exercising too hard and should slow down. If your heart is beating slower than your target heart rate, you should exercise a little harder.

When you begin your exercise program, aim for the lower part of your target zone (50 percent). As you get into better shape, slowly build up to the higher part of your target zone (75 percent). If exercising within your target zone seems too hard, exercise at a pace that is comfortable for you. You will find that, with time, you will feel more comfortable exercising and can slowly increase to your target zone.

Table 22.3. Target Heart Rates

Age	Target Heart Rate Zone 50-75%	Average Maximum Heart
20-30 years	98-146 beats per min.	195
31-40 years	93-138 beats per min.	185
41-50 years	88-131 beats per min.	175
51-60 years	83-123 beats per min.	165
61+ years	78-116 beats per min.	155

Stretching and Muscle Strengthening Exercises

Stretching and strengthening exercises such as weight training should also be a part of your physical activity program. In addition to using calories, these exercises strengthen your muscles and bones and help prevent injury.

Tips to a Safe and Successful Physical Activity Program

Make sure you are in good health. Answer the following questions before you begin exercising. (Source: British Columbia Department of Health)

- Has a doctor ever said you have heart problems?

- Do you frequently suffer from chest pains?

- Do you often feel faint or have dizzy spells?

- Has a doctor ever said you have high blood pressure?

- Has a doctor ever told you that you have a bone or joint problem, such as arthritis, that has been or could be aggravated by exercise?

- Are you over the age of 65 and not accustomed to exercise?

- Are you taking prescription medications, such as those for high blood pressure?

- Is there a good medical reason, not mentioned here, why you should not exercise?

If you answered "yes" to any of these questions, you should see your doctor before you begin an exercise program.

- Follow a gradual approach to exercise to get the most benefits with the fewest risks. If you have not been exercising, start at a slow pace and as you become more fit, gradually increase the amount of time and the pace of your activity.

- Choose activities that you enjoy and that fit your personality. For example, if you like team sports or group activities, choose things such as soccer or aerobics. If you prefer individual activities, choose things such as swimming or walking. Also, plan your activities for a time of day that suits your personality. If you are a morning person, exercise before you begin the rest of your day's activities. If you have more energy in the evening, plan activities that can be done at the end of the day. You will be more likely to stick to a physical activity program if it is convenient and enjoyable.

- Exercise regularly. To gain the most health benefits it is important to exercise as regularly as possible. Make sure you choose activities that will fit into your schedule.

- Exercise at a comfortable pace. For example, while jogging or walking briskly you should be able to hold a conversation. If you do not feel normal again within 10 minutes following exercise, you are exercising too hard. Also, if you have difficulty breathing or feel faint or weak during or after exercise, you are exercising too hard.

- Maximize your safety and comfort. Wear shoes that fit and clothes that move with you, and always exercise in a safe location. Many people walk in indoor shopping malls for exercise. Malls are climate controlled and offer protection from bad weather.

- Vary your activities. Choose a variety of activities so you don't get bored with any one thing.

- Encourage your family or friends to support you and join you in your activity. If you have children, it is best to build healthy habits when they are young. When parents are active, children are more likely to be active and stay active for the rest of their lives.

- Challenge yourself. Set short-term as well as long-term goals and celebrate every success, no matter how small.

Whether your goal is to control your weight or just to feel healthier, becoming physically active is a step in the right direction. Take advantage of the health benefits that regular exercise can offer and make physical activity a part of your lifestyle.

Additional Resources

The following organizations have materials on physical activity and weight control available to the public.

President's Council on Physical Fitness and Sports
701 Pennsylvania Avenue, NW
Suite 250
Washington, D.C. 20004
Phone: (202) 272-3421

National Heart, Lung, and Blood Institute
Information Center
P.O. Box 30105
Bethesda, MD 20824-0105
Phone: (301) 251-1222

American College of Sports Medicine
P.O. Box 1440
Indianapolis, IN 46206-1440
Phone: (317) 637-9200

Weight-Control Information Network
1 WIN WAY
BETHESDA, MD 20892-3665
Internet: WIN@matthewsgroup.com
Toll-free Number: (800) WIN-8098

The Weight-Control Information Network (WIN) is a service of the National Institute of Diabetes and Digestive and Kidney Diseases, part of the National Institutes of Health. Authorized by Congress (Public Law 103-43). WIN assembles and disseminates to health professionals and the general public information on weight control, obesity, and nutritional disorders, responds to requests for information; develops, reviews, and distributes publications; and develops communication strategies to encourage individuals to achieve and maintain a healthy weight.

Section 22.4

The Fatter Sex

©1993 Tufts University *Diet & Nutrition Letter*. Reprinted with Permission.

While it's common knowledge that men and women tend to gain weight after they marry, scientific findings suggest that overall, it's only men who fatten up as a direct result of having a ring placed on their fingers. In fact, they are twice as likely to be obese as never married or previously married men, say Cornell University researchers who looked over the records of more than 3,000 adults surveyed by the National Center for Health Statistics.

One reason may be that single men, who do not generally do much grocery shopping or cooking, eat more regularly or abundantly when women are around to put meals together for them. Then, too, unmarried men may intentionally manage their weight to be more attractive to potential marriage partners, but worry less about how they look after they "catch" a mate.

Women, on the other hand, are valued by their appearance more than men whether they are married or not, and therefore may remain more vigilant about their battle against the bulge even with a wedding band.

Paradoxically, excess weight is associated with illness and early death, whereas marriage, particularly for men, is associated with a lower rate of disease and a longer life. In other words, married men are better off healthwise than single men even though they are fatter. How can that be?

The researchers contend that certain effects of marriage may be so powerful they overcome the costs of the higher rate of obesity. They point to studies indicating that married men are more likely than the unmarried to get adequate sleep, avoid taking risks, sidestep substance abuse, and stay away from cigarettes. Another way of putting it: a pot belly may not be the greatest thing for a man's health, but not smoking and living sensibly all around appears to be more important to his overall well-being.

Section 22.5

Losing Weight Safely

FDA Consumer, Publication No. (FDA) 96-1231. This article originally appeared in the January-February 1996 *FDA Consumer*. The version below is from a reprint of the original article and contains revisions made in June 1996.

Americans trying to lose weight have plenty of company. According to a 1995 report from the Institute of Medicine (IOM), tens of millions of Americans are dieting at any given time, spending more than $33 billion yearly on weight-reduction products, such as diet foods and drinks.

Yet, studies over the last two decades by the National Center for Health Statistics show that obesity in the United States is actually on the rise. Today, approximately 35 percent of women and 31 percent of men age 20 and older are considered obese, up from approximately 30 percent and 25 percent, respectively, in 1980.

The words obesity and overweight are generally used interchangeably. However, according to the IOM report, their technical meanings are not identical. Overweight refers to an excess of body weight that includes all tissues, such as fat, bone and muscle. Obesity refers specifically to an excess of body fat. It is possible to be overweight without being obese, as in the case of a body builder who has a substantial amount of muscle mass. It is possible to be obese without being overweight, as in the case of a very sedentary person who is within the desirable weight range but who nevertheless has an excess of body fat. However, most overweight people are also obese and vice versa. Men with more than 25 percent and women with more than 30 percent body fat are considered obese.

Many people who diet fail to lose weight—or, if they do lose, fail to maintain the lower weight over the long term. As the IOM report, "Weighing The Options: Criteria for Evaluating Weight-Management Programs," points out, obesity is "a complex, multifactorial disease of appetite regulation and energy metabolism."

Because many factors affect how much or how little food a person eats and how that food is metabolized, or processed, by the body, losing weight is not simple. For example, recent studies suggest a role for genetic makeup in obesity. This area is still controversial, and more studies will be needed before scientists can say with certainty that a person's genes may set limits on how much weight can be lost and maintained.

Yet many people persist in seeking simple cures to this complex health problem. Lured by fad diets or pills that promise a quick and easy path to thinness, they end up disappointed when they regain lost weight.

"When it comes to weight loss, if something sounds too good—or too easy, or too delicious—to be true, it probably is," says Victor Herbert, M.D., J.D., professor of medicine and director of the Nutrition Center at the Mount Sinai School of Medicine and Bronx VA Medical Centers in New York City, and member of the board of directors of the National Council Against Health Fraud. "If a weight loss claim is sensational, it is not true; if it is true, it is not sensational."

No Shortcuts

"There are no shortcuts—no magic pills," adds Lori Love of the Food and Drug Administration's Center for Food Safety and Applied Nutrition. Losing weight sensibly and safely requires a multifaceted approach that includes setting reasonable weight-loss goals, changing eating habits, and getting adequate exercise. Appetite suppressants (diet pills) or other products may help some people over the short term, but they are not a substitute for adopting healthful eating habits over the long term.

The first step in losing weight safely is to determine a realistic weight goal. Table 22.1, developed by the U.S. Department of Agriculture and the Department of Health and Human Services, offers a range of suggested weights for adults based on their height.

A physician, dietitian or nutritionist also can help you set a reasonable goal. To reach the goal safely, plan to lose 1 to 2 pounds weekly by consuming approximately 300 to 500 fewer calories daily than usual (women and inactive men generally need to consume approximately 2,000 calories to maintain weight; men and very active women may consume up to 2,500 calories daily).

Moderation, Variety and Balance

After determining a reasonable goal weight, devise an eating plan based on the cornerstones of healthful eating—moderation, variety and balance, suggests Herbert.

"Moderation means not eating too much or too little of any particular food or nutrient; variety means eating as wide a variety as possible from each, and within each, of the five basic food groups; and balance refers to the balance achieved by following moderation and variety, as well as the balance of calories consumed versus calories expended," he explains. To lose weight, fewer calories should be consumed than expended; to maintain weight loss, the number of calories consumed and expended should be about the same.

Because fat is the most concentrated source of calories (9 calories per gram compared to 4 calories per gram for carbohydrate and protein), it is usually the focus of weight-maintenance and weight-loss diets. Limiting fat intake alone will likely limit calories, as well. Just as for the general population, weight-conscious consumers should limit fat intake to no more than 30 percent of total calories, according to the *Dietary Guidelines for Americans*.

Alcoholic beverages also are a source of calories (7 per gram of alcohol). Twelve ounces of regular beer, for example, provides 150 calories; the same amount of "light" beer, 105 calories. Five ounces of wine or 1.5 ounces of 80-proof distilled spirits provide 100 calories. But alcohol provides few, if any, nutrients, so if you drink alcoholic beverages and want to reduce your weight, consider reducing or eliminating your alcohol intake.

In selecting your diet, follow the five basic food groups and the recommended number of servings from each as incorporated into the Food Guide Pyramid developed by USDA and HHS. These groups are (1) bread, cereal, pasta, and rice; (2) vegetables; (3) fruits; (4) milk, yogurt and cheese; and (5) meat, poultry, fish, dry beans, eggs, and nuts. A sixth group (fats, oils and sweets) consists mainly of items that are pleasing to the palate but high in fat and/or calories; these should be eaten in moderation.

Avoid low-calorie fad diets that exclude whole categories of food such as carbohydrates (bread and pasta) or proteins (meat and poultry). These diets may be harmful because they generally do not include all nutrients necessary for good health. "Every fad diet that demands an unusual eating pattern, such as emphasizing only a few types of foods, deviates from one or more of the guidelines of moderation, variety and balance," says Herbert. "The greater the deviation, the more harmful the diet is likely to be."

Using the Food Label

To help consumers plan a healthful diet, FDA and USDA have revamped food labels. By law, most food labels now must display a Nutrition Facts panel containing information about how the food can fit into an overall daily diet. Nutrition Facts state how much saturated fat, cholesterol, fiber, and certain nutrients are contained in each serving. Serving sizes must now be based on standards set for similar kinds of food, so the nutritional value of similar products may be compared.

On the food label, Percent Daily Value shows what percentage of a given nutrient is provided in one portion for daily diets of 2,000 calories.

Whether or not a given food fits into a weight-loss diet depends on what other foods you eat that day. For most people, the goal is to select a variety of foods that together add up to approximately 100 percent of the Daily Value for total carbohydrate, dietary fiber, vitamins, and minerals; total fat, cholesterol and sodium each may add up to less than 100 percent.

This system permits a good deal of flexibility. No food is inherently "bad"; it is the total diet for the day that counts. You may compensate for an occasional rich dessert or serving of fried food by eating foods that are low in fat, oil or sugar for the rest of the day. However, high-fat foods should be limited, because they can quickly use up a day's supply of calories without providing high percentages of vital nutrients.

Look on the nutrition label for words such as "low," "light" or "reduced" to describe the calorie and fat content per serving. These foods must have significantly fewer calories or significantly less fat than similar products that do not make these claims.

Foods that claim to contain fewer calories or less fat than similar servings of similar products must show the difference on the label.

For example, on a container of low-fat cottage cheese, the label would show that a serving of the low-fat product contains 80 calories and 1.5 grams of fat while regular cottage cheese contains 120 calories and 5 grams of fat per serving.

Simple modifications in food selection and preparation allow you to include traditional favorites and snacks within the context of a healthful weight-loss diet; for example, select 1 percent or skim milk products instead of those made with whole milk, lean cuts of meat and poultry, and nonfat frozen yogurt instead of ice cream. Low-fat plain yogurt may be substituted for sour cream in dips, dressings or spreads; reduced-fat cheeses may be used instead of those made from whole milk. Broil, roast or steam foods instead of frying.

Load up on foods high in fiber, such as fruits, vegetables, legumes and whole grains. Fiber can be an important aid in weight mainte-nance because eating enough of it can help make a person feel full and thus not eat as much.

Also, include small portions of desserts or high-fat snacks rather than attempting to cut them out altogether. Eliminating favorite foods may result in cravings that can lead to binge eating and weight gain.

Exercise

Regular exercise is important for overall health as well as for los-ing and maintaining weight. There is evidence to suggest that body fat distribution affects health risks. For example, excess fat in the abdominal area (as opposed to hips and thighs) is associated with greater risk for high blood pressure, diabetes, early heart disease, and certain types of cancer. Vigorous exercise can reduce abdominal fat and thus lower the risk of these diseases.

The Dietary Guidelines for Americans recommends a half hour or more of moderate physical activity on most days, preferably every day. The activity can include brisk walking, calisthenics, home care, gar-dening, moderate sports exercise, and dancing. Regular exercise can help the body use up calories consumed daily, as well as excess calo-ries stored as fat. Weight-bearing exercises also help tone muscles and may reduce the risk of osteoporosis.

Over-the-Counter Diet Pills

The 1991/1992 Weight Loss Practices Survey, sponsored by FDA and the National Heart, Lung, and Blood Institute, found that 5 per-cent of women and 2 percent of men trying to lose weight use diet pills.

Products considered by FDA to be over-the-counter weight control drugs are primarily those containing the active ingredient phenylpropanolamine (PPA), such as Dexatrim and Acutrim. PPA is available OTC for weight control in a 75-mg controlled-release dosage form, when combined with a restricted diet and exercise.

Using diet pills containing PPA will not make a big difference in the rate of weight loss, says Robert Sherman of FDA's Office of OTC Drug Evaluation. "Even the best studies show only about a half pound greater weight loss per week using PPA combined with diet and exercise," he adds. Sherman cautions that the recommended dosage of these pills should not be exceeded because of the risk of possible adverse effects, such as elevated blood pressure and heart palpitations.

Since PPA is also used as a nasal decongestant in over-the-counter cough and cold products, consumers should read the labels of OTC decongestants to see if they contain PPA. They should not take PPA in two products labeled for different uses.

Sherman notes that FDA has received a small number of reports indicating that PPA use might be associated with an increased risk of stroke. A large-scale safety study was begun in September 1994 to explore the possibility. Based on available data, the agency does not believe that an increased risk of stroke is a concern when PPA is used at recommended dosages.

Rx Drugs

FDA has approved several prescription drugs for treating obesity. These include:

- Dexedrine and other amphetamines

- Ionamin and Adipex-P (phentermine) and other amphetamine derivatives

- Pondimin (fenfluramine hydrochloride) and Redux (dexfenfluramine), drugs not related to amphetamines.

The drugs appear to accomplish the same thing: They seem to help people on calorie-restricted diets adhere more closely to their diet, says Leo Lutwak, M.D., Ph.D., of FDA's division of metabolism and endocrine drug products. In studies of people on calorie-restricted diets, those who took the drugs lost more weight on average than those who took a placebo. The amount of weight lost varied but tended to be a loss of a fraction of a pound more per week.

The drugs' potential to promote long-term maintenance of weight loss has not been demonstrated except in the case of dexfenfluramine, which has been found effective and safe for use up to one year.

The drugs are "not magic pills," Lutwak warns. "They don't work unless you make dietary and exercise changes." FDA approved the drugs only for use with calorie-restricted diets.

The drugs face other restrictions. Except for dexfenfluramine, they should be used only for a few weeks. Dexfenfluramine can be used up to one year. Data on its safety and effectiveness beyond one year is not available.

Also, these drugs should be used only in people who are obese—not people looking to lose a few pounds, Lutwak says.

One reason is that the drugs are addictive and have the potential for abuse. Another is that the drugs have serious side effects, including high blood pressure and sleep disturbances. Also, certain drugs are not advised for people with certain medical conditions, such as phentermine for people with heart disease or high blood pressure, and fenfluramine and dexfenfluramine for people taking certain anti-depressants.

Weight-Loss Programs

Many people turn to weight-loss programs for help in planning a daily diet and changing lifestyle habits. The IOM report provides guidelines for evaluating the potential effectiveness of such programs.

"To improve their chances for success, consumers should choose programs that focus on long-term weight management; provide instruction in healthful eating, increasing activity, and improving self-esteem; and explain thoroughly the potential health risks from weight loss," according to the report. Consumers should also demand evidence of success. If it is absent or consists primarily of testimonials or other anecdotal evidence, "the program should be viewed with suspicion."

IOM recommends that potential clients be given a truthful, unambiguous, non-misleading statement about the program's approaches and goals, and a full disclosure of costs. The cost breakdown should include initial and ongoing costs, as well as the cost of extra products.

The basic tenet of weight loss—to eat fewer calories than you burn and to stay active—is easy to say but, like most lifestyle changes, not so easy to do. With realistic goals, and a commitment to losing weight slowly, safely and sensibly, the chances of long-term success improve dramatically.

Obesity a Disease

Obesity is now considered a disease—not a moral failing. According to a new report from the Institute of Medicine, "obesity is a heterogeneous disease in which genetic, environmental, psychological, and other factors are involved. It occurs when energy intake exceeds the amount of energy expended over time. Only in a small minority of cases is obesity caused by such illnesses as hypothyroidism or the result of taking medications, such as steroids, that can cause weight gain."

Public health concerns about this disease relate to its link to numerous other diseases that can lead to premature illness or death. The report notes that overweight individuals who lose even relatively small amounts of weight are likely to:

- lower their blood pressure (and thereby the risk of heart attack and stroke)

- reduce abnormally high levels of blood glucose (associated with diabetes)

- bring blood levels of cholesterol and triglycerides (associated with cardiovascular disease) down to more desirable levels

- reduce sleep apnea, or irregular breathing during sleep

- decrease the risk of osteoarthritis of the weight-bearing joints

- decrease depression

- increase self-esteem.

Of course, losing excess weight is also likely to improve appearance, which is a strong motivation for many people.

To order a copy of the IOM report, call (1-800) 624-6242 (in Washington, D.C., call 202-334-3313). The cost is $30 plus $4 shipping and handling.

—Marilynn Larkin

Marilynn Larkin is a writer in New York City.
Paula Kurtzweil, a member of FDA's public affairs staff, also contributed to this article.

Section 22.6

"Beer Belly" More Than a Figure of Speech

©1992 Tufts University *Diet & Nutrition Letter*. Reprinted with Permission.

It's no secret that the more frequently someone makes it through a six pack, the greater the chance that he (or she) will develop an unsightly beer belly. But it's not just the extra calories in beer, or any other alcoholic beverage for that matter, that adds flab. The latest word is that alcohol also appears to slow the rate at which the body burns fat, thereby making it more likely to "stick to" the gut-or thighs or buttocks.

Swiss scientists found that out when they instructed a group of young men to drink enough alcoholic beverages for a day to add 25 percent more calories than usual to their diets and, during a separate 24-hour period, replaced 25 percent of their calories with alcohol. Either way, the men's bodies burned about a third less fat than on days when they drank no alcohol at all.

The upshot: habitually drinking beer, wine, or any other form of alcohol may shift metabolism such that fat is more likely to end up on the belly, hips, or thighs than broken down and "sent" out of the body.

Section 22.7

Choosing a Safe and Successful Weight-Loss Program

NIH Publication No. 94-3700. NIDDK Web Document, (http://www.niddk.nih.gov/nutritiondocs.html). This statement was developed with the advice of the National Task Force on Prevention and Treatment of Obesity, a subcommittee of the National Digestive Diseases Advisory Board. December 1993.

Almost any of the commercial weight-loss programs can work, but only if they motivate you sufficiently to decrease the amount of calories you eat or increase the amount of calories you burn each day (or both). What elements of a weight-loss program should an intelligent consumer look for in judging its potential for safe and successful weight loss? A responsible and safe weight-loss program should be able to document for you the five following features:

- The diet should be safe. It should include all of the Recommended Daily Allowances (RDAs) for vitamins, minerals, and protein. The weight-loss diet should be low in calories (energy) only, not in essential foodstuffs.

- The weight-loss program should be directed toward a slow, steady weight loss unless your doctor feels your health condition would benefit from more rapid weight loss. Expect to lose only about a pound a week after the first week or two. With many calorie-restricted diets there is an initial rapid weight loss during the first one to two weeks, but this loss is largely fluid. The initial rapid loss of fluid also is regained rapidly when you return to a normal-calorie diet. Thus, a reasonable goal of weight loss must be expected.

- If you plan to lose more than 15 to 20 pounds, have any health problems, or take medication on a regular basis, you should be evaluated by your doctor before beginning your weight-loss

579

program. A doctor can assess your general health and medical conditions that might be affected by dieting and weight loss. Also, a physician should be able to advise you on the need for weight loss, the appropriateness of the weight-loss program, and a sensible goal of weight loss for you. If you plan to use a very-low-calorie diet (a special liquid formula diet that replaces all food intake for one to four months), you definitely should be examined and monitored by a doctor.

- Your program should include plans for weight maintenance after the weight loss phase is over. It is of little benefit to lose a large amount of weight only to regain it. Weight maintenance is the most difficult part of controlling weight and is not consistently implemented in weight-loss programs. The program you select should include help in permanently changing your dietary habits and level of physical activity, to alter a lifestyle that may have contributed to weight gain in the past. Your program should provide behavior modification help, including education in healthy eating habits and long-term plans to deal with weight problems. One of the most important factors in maintaining weight loss appears to be increasing daily physical activity, often by sensible increases in daily activity, as well as incorporating an individually tailored exercise program.

- A commercial weight-loss program should provide a detailed statement of fees and costs of additional items such as dietary supplements.

Obesity affects about one in four adult Americans, and during any one year, over half of Americans go on a weight-loss diet or are trying to maintain their weight. For many people who try to lose weight, it is difficult to lose more than a few pounds and few succeed in remaining at the reduced weight. The difficulty in losing weight and keeping it off leads many people to turn to a professional or commercial weight-loss program for help. These programs are quite popular and are widely advertised in newspapers and on television. What is the evidence that any of these programs is worthwhile, that they will help you lose weight and keep it off and that they will do it safely?

Obesity is a chronic condition. Too often it is viewed as a temporary problem that can be treated for a few months with a strenuous diet. However, as most overweight people know, weight control must be considered a life-long effort. To be safe and effective, any weight-loss program must address the long-term approach or else the program is largely a waste of money and effort.

Chapter 23

Exercise

Chapter Contents

Section 23.1

Anabolic Steroids: A Threat to Body and Mind

DHHS Pub. No. (ADM) 91-1810.

The Price of Perfection

Shock waves went through the sports world when Canadian track superstar Ben Johnson was denied his gold medal at the 1988 Olympics after tests showed he had taken anabolic steroids. The incident called international attention to the use of anabolic steroids among world-class athletes to gain competitive advantage.

Still, athletes and nonathletes alike persist in taking them. Teenagers are taking anabolic steroids not just to excel in sports but to enhance their self-images by perfecting their physiques. There are even reports of male adults in physically demanding professions like law enforcement using them to appear tougher and more formidable.

As the drug grows in popularity so does awareness of the serious side effects it may cause. One of the most alarming is the threat of AIDS. HIV—human immunodeficiency virus—can be transmitted if shared needles are used to inject the drug.

But potential harm to physical and psychological health is only one aspect of this troubling trend.

A Question of Values

The nonmedical use of anabolic steroids raises more ethical and moral issues. Engaging in steroids use is illegal. Users are likely to find themselves acquiring these drugs through illicit—and expensive—channels. The heavy demand for anabolic steroids has given rise to a black market, with sales estimated at as much as $400 million a year. Moreover, supplies, which are often illegally manufactured and do not meet established standards, may be contaminated.

Athletes who use these drugs are cheating. They gain an unfair advantage over opponents and violate the ban on steroids imposed by most major sports organizations.

Another Addictive Substance?

Can anabolic steroids be added to the list of addictive drugs? Early signs point to addictive patterns among users. At the very least, users demonstrate an unwillingness to give up anabolic steroids even in the face of possibly dire consequences to their health.

Stopping the Trend

As the health risks of anabolic steroids become more apparent, efforts to curtail their use—through education, legislation, and medical practices—are intensifying.

For those already hooked, kicking the steroids habit is the best chance to escape devastating side effects. For potential users, the solution, of course, is to never take the drug at all. There are other ways to be a winner athletically and socially without harming health and without cheating.

Using Anabolic Steroids

Valid Medical Uses

Steroids are drugs derived from hormones. Anabolic steroids comprise one group of these hormonal drugs. In certain cases, some may have therapeutic value.

The U.S. Food and Drug Administration has approved the use of selected anabolic steroids for treating specific types of anemia, some breast cancers, osteoporosis, endometriósis, and hereditary angioedema, a rare disease involving the swelling of some parts of the body.

Some medical specialists believe that anabolic steroids can improve the appetite and improve healing after surgery, but the FDA has withdrawn approval for such uses since the claims are vague and largely unsubstantiated.

What Are Anabolic Steroids?

Anabolic steroids—or more precisely, anabolic/androgenic steroids—belong to a group known as ergogenic, or so-called "performance-enhancing," drugs. They are synthetic derivatives of testosterone, a natural male hormone.

"Anabolic" means growing or building. "Androgenic" means "masculinizing" or generating male sexual characteristics.

Most healthy males produce between 2 and 10 milligrams of testosterone a day. (Females do produce some testosterone, but in trace amounts.) The hormone's anabolic effects help the body retain dietary protein, thus aiding growth of muscles, bones, and skin.

The androgenic characteristics of testosterone are associated with masculinity. They foster the maturing of the male reproductive system in puberty, the growth of body hair and the deepening of the voice. They can affect aggressiveness and sex drive.

Do They Really Work?

Anabolic steroids are designed to mimic the bodybuilding traits of testosterone while minimizing its "masculinizing" effects. There are several types, with various combinations of anabolic and androgenic properties. The International Olympics Committee to date has placed 17 anabolic steroids and related compounds on its banned list.

Athletes who have used anabolic steroids—as well as some coaches, trainers, and physicians—do report significant increases in lean muscle mass, strength, and endurance. But no studies show that the substances enhance performance.

Anabolic steroids do not improve agility, skill or cardiovascular capacity. Some athletes insist that these substances aid in recovery from injuries, but no hard data exists to support the claim.

Sports Organizations Outlawing Anabolic Steroids

The International Olympics Committee banned steroids use by all athletes in its member associations in 1975. Since then most major amateur and professional organizations have put the drugs on their list of banned substances. They include:

- National Football League
- National Collegiate Athletic Association
- International Amateur Athletic Federation
- International Federation of Body Builders

A Brief History

Winning Through Doping

The drive to compete—and to win—is as old as humankind. Throughout history, athletes have sought foods and potions to transform their bodies into powerful, well-tuned machines.

Greek wrestlers ate huge quantities of meat to build muscle, and Norse warriors—the Berserkers—ate hallucinogenic mushrooms to gear up for battle.

The first competitive athletes believed to be charged with "doping"—taking drugs and other nonfood substances to improve performance—were swimmers in Amsterdam in the 1860s. Doping, with anything from strychnine and caffeine to cocaine and heroin, spread to other sports over the next several decades.

Enter Anabolic Steroids

The use of anabolic steroids by athletes is relatively new. Testosterone was first synthesized in the 1930s and was introduced into the sporting arena in the 1940s and 1950s. When the Russian weightlifting team—thanks, in part, to synthetic testosterone—walked off with a pile of medals at the 1952 Olympics, an American physician determined that U.S. competitors should have the same advantage.

By 1958 a U.S. pharmaceutical firm had developed anabolic steroids. Although the physician soon realized the drug had unwanted side effects, it was too late to halt its spread into the sports world.

Early users were mainly bodybuilders, weightlifters, football players, and discus, shot put, or javelin throwers—competitors who relied heavily on bulk and strength.

During the 1970s demand grew as athletes in other sports sought the competitive edge that anabolic steroids seemed to provide.

By the 1980s, as nonathletes also discovered the body-enhancing properties of steroids, a black market began to flourish for the illegal production and sale of the drugs for nonmedical purposes.

The Position of the Medical Community

The American Medical Association condemns the use of anabolic steroids by athletes. Other medical associations have joined with the AMA in deploring steroids abuse, including the:

- American Academy of Pediatrics
- American College of Sports Medicine
- American Osteopathic Academy of Sports Medicine

Abusing Anabolic Steroids

Who Takes Them—And Why?

Today it is not only the college football player or the professional weightlifter or the marathon runner who may use anabolic steroids.

585

It may be an 18-year-old who loathes his skinny body. Or a 15-year-old in a hurry to reach maturity.

Or a policeman who wants more muscle power on the job.

And the use of anabolic steroids is not confined to males. Professional and amateur female athletes—track and field competitors, swimmers, bodybuilders—feel the pressure to triumph, too.

Increasing numbers of adolescents are turning to steroids for cosmetic reasons. In a 1986 survey, as many as 45 percent of 200 high school users cited appearance as a primary reason for taking steroids.

Young people who use steroids defy easy categorizing. They come from cities and rural areas, from poor families and wealthy ones. They are of all races and nationalities. The common link among them is the desire to look, perform and feel better—at almost any cost. Users—and especially the young—are apt to ignore or deny warnings about health risks. If they see friends growing taller and stronger on steroids, they want the same benefits. They want to believe in the power of the drug.

How Prevalent Is Use?

Surveys and anecdotal evidence indicate that the rate of nonmedical steroids use may be increasing.

In 1990, a NIDA survey of high school seniors showed that nearly 3 percent—5 percent of males and 0.5 percent of females—reported using steroids at some time in their lives.

The same survey showed that steroids were used within the last year by nearly as many students as crack cocaine and by more students than the hallucinogenic drug PCP.

Use among college females appears to have increased somewhat. A study of 11 universities in 1984 found that steroids users were reported in only one women's sport—swimming—at a rate of 1 percent. In a follow-up survey in 1988, 1 percent of women in track and field and basketball also reported taking steroids.

Use among adult or professional athletes has not been well documented, although anecdotal evidence clearly supports the suggestion that anabolic steroids have enjoyed popularity among football players, weightlifters, wrestlers, and track and field competitors, among others.

A Glossary of Terms

Drug and steroids use in sports has spawned a glossary of its own:

- *Blending*—Mixing different drugs.
- *Bulking up*—Increasing muscle mass through steroids.
- *Cycling*—Taking multiple doses of steroids over a specified period of time, stopping for a time and starting again.
- *Doping*—Using drugs and other nonfood substances to improve athletic performance and prowess.
- *Ergogenic drugs*—Performance-enhancing substances.
- *Megadosing*—Taking massive amounts of steroids, by injection or pill.
- *Plateauing*—When a drug becomes ineffective at a certain level.
- *Roid rages*—Uncontrolled outbursts of anger, frustration or combativeness that may result from using anabolic steroids.
- *Shotgunning*—Taking steroids on a hit-or-miss basis.
- *Stacking*—Using a combination of anabolic steroids, often in combination with other drugs.
- *Tapering*—Slowly decreasing steroids intake.

Megadosing

Anabolic steroids are usually taken in pill form. Some that cannot be absorbed orally are taken by injection. The normal prescribed daily dose for medical purposes usually averages between 1 and 5 milligrams.

Some athletes, on the other hand, may take up to hundreds of milligrams a day, far exceeding medically recommended dosages. Operating on the erroneous more-is-better theory, some athletes indulge in a practice known as "stacking." They take many types of steroids, sometimes in combination with other drugs such as stimulants, depressants, pain killers, anti-inflammatories, and other hormones.

Many users "cycle," taking the drugs for 6 to 12 weeks or more, stopping for several weeks and then starting another cycle. They may do this in the belief that by scheduling their steroids intake, they can manipulate test results and escape detection. It is not uncommon for athletes to cycle over a period of months or even years.

Health Hazards

Raising a Red Flag

Although controlled studies on the long-term outcome of megadosing with anabolic steroids have not been conducted, extensive research on prescribed doses for medical use has documented the potential side effects of the drug, even when taken in small doses. Moreover, reports by athletes, and observations of attending physicians, parents, and coaches do offer substantial evidence of dangerous side effects.

Some effects, such as rapid weight gain, are easy to see. Some take place internally and may not be evident until it is too late. Some are irreversible.

The Dangers

Dangers to Men. Males who take large doses of anabolic steroids typically experience changes in sexual characteristics. Although derived from a male sex hormone, the drug can trigger a mechanism in the body that can actually shut down the healthy functioning of the male reproductive system. Some possible side effects:

- Shrinking of the testicles
- Reduced sperm count
- Impotence
- Baldness
- Difficulty or pain in urinating
- Development of breasts
- Enlarged prostate

Dangers to Women. Females may experience "masculinization" as well as other problems:

- Growth of facial hair
- Changes in or cessation of the menstrual cycle
- Enlargement of the clitoris
- Deepened voice
- Breast reduction

Dangers to Both Sexes. For both males and females, continued use of anabolic steroids may lead to health conditions ranging from merely irritating to life-threatening. Some effects are:

- Acne
- Jaundice
- Trembling
- Swelling of feet or ankles
- Bad breath

- Reduction in HDL, the "good" cholesterol
- High blood pressure
- Liver damage and cancers
- Aching joints
- Increased chance of injury to tendons, ligaments, and muscles

Special Dangers to Adolescents

Anabolic steroids can halt growth prematurely in adolescents. Because even small doses can irreversibly affect growth, steroids are rarely prescribed for children and young adults, and only for the severely ill.

The Office of the Inspector General in the U.S. Department of Health and Human Services has gathered anecdotal evidence that preteens and teens taking steroids may be at risk for developing a dependence on the drugs and on other substances as well.

The Threat of AIDS

People sometimes take injections of anabolic steroids to augment oral dosages, using large-gauge, reusable needles normally obtained through the black market. If needles are shared, users run the risk of transmitting or contracting the HIV infection that can lead to AIDS.

The Psychological Effects

Scientists are just beginning to investigate the impact of anabolic steroids on the mind and behavior. Many athletes report "feeling good" about themselves while on a steroids regimen. The downside, according to Harvard researchers, is wide mood swings ranging from periods of violent, even homicidal, episodes known as "roid rages" to bouts of depression when the drugs are stopped.

The Harvard study also noted that anabolic steroids users may suffer from paranoid jealousy, extreme irritability, delusions, and impaired judgment stemming from feelings of invincibility.

Are Anabolic Steriods Addictive?

Evidence that megadoses of anabolic steroids can affect the brain and produce mental changes in users poses serious questions about possible addiction to the drugs.

While investigations continue, researchers at Yale University have found that long-term steroids users do experience many of the characteristics of classic addiction: cravings, difficulty in ceasing steroids use and withdrawal symptoms.

Pennsylvania State University researchers studied a group of high school seniors who had developed a psychological, if not physical, dependence on anabolic steroids. Adolescent users exhibit a prime trait of addicts—denial. They tend to overlook or simply ignore the physical dangers and moral implications of taking illegal substances.

Certain delusional behavior that is characteristic of addiction can occur. Some athletes who "bulk up" on anabolic steroids are unaware of body changes that are obvious to others, experiencing what is sometimes called reverse anorexia.

Supply and Demand: The Black Market

Many users maintain their habit with anabolic steroids acquired through a highly organized black market handling up to $400 million worth of the drugs a year.

Until recently most underground steroids were legitimately manufactured pharmaceuticals that were diverted to the black market through theft and fraudulent prescriptions. More effective law enforcement coupled with greater demand forced black marketers to seek new sources.

Now black-market anabolic steroids are either made overseas and smuggled into the United States or are produced in clandestine laboratories in this country. These counterfeit drugs may present greater health risks because they are manufactured without controls and thus may be impure, mislabeled, or simply bogus.

Sales are made in gyms, health clubs, on campuses, and through the mail. Users report that suppliers may be drug dealers or they may be trainers, physicians, pharmacists, or friends.

It's not hard for users to buy the drugs or to learn how to use them. Many of them rely on an underground manual, a "bible" on steroids that circulates around the country.

Safe—And Healthy—Alternatives

Anabolic steroids may have a reputation for turning a wimp into a winner or a runt into a hulk, but the truth is that it takes a lot more to be a star athlete.

Athletic prowess depends not only on strength and endurance, but on skill and mental acuity. It also depends on diet, rest, overall mental and physical health, and genes. Athletic excellence can be, and is, achieved by millions without reliance on dangerous drugs.

Fighting Back

Testing

The major national and international sports associations enforce their ban against anabolic steroids by periodic testing. Testing, however, is controversial.

Some observers say the tests are not reliable, and even the International Olympic Committees tests, considered to be the most accurate, have been challenged. Athletes can manipulate results with "masking agents" to prevent detection, or they can take anabolic steroids that have calculable detection periods.

Despite the problems, testing remains an important way of monitoring and controlling the abuse of steroids among athletes. Efforts are underway to make testing more accurate.

Treatment

Treatment programs for steroids abusers are just now being developed as more is learned about the habit.

Medical specialists do find persuasion is an important weapon is getting the user off the drug. They attempt to present medical evidence of the damage anabolic steroids can do to the body. One specialist notes that medical tests, such as those that show a lowered sperm count, can motivate male athletes to cease usage.

One health clinic considers the anabolic steroids habit as an addiction and structures treatment around the techniques used in traditional substance abuse programs. It focuses on acute intervention and a long-term follow-up, introducing nonsteroid alternatives that will maintain body fitness as well as self-esteem.

Legislation

Both Federal and State governments have enacted laws and regulations to control anabolic steroids abuse.

In 1988, Congress passed the Anti-Drug Abuse Act, making the distribution or possession of anabolic steroids for nonmedical reasons a Federal offense. Distribution to minors is a prison offense.

In 1990, Congress toughened the laws, passing legislation that classifies anabolic steroids as a controlled substance. The new law also increases penalties for steroids use and trafficking. To halt diversion of anabolic steroids onto the black market, the law imposes strict production and recordkeeping regulations on pharmaceutical firms.

Over 25 states have passed laws and regulations to control steroids abuse, and many others are considering similar legislation.

Education

Prevention is the best solution to halting the growing abuse of anabolic steroids. The time to educate youngsters is before they become users.

Efforts must not stop there, however. Current users, as well as coaches, trainers, parents, and medical practitioners need to know about the hazards of anabolic steroids. The young need to understand that they are not immortal and that the drugs can harm them. An education campaign must also address the problem of covert approval by some members of the medical and athletic communities that encourages steroids use.

The message needs to be backed up by accurate information and spread by responsible, respected individuals.

For Further Information

NIDA Hotline
1-800-662-HELP

Operated by the National Institute on Drug Abuse, this is a confidential information and referral line that directs callers to drug abuse treatment centers in their local community.

NCADI
1-800-729-6686

The National Clearinghouse for Alcohol and Drug Information (NCADI) provides information on all drugs, including alcohol. Free materials on drug abuse are also available. If you wish to write NCADI, the address is P.O. Box 2345, Rockville, MD 20852.

Resources

American College of Sports Medicine, "Position Stand on The Use of Anabolic/Androgenic Steroids in Sports," 1984.

American Osteopathic Academy of Sports Medicine, "Policy Statement and Position Paper: Anabolic/ Androgenic Steroids and Substance Abuse in Sport," May 1989.

Buckley, W.E.; Yesalis, C.E.; Vicary J.R.; Streit, A; Katz D.L.; Wright, J.E., "Indications of Psychological Dependence Among Anabolic/Androgenic Steroids Abusers." Adaptation from a paper, "Anabolic steroids Use: Indications of Habituation Among Adolescents," *Journal of Drug Education*, 1989.

Carolan, N.J., "The Treatment of the Anabolic steroids Addict," Unpublished paper, 1991.

Cicero, T.J., and O'Connor, L.H., "Abuse Liability of Anabolic Steroids and Their Possible Role in the Abuse of Alcohol, Morphine and Other Substances," *NIDA Research Monograph 102*, 1990.

Dyment, P.G., and Goldberg, B., Committee on Sports Medicine, "Anabolic Steroids and the Adolescent Athlete," *Pediatrics*, January 1989.

Frankle, M.A., "Anabolic-Androgenic Steroids: A Guide for the Physician," *The Journal of Musculoskeletal Medicine*, November 1989.

Friedl, K.E., "Reappraisal of the Health Risks Associated with the Use of High Doses of Oral and Injectable Androgenic Steroids," *NIDA Research Monograph 102*, 1990.

Hecht, A., "Anabolic Steroids: Pumping Trouble," FDA Consumer, September 1984.

International Federation of Bodybuilders, "The Battle Against Steroids Goes On: Position Paper of the I.F.B.B," 1990.

Kashkin, K.B., and Kleber, H.D., "Hooked on Hormones? An Anabolic Steroid Addiction Hypothesis," *Journal of the American Medical Association*, December 1989.

Katz, D.L., and Pope, H.G., "Anabolic/Androgenic Steroid-Induced Mental Status Changes," *NIDA Research Monograph 102*, 1990.

Kennedy, N., "Steroid Studies: Estimated Percentages of Use," Appendix B of the Research Subcommittee of the Interagency Task Force on Anabolic Steroids, National Institute on Drug Abuse, 1990.

Lombardo, J.A., "Anabolic/Androgenic Steroids," *NIDA Research Monograph 102*, 1990.

Miller, R.W., "Athletes and Steroids: Playing a Deadly Game," *FDA Consumer*, November 1987.

National Institute on Drug Abuse, "Anabolic Steroids: Is Bigger Better or Just Big Trouble?," *NIDA Notes*, Spring/Summer 1989.

National Institute on Drug Abuse, "Study of Athletes Shows Aggression and Other Psychiatric Side Effects From Steroid Use," *NIDA Notes*, Spring/Summer 1989.

Norris, J.A., "FDA Warns: Steroids May Be Hazardous to Your Health," *Schools Without Drugs: The Challenge*, U.S. Department of Education, November 1987.

Office of Inspector General, U.S. Department of Health and Human Services, "Adolescents and Steroids: A User Perspective," August 1990.

Office of Inspector General, U.S. Department of Health and Human Services, "Adolescent Steroid Use," 1990.

Stehlin, D., "For Athletes and Dealers, Black Market Steroids Are Risky Business," *FDA Consumer*, 1987.

U.S. Food and Drug Administration, "The Blackmarketing of Anabolic, Ergogenic and Related Prescription Drugs for Athletic Enhancement: An FDA Overview," *FDA Consumer*, 1987.

U.S. General Accounting Office, "Drug Misuse: Anabolic Steroids and Human Growth Hormone," August 1989.

Yesalis, C.E.; Anderson, W.A.; Buckley, W.E.; and Wright, J.E., "Incidence of Non-Medical Use of Anabolic Steroids," *NIDA Research Monograph 102*, 1990.

Section 23.2

Steroid Substitutes

"No-Win Situation for Athletes," *FDA Consumer*, December 1992.

German sprinters Katrin Krabbe and Grit Breuer never made it to the 1992 Summer Olympics in Barcelona, Spain.

United States hammer thrower Jud Logan and shot putter Bonnie Dasse went but were sent home early.

Also sent home from the Olympics were Wu Dan, a Chinese women's volleyball player; Madina Biktagirova, a Unified Team marathoner; and Andrew Davies and Andrew Saxton, both British weight lifters.

All tested positive for banned drugs, but, surprisingly to some fans, none of the drugs were anabolic steroids.

Krabbe, Breuer, Logan, Dasse, Davies, and Saxton tested positive for clenbuterol, a veterinary drug. Dan tested positive for strychnine, a poison that is a stimulant in small doses; and Biktagirova tested positive for norephedrine, a mild stimulant. Though the three drugs are not steroids, all are abused in sports because athletes believe they enhance performance.

From athletes in international competition to college and high school athletes to the teenager who simply wants to "bulk up," people of all ages and abilities have found alternatives to replace anabolic steroids.

Regulated by the Drug Enforcement Administration, anabolic steroids were placed in the Controlled Substances Act's Schedule III (which includes some narcotic drugs, stimulants and depressants) by the Anabolic Steroids Act of 1990. Unlawful distribution and possession with the intent to distribute anabolic steroids is a federal crime, punishable by up to five years in prison.

Since the law was enacted, many athletes have avoided anabolic steroids because of the penalties associated with their abuse, says Donald Leggett, a compliance officer in the Food and Drug Administration's Center for Drug Evaluation and Research. "They have looked at other chemicals that perform in a similar fashion but are not technically regulated as or called anabolic steroids."

Those alternatives include prescription, veterinary, investigational, and unapproved drugs, and dietary supplements.

Dietary supplements are regulated as foods. No data has been submitted to FDA to prove bodybuilding claims for these substances, and the short- and long-term effects of their use are unknown.

"Many alternatives are labeled as 'dietary supplements' even though they make anabolic and other athletic enhancement claims. Such attempts to market directly to the public may represent a circumvention of the safety and efficacy provisions required of drugs. Thus, the short- and long-term effects of their use are generally unknown," Leggett says.

When supplement manufacturers make bodybuilding and drug-type claims, FDA can, and often does, issue warning letters to the manufacturer or prosecute for consumer fraud. FDA's Center for Drug Evaluation and Research recently won several court cases involving consumer fraud by supplement manufacturers, Leggett says.

The consumer is defrauded by believing these supplements will build muscles or promote testosterone production, when in fact they do no such thing, he says.

In a study, published in the Aug. 26, 1992, *Journal of the American Medical Association*, of bodybuilding magazine advertisements, Rossanne M. Philen, M.D., and colleagues, report that they counted 89 supplement brands, 311 products, and 235 ingredients, most of which were unspecified amino acids. More than 22 percent of the products had no ingredients listed in their advertisements.

The study also found that many steroid-type ingredients, called sterols, were being advertised. With the exception of ecdysterone, the sterols were all plant derivatives. Ecdysterone is an insect hormone with no known use in humans.

The abuse of many of these ingredients, as well as prescription, veterinary, investigational, and unapproved drugs, concerns FDA.

Agency investigators have collected more than 3,000 drug samples from the black market over a 10-year period, according to Leggett. Many of those samples, he says, were not steroids but other, potentially more dangerous, prescription drugs.

Some steroid alternatives popular among athletes include the investigational drugs clenbuterol and gamma hydroxybutyric acid, or GHB, and approved prescription drugs such as human growth hormone and erythropoietin, better known as EPO.

Clenbuterol

Clenbuterol is used in several European countries by animal trainers to build muscle mass and strength in exhibition livestock. It has never been approved for any use in the United States.

Athletes use clenbuterol because they think it has the same mass and strength-building capability in people as it does in animals.

But clenbuterol also has serious, immediate side effects in humans. In Spain, between March and July 1990, 135 people became ill after eating beef liver that contained clenbuterol residues. Their symptoms included fast heart rate, muscle tremors, headache, dizziness, nausea, fever, and chills. Symptoms appeared from 30 minutes to six hours after they ate the liver and lasted for nearly two days.

Like most other steroid alternatives, the long-term effects of clenbuterol are not fully known. But, Leggett says, some serious cardiovascular complications may result from their use.

In many instances, veterinary drugs are used simply because they are easier than human drugs to obtain, Leggett says. "Historically, there are places in this country, particularly in rural areas, where just about anyone could walk in and purchase a veterinary equivalent of a [human] drug that would require a doctor's prescription."

Gamma Hydroxybutyric Acid

Gamma hydroxybutyric acid, better known as GHB, is another steroid alternative used widely by teenagers and athletes of all abilities.

GHB is an investigational new drug that powerfully and rapidly induces sleep and depresses the central nervous system in animals and humans, according to Leggett.

The drug has been illegally marketed as a steroid alternative both openly and "in the back room" in gyms, spas, and health food stores and advertised in bodybuilding magazines. Promoters claim it stimulates production of human growth hormone and thus produces muscle mass and weight loss. It has also been promoted as a sleep aid and touted as a street drug.

But GHB is extremely dangerous.

A Duluth, Ga., teenager, getting ready for his high school prom on May 11, 1990, drank a concoction of water and Somatomax PM, a powdery substance containing GHB his friend had bought at a health food store. Instead of getting the "high" he had expected, he was in a coma 20 minutes after taking the drink. Fortunately, his parents soon found him, and with emergency treatment he recovered.

There were 80 hospitalizations from GHB use reported through November 1990, according to a national Centers for Disease Control study published in the Nov. 30, 1990, issue of *Morbidity and Mortality Weekly Report.*

Patients reported that within 15 to 60 minutes of taking one-half to three teaspoons of GHB, they developed symptoms such as vomiting, drowsiness, dizziness, tremors, seizure-like movements, unconsciousness, slowed heartbeat, lowered blood pressure, breathing difficulty, and breathing cessation. Patients recovered, usually with emergency room care, in 2 to 96 hours. There have been no reported deaths.

Human Growth Hormone

Human growth hormone, or HGH, is another popular steroid alternative. Produced naturally by the human body, HGH's only approved medical use is to treat pituitary dwarfism, but it is under investigation to treat other disorders.

Human growth hormone, manufactured using recombinant DNA technology, is identical to the natural hormone. Some athletes believe that HGH promotes muscle growth and muscle strength although researchers have not confirmed these claims.

Lyle Alzado, a former Los Angeles Raiders defensive lineman, said in a July 4, 1991, *New York Times* article that human growth hormone has become the drug of choice for today's athlete, primarily because it is undetectable in drug tests. Alzado died May 14, 1992, from a rare form of brain cancer, central nervous system lymphoma, which he attributed to his prolonged use of steroids and HGH.

Too much human growth hormone, produced by a hyperactive pituitary gland or a tumor, is the cause of acromegaly, a condition characterized by excessive growth of the bones of the hands, feet and face. Acromegaly is ultimately fatal because of resulting heart disease and other metabolic problems.

Erythropoietin

Erythropoietin, or EPO, is another steroid alternative used in the international sports community although it has seen limited abuse in the United States.

EPO, approved for treating anemias associated with chronic renal failure and zidovudine (AZT) therapy in HIV-infected patients, stimulates bone marrow to produce red blood cells. The hormone appeals to athletes because they tire less easily when taking it and because it is undetectable by tests presently used.

"It [EPO] increases the red blood cell count, and therefore the athlete is able to absorb more oxygen and increase stamina—the oxygen-carrying capacity of the blood system is just unbelievable," Leggett says.

But EPO use is not without risk. As the body's red blood cell count rises and the blood thickens, blood clots, heart attack, or stroke could result.

Abuse of EPO is especially risky among marathoners and long-distance bicyclists. As these athletes compete, Leggett explains, they lose body fluids, including blood fluids. Reducing blood fluids concentrates the already abnormally high red blood cell count, which can lead to polycythemia, an abnormal increase in circulating red blood cells.

"EPO can turn their blood to the consistency of Jell-O," he says.

Severe Penalties

Here are some potential health effects of drugs and other substances—ranging from the mildest to the most severe—used as alternatives to anabolic steroids.

- greasy skin
- headache
- severe acne
- premature balding
- bloating associated with water retention
- dizziness
- chills
- drowsiness
- nausea
- vomiting
- muscle tremors
- fever

- fast heart rate
- slowed heart rate
- bloody diarrhea
- seizure-like movements
- lowered blood pressure
- breathing difficulty
- breathing cessation
- blood clots
- cardiovascular problems
- liver disease
- cancer
- heart attack
- stroke
- death

Deadly Potential

FDA is particularly concerned with athletes' abuse of prescription drugs because they usually take the drugs without a physician's supervision and in higher doses than recommended for their limited medical uses.

"We consider these things to have the potential for hazard when they're not monitored or taken in accordance with the supervision of a licensed practitioner," Leggett says.

"Many of these people take way above and beyond the directions for use simply because they feel 'the more the better.' That was true of anabolic steroids, too. The people who are taking these drugs are essentially saying, 'If one teaspoon is recommended, I'm going to take five and grow five times as fast.'"

With that philosophy, the potential for an overdose is very high—and so is the potential for death.

FDA is also concerned about the prescription, veterinary, investigational, and unapproved drugs used as steroid alternatives primarily because little is known of the short- and long-term effects these drugs may have on humans, especially when taken in higher-than-recommended doses or in combination with other drugs.

Comparing anabolic steroids to those steroid alternatives, Leggett says, "We approved all of these anabolic steroids for domestic use in treating diseases like anemias, osteoporosis, and certain cancers. We know what to expect from their label dosage and overdoses.

"We have no idea what a normal dosage or overdose is for many of the steroid alternatives or what might be their effect. This is because we've never seen any clinical studies reflecting their use in humans. So, we're completely without a baseline there."

Some short term reactions from using steroid alternatives are similar to those associated with anabolic steroid abuse. These reactions include: bloody diarrhea, nausea, vomiting, severe acne, premature balding, bloating associated with water retention, and greasy skin.

"Those are all soft effects, which may or may not be very serious," Leggett says. "But if the preliminary effects from using steroid alternatives are similar to those associated with anabolic steroid abuse, then there is the potential for some of the long-term effects, too. Effects long-term steroid abusers experience include cardiovascular problems, liver disease, certain cancers."

Clenbuterol, gamma hydroxybutyric acid, human growth hormone, and erythropoietin, all banned in international competition, are some of the more popular steroid alternatives athletes are now abusing. But, Leggett says, this list is likely to grow as athletes experiment with different and new chemicals.

As athletes strive for bigger, more muscular bodies through chemicals, Leggett, expecting the worst, says, "I'm sure they'll come up with something someday that's even more disastrous than the few [drugs] we've seen in recent years."

— by Kevin L. Ropp

Kevin L. Ropp is a staff writer for *FDA Consumer*.

Section 23.3

Flattening Your Tummy

"A flat, sexy stomach in 5 minutes flat!" (Yeah, right!)

It's a good time to be selling a machine that exercises the abdominal muscles. An estimated 2.75 million devices for reshaping the midsection were sold in 1995 at a total cost of $145 million.

Abs frenzy is absolutely inescapable. Four of the 10 most frequently shown cable TV infomercials feature ab machines, so it's impossible to channel-surf for more than a short while without seeing an ad for a gadget that will "tighten and tone your abs" or provide "firmer abs in just minutes a day." By the same token, you can browse magazine racks and find a slew of stories on how to "revamp your abs" or "ripple your gut."

Better—But Not Necessarily Flatter—Bodies

Alas, all the abdominal exercises in the world cannot give you a washboard stomach. That's because they don't spot-reduce the layer of fat many people have between the ab muscles and the skin. The only way to get rid of fat is to burn more calories than you consume. Even then, there's no guarantee that the tummy is where the fat will come off.

"Some people who get rid of fat when they burn calories lose everything from their arms and legs but not much from their bellies," says Miriam Nelson, PhD, an exercise physiologist at the Jean Mayer USDA Human Nutrition Research Center on Aging at Tufts. In other words, to a certain extent, washboard abs are born, not made. "Those flat-bellied Hollywood people you read about who do 500 stomach crunches a day—a lot of them have pretty darn good-looking bodies to begin with," Dr. Nelson comments.

That doesn't mean abdominal exercises are a waste of time, however. "Notoriously, in most people, the abdominal muscles are very weak and underdeveloped," Dr. Nelson says. "Those muscles should be stronger, more conditioned. They're part of the scaffolding for the spine, and when they're in good shape they help prevent or minimize back pain, a problem for many people." Toned abdominal muscles also improve posture, which prevents the body from sagging with the belly swayed out in front.

But you don't need to spend money on special equipment to perform an ab workout. "Different kinds of sit-ups will work your abs just fine," Dr. Nelson says. "And they're free."

Moreover, she explains, some machines don't actually work the abdominals. Some end up toning muscles in the arms or hips more than those in the stomach. Most machines that do work the abdominal muscles don't work the opposing muscles in the lower back.

A machine that trains just one set of muscles is not a bad thing in and of itself, Dr. Nelson says. But if you focus only on training the abdominals, your back is going to slump more and your posture will worsen. And that could lead to discomfort.

Evaluating Popular Ab-Shaping Machines

Not everybody feels motivated enough to get down on the living room floor and start doing sit-ups. Some people become more committed to exercise if they invest in a piece of body-toning equipment. For those who think they might like to buy a stomach-crunching aid, exercise physiologist Dr. Nelson and certified personal trainer Michael Wood, also of the physiology laboratory at Tufts's Human Nutrition Research Center, evaluated some of the most popular ab-training gadgetry on the market:

Ab Roller Plus, $89.95. This contraption rolls forward with you as you lift off the ground, making it easier to initiate sit-ups from the stomach rather than from the arms. Therefore, it targets the abdominal muscles effectively. It also allows for a smooth arc as you raise yourself, taking strain off the neck.

AbWorks by NordicTrack, $119.95. A padded board with bars that help the arms and feet stay in position, this machine lets you maintain a pelvic tilt with relative ease and thereby targets the abdominals without wasted motion. It also prevents unnecessary strain by supporting the head and neck. An added bonus: The machine allows you to do different kinds of sit-ups to focus on different areas of the stomach. Caution: Watch the instructional video that comes with AbWorks before starting. If you use the equipment incorrectly, you'll end up exercising the arms, not the abs.

EZ Krunch Abdominal Exerciser. $29.95. This machine is "total junk" that's "cumbersome to use" and causes "a lot of wasted movement," say experts Dr. Nelson and Mr. Wood. Held between the thighs while you sit and pushed down with a gizmo that looks like a truncated pogo stick, it works the triceps at the back of the upper arm rather than the abdominals. It exercises the hips more than the abs, too.

PowerTek Power Abs System, $29.95. A gadget that you literally pull against your stomach, the Power Abs System works the biceps on the front of the upper arms much more than the abdominals. Rather than putting the abdominal muscles through their full range of motion, it simply forces you to hold in your stomach.

Weider AbShaper, $49.95. Essentially a pad with bars for the hands, this machine lifts as you do, supporting the neck and freeing it of strain. That allows you to focus fully on crunching the abdominals as you make the contraction.

Toning the Abs for Free

For our readers who want above-average abs without slimming their wallets, here's a basic sit-up, or stomach crunch, that will do the trick. Also presented is an exercise for the lower back, a good addition to any ab-training workout you choose.

Bent-Knee Sit-Up: Lie on your back with your knees bent and your feet flat on the floor, several inches apart. Keep your hands palms down on your thighs. (When you do sit-ups with your hands clasped behind your head, you tend to pull yourself up by the neck, which causes neck pain and leaves the abdominals without a real workout.) Gently tuck in your chin. Then lift your shoulders 3 or 4 inches off the floor while sliding your palms upward toward your knees. (Your shoulders don't need to go higher because the abdominal muscles do not have a wide range of motion.) Hold for a moment; think of your stomach as a sponge that you're squeezing. Then return slowly to the starting position.

You are doing the sit-ups correctly if you feel your abdominal muscles quiver as you hold the crunch. If you feel more strain in your hips or arms than in your belly, you're not using your abdominals to their fullest capacity.

Back Extension (a companion exercise to any abdominal workout): Put on ankle weights to anchor your feet to the ground. Then lie face down with two pillows under your pelvis (hips). With your arms straight out in front of your head, slowly lift your back 4 to 5 inches off the floor. Keep your back straight; don't arch it. Hold, then slowly lower your back. Repeat. When it becomes too easy to do 8 to 12 repetitions at a time, increase the number of repetitions. Do not increase the weight on your ankles for this exercise.

You Can Flatten Your Tummy (to Some Degree)

What makes a man look good has changed more than a little since Henry VIII was depicted eating a leg of game meat in a gesture of girthful might. Today, as anybody thumbing through the pages of *GQ* or *Esquire* or visiting "Melrose Place" can tell you, pot bellies are most decidedly "out." And men are getting the message.

Consider that a product called Belly Buster, a cream you're supposed to rub on your stomach to melt away fat, is outselling Thin Thighs, a similar item women use in the vain hope that a "magic" potion could ever change the body's contours. And in an informal survey in Redbook magazine, six out of 10 men made pot belly-lamenting comments ranging from "I'd like to have a tighter stomach" to "I hate my abdominals" to "Everything I eat goes to my gut."

The naked truth is that many men, even those in good physical shape, are predisposed to have a little squeezability around the middle. It's simply a biology-is-destiny effect that cannot be beaten without torturous, time-consuming exercise regimens that few men, save the Fabios of the world, need put themselves through. But there are a couple of things a man (or woman) can do to help turn a pot into more of a pan, if you will.

One is not to eat too many calories at once, especially in the evening. Eating a lot at the same time can cause abdominal distension. And when it's followed by sleep, the abdominal muscles relax and stretch like an overused rubber band—to the point that a pot belly can eventually develop. Another step is to exercise the abdominal and lower back muscles a couple of times a week. It's not that working those areas will shrink a big belly by burning fat there. There's no such thing as spot reducing. When you burn fat through exercise (or eating fewer calories) you burn it all over the body, not just in the place you would like to target. But performing exercises that strengthen the muscles in the abdomen and lower back will improve posture and thereby make the stomach stick out less.

"If there's a lot of poundage out in front" explains J. Anthony Spataro, PhD, of the New Mexico Department of Public Health, "the back will sway backward and the belly will protrude forward. But strengthening the right muscles will make the pot belly appear less prominent as well as reduce the risk of suffering lower back problems." Good strengthening exercises for the lower back include back extensions—lying face down with two pillows under your hips and, with your arms stretched out in front of you, lifting your back four to five inches off the floor. For the abdominals, bent-knee sit-ups will do the trick.

Special Advice for Pot-Bellied Joggers

Some people who jog on a regular basis develop pot bellies because all that bouncing up and down and "jiggling around" can stretch the muscles in the stomach, Dr. Spataro says. They may also develop spare tires because of changes in posture that occur with running, which, as in people who have a lot of fat around the middle, can cause the back to sway out backward and the belly to protrude forward. The way to counter the effect is to follow the same advice as anyone else with a pot belly: make a habit of strengthening the abdominal and lower back muscles.

Joggers should also exercise and stretch the hamstring muscles at the backs of the upper thighs. The hamstrings are important, Dr. Spataro explains, because they exert a pull all the way up through the back. And as they contract or tighten while you run, you are pulled out of position in such a way that your back tilts backward and your hips are displaced forward. The effect, again, is a protruding belly (along with a shortened gait and potential back problems).

Good strengthening exercises for hamstrings include knee flexions, which involve standing behind a chair with ankle weights strapped on and bending each leg at the knees. As for hamstring stretches, which help keep those muscles elongated so you get a full stride and don't develop back problems that cause the stomach to sag outward, one way they can be accomplished is by trying to touch your toes without bending your knees.

"It doesn't matter if you are not able to reach your toes," Dr. Spataro says. "Just bend from the waist (with your legs together) and let your arms go down as far as possible. If you can only get as far as your calves, you're still stretching your hamstrings." Dr. Spataro recommends holding for 10 seconds, then coming back up for 10 seconds and repeating the process four or five more times. He also advises that for both safety and effectiveness, you go slowly and deliberately rather than bounce.

"I don't think most runners are stretchers," Dr. Spataro says. "They don't want to be bothered. But stretching after a run is important, not just for the belly but also to avoid back pain. I'm a terrible stretcher myself," Dr. Spataro, an exercise physiologist, concedes. "But I just turned 52 and I'm developing sort of a pot, so I need to get started."

Section 23.4

Have You Been Doing the Other Kind of Exercise?

Summertime and the aerobics are easy. When the weather is warm many people are much more inclined to get out there and jog, swim, walk briskly, play a rigorous game of tennis or soccer, or engage in other forms of aerobic activity. Such fast-paced action is important because in the process of making you huff and puff it strengthens your heart and the rest of your cardiovascular system, so you will be much less likely to fall victim to heart disease.

What's great about aerobic activity—besides lowering your risk of becoming a heart attack victim—is that nobody has to show you how to do it. Everyone knows, at the very least, how to put one foot in front of the other and work up a good sweat while going at it. Not so with a type of exercise that is as important to health but is just beginning to garner the attention it deserves: isotonics, also known as strength training, weight training, or resistance training.

Isotonics is crucial to being in the best of health because it builds up muscle mass. The more muscle you have, the stronger you are, so that you can carry heavy packages or perform other tasks without becoming winded. "The gratification is immediate," says Tufts University exercise physiologist William Evans, PhD. "You get stronger by the second week. In just 12 weeks you can double or triple your strength."

Increased muscle mass also raises the body's metabolic rate, which means you burn "extra" calories. The reason is that muscle requires more calories than body fat to sustain itself. People who have a higher proportion of muscle to fat can therefore eat more calories without gaining weight. To look at it another way, they can lose weight without eating a lot less. "Increasing amounts of evidence show that building muscle through strength training is just as important for weight loss as aerobics," says Dr. Evans.

Another benefit of greater muscle mass is that it decreases the risk for developing diabetes. As Dr. Evans explains, the more muscle mass in the body, the less insulin it takes to get sugar, or glucose, out of the blood and into the tissues, where it's needed for energy. Thus, the body is less likely to "run out of" insulin, so to speak—which is another way of saying the chance of developing adult-onset diabetes is lessened.

Other bonuses of engaging in isotonics: it can improve the ratio of "good" HDL-cholesterol to "bad" LDL-cholesterol, thus protecting against heart disease, and it increases bone density, protecting against the fractures associated with osteoporosis in later life. A study conducted at Tufts shows that it may even help mitigate the effects of rheumatoid arthritis.

Of course, strength training needs to be taught to some degree. It is not something that comes naturally, although it does become a habit before long because it leads to a more able body so quickly that people tend to stick with it.

Getting down to Brass Tacks

While performing isotonics isn't exactly second nature, it is not a complicated set of activities meant only for the super-fit crowd. You don't have to join a gym or buy a set of barbells. And you can do it right in your own home.

The meaning behind the term isotonics is not complicated either. All you're doing when you perform an isotonic, or resistance-training, routine is getting specific muscles in different parts of the body to work harder than usual by pushing them against more weight than they are accustomed to. The more weight you can push or lift over time (the more "resistance" you can overcome), the stronger the muscles doing the pushing and the bigger the muscle mass.

For many people, in fact, strength training can begin with pushing against the weight of their own bodies without any equipment. One strength-training activity that challenges muscles to "lift" or "push against" the body's weight is the pushup. Every time you lift your body off the floor (and thereby overcome the resistance of its weight), you are strengthening the muscles in your arms, chest, shoulders, and back.

After a while, anyone who practices push-ups is probably going to do them with ease. If the activity becomes too easy and no longer presents a challenge, however, it no longer does the trick of making the muscles stronger than they were. How do you know when an isotonic exercise has become too easy? When you've strengthened a muscle or a group of muscles to the point that you can do more than 8 to 12 repetitions without resting for more than a few seconds in between; the particular muscles you are working on should feel almost thoroughly exhausted by the time you reach repetition 12. At that point, you need to find another activity to challenge those muscles or do something to make the activity harder to accomplish. In the case of push-ups, that something might be to strap a pack onto your back.

Muscle groups throughout the upper and lower body can be safely strengthened using the up-to-12-times-in-a-row approach. Upper body muscles are comprised of those in the arms, shoulders, and chest (such as the biceps on the inside of the upper arm, the triceps on the outside of the upper arm, and the deltoids in the shoulders) and those in the abdomen. Lower-body muscles are the gluteals or buttocks muscles, those in the front part and the back part of the thighs (the quadriceps and hamstrings, respectively), and those on the inside and outside of the hips (the hip abductors and the hip adductors). Many different kinds of isotonic exercises can increase the mass—and the strength—of each of these muscle groups. Illustrated here are some of the most basic exercises (not necessarily the easiest, just easy to learn) focused on the muscles people use most often in daily activities. That is, they give the most noticeable improvement in strength for the effort.

You can use weights in the form of jugs with handles or can-shaped cylinders or store-bought weight cuffs. The kind of weight you use doesn't matter as long as it isn't too heavy for you yet heavy enough to challenge your muscles to push past their starting strength. If you buy commercial weights at a sporting goods store, a good bet is to buy hand weights (free weights) for the upper body and ankle weights, or cuffs, for the lower. Be sure the weights have a range of two and a half to three times the weight you can lift presently, since that is approximately the increase in ability you can expect if you adhere faithfully to a weight-training program for three months. If you can currently lift 10 pounds, buy a set of weights that goes up to the 25 or 30 pounds you will be able to lift in about three months. If you can currently lift 20 pounds, buy a set that tops out at 50 to 60 pounds.

Those who do not want to spend any money on weight training can make weights from, say, milk containers (with handles to make lifting safer) and plastic bags filled with sand that they can strap to their ankles. A sedentary woman who has not done much exercising for many years may want to start with a one-gallon milk container filled with water, which weighs about 8 pounds. Men, who generally start out with more muscle than women, may want to fill a one-gallon container with sand, or if that's too light (or becomes too light) with lead shot, available at hardware stores.

How Often, and for How Long?

Happily, weight training will intrude only a little on your life, even less than aerobics. If you're committed to exercising both your upper and lower body at every session, all you need is two to three sessions a week, 30 to 40 minutes each, for a total of about an hour or two every seven days (or, at most, 1 percent of your time). During a session, you'll want to go through each exercise about three times. For instance, you should not do 8 to 12 arm curls and then go on to the next activity thinking you're done with arm curls for the day. You should do three "sets" of 8 to 12 arm curls, waiting a little between each set, and then go on to the next exercise. Alternatively, you may want to perform one set of 8 to 12 arm curls followed by one set of all your other exercises and then repeat that multi-exercise sequence two times.

Regardless of which exercise you do, it's important to perform each repetition slowly, taking as many as six to nine seconds. "A lot of people go too fast," Dr. Evans says. "When you do that you are not training your muscle—as well as the joint connected to the muscle—through its entire range of motion, so you're not increasing its strength and flexibility as much as possible." Breathing properly is important too. Inhale before you lift or push, exhale as you lift, and inhale again as you slowly return to the starting position. What you should not do is swing a weight fast or bounce at the end of a repetition. You should also not exercise the same muscle groups in more than one session per day. You need to give the muscles sufficient time to recover.

Safety's sake requires, in addition, a 10-minute warm-up before each exercise session. The first five minutes should consist of low-intensity aerobics; walking around serves the purpose. The second five should consist of gentle and relaxing stretching maneuvers, such as sitting on the floor and extending a leg straight out in front of you (with the other leg bent in toward the outstretched one), grabbing your ankle with your hands, slowly pulling your body forward as far as possible (keeping the leg straight all the while), and then holding the position for 10 to 15 seconds. Always keep your back as straight as possible while stretching; bending it can trigger an injury in those prone to back trouble.

Devoting the extra 10 minutes to a warm-up will render your muscles, tendons, and ligaments more pliant—that is, less like cold rubber bands that "snap" and tear easily. The same warm-up, incidentally, is recommended for aerobic exercise, which is why some people combine their aerobic and isotonic exercise sessions; it's a way of "killing" two work-out activities with one warm-up "stone." The recommended order: warm-up, aerobics, isotonics, and a five-minute cool down or five minutes of walking around to keep from shifting the body too abruptly back into low gear.

It should be pointed out that aerobics improve isotonic capacity and vice versa. It makes sense. When you engage in any type of aerobic activity you are getting your muscles to work for you and thereby preparing them for the rigors of isotonics, and when you build muscle through isotonics you are priming your body to perform better at aerobics. That's because the more muscle mass you have, the more oxygen you are able to take in and pump to all your tissues to fuel movements such as running and walking. In fact, how much oxygen you can take in—the deeper you can breathe and the better your heart can pump—is the measure of your aerobic capacity.

Aerobics and isotonics also have a synergistic effect in making you feel and look better. Aerobics primarily burn fat, while isotonics tone and build muscle. The two together are an unbeatable body-beautiful combination, but you have to keep at it for life because the benefits of exercise can't be stored. Once you stop training, you start returning to your pre-exercise fitness levels within a couple of weeks.

A note for men 40 and above and women who are at least 50 as well as for those with diabetes, heart disease, or high blood pressure: See your doctor before you start a fitness regimen. That may sound like a pain in the neck if you want to get going quickly, but a physician can make sure you don't take on too much too fast and thereby damage rather than improve your health.

Not for the Spandex Crowd Only

You may believe a weight-training regimen is not for you. Perhaps you're a young woman who does not want to build up muscle for fear of losing your feminine physique or a silver-haired grandfather who feels he doesn't have the energy to start a strength-training program. But both ways of thinking are unfounded. Says Dr. William Evans, "To start looking like Arnold Schwarzenegger, you'd need to work out five or six hours every single day rather than the hour to hour and a half per week that's recommended, so women need not worry." Even women who do work out a good deal needn't be too concerned about developing bulging biceps. Men are much more apt than women to develop large muscles through isotonics, presumably because of the hormone testosterone.

As for being too old to engage in strength training, one could argue that at any age you're too old not to. Consider that between the ages of 20 and 70, the typically sedentary American loses about 30 percent of the total number of muscle cells in the body (which comes to about six to seven pounds of lean body mass per decade). The muscle cells that do remain shrink and begin to atrophy. So even if you do not gain any weight over the years, you could be becoming fatter: the pounds you lose as muscle, or lean body mass, are made up for with flab. And a lot of it.

The average sedentary 25-year-old woman is about 25 percent fat. But by the time she reaches age 65, fat accounts for some 43 percent of her makeup. Sedentary men go from being about 18 percent fat at age 25 to 38 percent fat by the time they start collecting Social Security. Dr. Evans calls the age-related shift in the proportion of fat muscle sarcopenia, which means flesh poverty.

Isotonics can, to a large degree, reverse that trend, not by replacing lost muscle but by building up the muscle cells that remain. In other words, age-related muscle loss and all the attendant problems to which it contributes is not a fact of life that has to be accepted passively. Anyone, whether 20, 60, or 80, whether man or woman, can build up muscle strength. Dr. Evans even has a 101-year-old patient who has been on a weight-training program since he was 97. He now has the strength of a (sedentary) 60-year-old.

For more information on strength training as well as exercise in general, we recommend *Biomarkers: The 10 Determinants of Aging You Can Control,* by William Evans, PhD, and Irwin Rosenberg, MD (Simon & Schuster, $12.00 in paperback 1-800-223-2336) or the *American College of Sport Medicine's ACSM Fitness Book* (Leisure Press, $11.95, 1-800-747-4467). Some people may want to acclimate themselves to a strength-training program by paying for a couple of sessions with a Y or health-club instructor who is certified by the American College of Sport Medicine or has a college degree in exercise physiology or physical education. Many clubs offer training in the proper use of free weight and the like even for individuals who choose not to purchase year-round membership.

Bent-knee push-ups. Some people don't start out with the strength to do straight-knee push-ups. If that's the case, we recommend this easier version, in which you raise your body from head to knee rather than from head to toe. After a while, you will be able to move on to the more taxing straight-knee style.

Arm curl (biceps curl). You can do this holding a weight or wearing a wrist weight (as shown). Bend your elbow and "curl" the weight to shoulder level. Slowly return to the starting position.

Chest and shoulder exercise (for the deltoid). Make sure you are sitting upright. Raise your arm slowly forward and up until your elbow is straight. Stop when your arm is fully extended above your head and then return slowly to the starting position.

Upper-arm (triceps) exercise. Hold a weight in each hand and raise both arms over your head. Bend one elbow back as you lower one hand behind your head. Raise it back overhead, joining the other hand. Now do the same with your other arm. Keep alternating.

Knee extension (for the quadriceps). Cuff or strap a weight to your ankle. Extend your leg so it's as straight out in front of you as possible. Lower your leg back to its starling position, but rest no more than one second before repeating. After eight to 12 repetitions (one set), switch to the other leg.

Chapter 24

Tobacco, Alcohol, and Drugs

Chapter Contents

Section 24.1

Cigarette Smoking-Related Mortality

NIH web document e-pub (http://www.cdc.gov/ncctphp/osh/mortali.htm). Office on Smoking and Health, National Center for Chronic Disease Prevention and Health Promotion, Centers for Disease Control and Prevention, July 1996.

Cigarette smoking is the single most preventable cause of premature death in the United States. Each year, more than 400,000 Americans die from cigarette smoking. In fact, one in every five deaths in the United States is smoking related. Every year, smoking kills more than 276,000 men and 142,000 women.[1]

About 10 million people in the United States have died from causes attributed to smoking (including heart disease, emphysema, and other respiratory diseases) since the first Surgeon General's report on smoking and health in 1964—2 million of these deaths were the result of lung cancer alone.[2]

Between 1960 and 1990, deaths from lung cancer among women have increased by more than 400 percent,-exceeding breast cancer deaths in the mid-1980s.[3] The American Cancer Society estimated that in 1994, 64,300 women died from lung cancer and 44,300 died from breast cancer.[4]

Men who smoke increase their risk of death from lung cancer by more than 22 times and from bronchitis and emphysema by nearly 10 times. Women who smoke increase their risk of dying from lung cancer by nearly 12 times and the risk of dying from bronchitis and emphysema by more than 10 times. Smoking triples the risk of dying from heart disease among middle-aged men and women.[1]

Every year in the United States, premature deaths from smoking rob more than five million years from the potential lifespan of those who have died.[1]

On average, smokers die nearly seven years earlier than nonsmokers.[2]

Annually, exposure to secondhand smoke (or environmental tobacco smoke) causes an estimated 3,000 deaths from lung cancer among American adults.[5] Scientific studies also link secondhand smoke with heart disease.

Table 24.1. Causes of Death

Disease	Men	Women	Overall
Cancers			
Lung	81,179	35,741	116,920
Lung from ETS	1,055	1,945	3,000
Other	21,659	9,743	31,402
Total	103,893	47,429	151,322
Cardiovascular Diseases			
Hypertension	3,233	2,151	5,450
Heart Disease	88,644	45,591	134,235
Stroke	14,978	8,303	23,281
Other	11,682	5,172	16,854
Total	118,603	61,117	179,820
Respiratory Diseases			
Pneumonia	11,292	7,881	19,173
Bronchitis/Emphysema	9,234	5,541	14,865
Chronic Airway Obstruction	30,385	18,579	48,982
Other	787	668	1,455
Total	51,788	32,689	84,475
Diseases Among Infants	1,006	705	1,711
Burn Deaths	863	499	1,362
All Causes	**276,153**	**142,537**	**418,690**

References

1. Centers for Disease Control and Prevention. Smoking-attributable mortality and years of potential life lost—United States, 1990. *Morbidity and Mortality Weekly Report* 1993;42(33):645-8.

2. Centers for Disease Control and Prevention. Office on Smoking and Health, unpublished data, 1994.

3. Centers for Disease Control and Prevention. Mortality trends for selected smoking-related and breast cancer—-United States, 1950-1990. *Morbidity and Mortality Weekly Report* 1993;42(44):857, 863-6.

4. American Cancer Society. *Cancer Facts & Figures—1996*. Atlanta (GA): American Cancer Society, 1996.

5. U.S. Environmental Protection Agency. *Respiratory Health Effects of Passive Smoking: Lung Cancer and Other Disorders*. Washington (DC): U.S. Environmental Protection Agency, Office of Health and Environmental Assessment, Office of Research and Development. EPA/600/6-90/006F. December 1992.

Section 24.2

Substance Abuse: Alcohol and Other Drugs

NIH web document http://www.healthfinder.gov/tours/subabuse.htm.

General Questions

What is substance abuse?

Abuse of alcohol, tobacco, and drugs has pervasive effects and is linked to death, unintentional injury (particular automobile crashes), chronic disease, school failure, unintended pregnancy, HIV infection, violent and abusive behavior, and all sorts of other psychological and social problems.

Substance abuse encompasses over-the-counter and prescription drugs, as well as illicit drugs and can involve household and other products, such as aerosol sprays.

How big a health problem is substance abuse?

Alcohol, tobacco, and drug use contributes significantly to the Nation's health care bill as well as the deficit.

Former Secretary of Health, Education, and Welfare Joseph A. Califano, Jr. (currently chairman and president of the Center on Addiction and Substance Abuse at Columbia University) estimates that in 1993, the cost to society of alcohol, tobacco, and other drugs was nearly $400 billion—about $1,608 for every man, woman and child in the Nation.[1]

Alcohol and other drug use has been implicated as a factor in many of this country's most serious and expensive problems, including violence, injury, child and spousal abuse, HIV/AIDS and other sexually transmitted diseases, teen pregnancy, school failure, car crashes, escalating health care costs, low worker productivity, and homelessness.[2]

A large part of the national health care bill is for alcohol, tobacco, and other drug-related medical expenses. For example, 25 to 40 percent

619

of all Americans in general hospital beds (that is not in a maternity or intensive care unit bed) are being treated for complications of alcoholism.[1]

Twenty-eight percent of all admissions to one large metropolitan hospital's intensive care units (ICUs) were related to ATD problems (9 percent alcohol, 14 percent tobacco, and 5 percent other drugs). The ATD-related admissions were much more severe than the other 72 percent of admissions, requiring 4.2 days in ICU versus 2.8 days as well as much more expensive—about 63 percent greater than the average cost for other ICU admissions.[1,2]

Health care costs related to substance abuse are not limited to the abuser. Children of alcoholics average 62 percent more hospital days than do other children. These increased hospital days result from 24 percent more inpatient admissions and 29 percent longer stays when admitted.[3]

The Center on Addiction and Substance Abuse at Columbia University estimates that at least 1 of every 5 dollars Medicaid spends on hospital care and 1 in every 5 Medicaid hospital days are attributable to substance abuse.[1]

Alcohol is the drug most frequently used by 12- to 17-year-olds—and the one that causes the most negative health consequences. More than 4 million adolescents under the legal drinking age consume alcohol in any given month. Alcohol-related car crashes are the number one killer of teens. Alcohol use also is associated with homicides, suicides, and drownings—the other three leading causes of death among youth.[2]

1. Center on Addiction and Substance Abuse, Columbia University, *The Cost of Substance Abuse to America's Health Care System, Report 1: Medicaid Hospital Costs*, 1993.

2. *Center for Substance Abuse Prevention's Discussion Paper on Preventing Alcohol, Tobacco, and Other Drug Problems*, 1993.

3. Children of Alcoholics Foundation, *Children of Alcoholics in the Medicaid System: Hidden Problems, Hidden Costs*, 1990.

Can substance abuse be prevented?

Different ATD prevention programs yield economic benefits at various times. For example, if alcohol- and drug-taking behavior is reduced among pregnant women, the payoff will be realized within a year. In contrast, the benefits of a successful preschool program may not accrue to society for a decade or more—when these youngsters become adolescents and begin making choices about ATD use.

What types of prevention activities can be carried out?

There is no limit to the types of individuals and organizations or to the activities that help prevent substance abuse. Visit the National Clearinghouse for Alcohol and Drug Information (http://www.health. org/mpw.fact/mpw.fact.htm) for specific activities to be carried out by health care professionals, individuals (including older Americans, Hispanics/Latinos, American Indians/Alaska Natives, African Americans, and Asian/Pacific Islander Americans), media, business, youth-serving groups; parents, guardians, and caretakers; community groups, faith communities, colleges and universities, the judiciary, State and local governments, victims of natural disasters, family members and providers of people with disabilities, juvenile justice and child welfare, patrons of the arts, and schools.

Treatment

Can substance abuse be treated?

Treatment is a very effective means of tackling America's substance abuse problem because it saves lives and money. Treatment reduces crime, the rate of recidivism to the prison system, health care costs and costs to business, including decreased productivity, higher insurance premiums and increased medical claims.

- Substance abuse treatment, like many other medical treatments, is most successful when it provides a continuum of care, allowing patients to be treated in the most appropriate manner and at the proper intensity for their condition.

- Drug abuse among young people—especially marijuana use—is on the rise. We need to send clear and consistent messages to young people that drug use is dangerous, illegal and wrong.

- Including treatment in the criminal justice system, either as an integral part or as an alternative where appropriate, is an effective means of reducing recidivism rates for drug users.

- Culturally and/or gender-specific treatment programs are crucial in meeting the needs of cultural minorities and women, including those who are pregnant or have young children.

Specific Topics

How can I tell if a friend or a loved one has a problem with alcohol, marijuana, or other illicit drugs?

Sometimes it is tough to tell. Most people won't walk up to someone they're close to and ask for help. In fact, they will probably do everything possible to deny or hide the problem. But, there are certain warning signs that may indicate that a family member or friend is using drugs and drinking too much alcohol.

If your friend or loved one has one or more of the following signs, he or she may have a problem with drugs or alcohol:

- Getting high on drugs or getting drunk on a regular basis

- Lying about things, or the amount of drugs or alcohol they are using

- Avoiding you and others in order to get high or drunk

- Giving up activities they used to do such as sports, homework, or hanging out with friends who don't use drugs or drink

- Having to use more marijuana or other illicit drugs to get the same effects

- Constantly talking about using drugs or drinking

- Believing that in order to have fun they need to drink or use marijuana or other drugs

- Pressuring others to use drugs or drink

- Taking risks, including sexual risks and driving under the influence of alcohol and/or drugs

- Feeling run-down, hopeless, depressed, or even suicidal

- Suspension from school for an alcohol- or drug-related incident

- Missing work or poor work performance because of drinking or drug use

Many of the signs, such as sudden changes in mood, difficulty in getting along with others, poor job or school performance, irritability, and depression, might be explained by other causes. Unless you observe drug use or excessive drinking, it can be hard to determine the cause of these problems. Your first step is to contact a qualified alcohol and drug professional in your area who can give you further advice.

How can I tell if I have a problem with drugs or alcohol?

Drug and alcohol problems can affect every one of us regardless of age, sex, race, marital status, place of residence, income level, or lifestyle.

You may have a problem with drugs or alcohol if:

- You can't predict whether or not you will use drugs or get drunk.

- You believe that in order to have fun you need to drink and/or use drugs.

- You turn to alcohol and/or drugs after a confrontation or argument, or to relieve uncomfortable feelings.

- You drink more or use more drugs to get the same effect that you got with smaller amounts.

- You drink and/or use drugs alone.

- You remember how last night began, but not how it ended, so you're worried you may have a problem.

- You have trouble at work or in school because of your drinking or drug use.

- You make promises to yourself or others that you'll stop getting drunk or using drugs.

- You feel alone, scared, miserable, and depressed.

If you have experienced any of the above problems, take heart, help is available. More than a million Americans like you have taken charge of their lives and are living healthy and drug-free.

How can I get help?

You can get help for yourself or for a friend or loved one from numerous national, State, and local organizations, treatment centers, referral centers, and hotlines throughout the country. There are various kinds of treatment services and centers. For example, some may involve outpatient counseling, while others may be 3- to 5-week-long inpatient programs.

While you or your friend or loved one may be hesitant to seek help, know that treatment programs offer organized and structured services with individual, group, and family therapy for people with alcohol and drug abuse problems. Research shows that when appropriate treatment is given, and when clients follow their prescribed program, treatment can work. By reducing alcohol and/or drug abuse, treatment reduces costs to society in terms of medical care, law enforcement, and crime. More importantly, treatment can help keep you and your loved ones together.

Remember, some people may go through treatment a number of times before they are in full recovery. Do not give up hope.

Each community has its own resources. Some common referral sources that are often listed in the phone book are:

- Local emergency health clinics, or community treatment services

- City/local health departments

- Alcoholics Anonymous, Narcotics Anonymous, or Al-Anon/ Alateen Hospitals

What are important messages for teenagers?

- Know the law. Methamphetamines, marijuana, hallucinogens, crack, cocaine, and many other substances are illegal. Depending on where you are caught, you could face high fines and jail time. Alcohol is illegal to buy or possess if you are under 21.

- Be aware of the risks. Drinking or using drugs increases the risk of injury. Car crashes, falls, burns, drowning, and suicide are all linked to drug use.

- Keep your edge. Drug use can ruin your looks, make you depressed, and contribute to slipping grades.

- Play it safe. One incident of drug use could make you do something that you will regret for a lifetime.

- Do the smart thing. Using drugs puts your health, education, family ties, and social life at risk.

- Get with the program. Doing drugs isn't "in" anymore.

- Think twice about what you're advertising when you buy and wear T-shirts, hats, pins, or jewelry with a pot leaf, joint, blunt, beer can, or other drug paraphernalia on them. Do you want to promote something that can cause cancer? make you forget things? or make it difficult to drive a car?

- Face your problems. Using drugs won't help you escape your problems, it will only create more.

- Be a real friend. If you know someone with a drug problem, be part of the solution. Urge your friend to get help.

- Remember, you DON'T NEED drugs or alcohol. If you think "everybody's doing it," you're wrong! Over 86 percent of 12-17 year-olds have never tried marijuana; over 98 percent have never used cocaine; only about half a percent of them have ever used crack. Doing drugs won't make you happy or popular or help you to learn the skills you need as you grow up. In fact, doing drugs can cause you to fail at all of these things.

To Learn More about Substance Abuse, Read:

- President Clinton's 1996 National Drug Control Strategy and Methamphetamine Strategy: http://www.health.org/pubs/factsht/prmeth.htm

- Treatment Improvement Protocols from the Center for Substance Abuse Treatment: http://text.nlm.nih.gov/

- Fetal Alcohol Syndrome: http://www.nofas.org/

- Center on Addiction and Substance Abuse: http://www.casacolumbia.org/home.htm

- Higher Education Center for Alcohol and Other Drug Prevention: http://www.edc.org/hec

- Mothers Against Drunk Driving: http://www.madd.org

- National Institute on Drug Abuse: http://www.nida.nih.gov/

- Drug Search—Get factual information about the effects of alcohol, tobacco, and drugs, or browse the slang dictionary of drug terms.: http://www.lec.org/DrugSearch/index.html

For More Resources to Write or Call:

www.health.org/pubs/strafact/

National Institute on Drug Abuse (NIDA)
5600 Fisher's Lane, Rockville, Md 20857
(301) 443-1124

Part Seven

Gender, No Guarantee of Immunity

Chapter 25

Breast Cancer, Osteoporosis, and Eating Disorders

Seymour Kramer noticed a patch of what looked like blood on his pajama top three years ago and thought he had cut himself. But he wasn't scratched. His doctor tested the discharge and told the New Jersey man he had breast cancer.

Dan, 70, a retired Michigan engineer who asked that his last name not be used, was pulling weeds three years ago. For no apparent reason, he fractured two vertebrae. Doctors told him his bones were wasting away. He has osteoporosis.

As a teenager, Gary Grahl was obsessed with having a trim, "athletic" body. The Wisconsin resident shunned food and exercised excessively. Sometimes he'd do situps and pushups for three hours before school. He ate little and shrank from 160 to an unhealthy 104 pounds. Over a six-year period, he was hospitalized four times. Now 26, Grahl says he is "completely recovered" from his eating disorder.

What do these men have in common? They all suffer from illnesses typically thought of as "women's diseases." Breast cancer, osteoporosis, and eating disorders all occur in men, too, though their prevalence is much greater in the female population. As a result, many men, unaware that the diseases affect both sexes, may fail to recognize symptoms. Likewise, doctors and families often don't suspect these illnesses. This can delay therapy and make disorders difficult to treat.

Medical experts say men may shy away from seeking medical treatment for disorders they feel are unmasculine. In support groups, men

---

FDA Consumer, July/August 1995.

use terms like "very scared" and "ashamed" to describe initial feelings about their illnesses. Others express frustration at the difficulty in finding information and therapy.

Osteoporosis

High on the list of such conditions is osteoporosis. Though women are four times more likely to acquire it, about five million men in this country have osteoporosis, according to the National Osteoporosis Foundation. A disorder which bones become weakened, Osteoporosis is sometimes called the "silent disease" because it has no symptoms. It often manifests itself in fractures of the hip, wrist, spine, and other bones. Among both sexes, it is responsible for 1.5 million fractures a year.

Scientists are still piecing together just how osteoporosis develops, but it is well known that a key factor is deficiency of the mineral calcium. Leo Lutwak, M.D., Ph.D., a medical officer in FDA's Center for Drug Evaluation and Research, emphasizes that calcium intake over a person's lifetime is crucial to preventing bone loss. Ideally, he says, a diet adequate in calcium starting in childhood "can maximize peak bone mass," helping to ensure strong bones and make osteoporosis less likely. The revised food label that went into effect in 1994 can help consumers pinpoint calcium-rich foods (see the May 1993 issue of *FDA Consumer*).

About 99 percent of the body's calcium is stored in bones and teeth. Bone is continually being broken down and rebuilt. If the amount of calcium absorbed equals the amount lost, a state of balance occurs. When calcium absorption is greater than losses, the body accrues a "positive balance" that it can use for bone growth and repair. But when dietary intake of calcium can't meet the body's needs, the body draws the mineral from bones to allow a constant bloodstream supply. Ultimately, the breakdown process can exceed deposits, causing a possible reduction in bone mass and density.

Osteoporosis is seen less often in men than in women for several reasons. Men generally have greater bone mass than women, and in males, bone loss begins later and advances more slowly. But men do have a hormonal drop-off in testosterone similar to women's reduction of estrogen after menopause. Testosterone may diminish as a result of hypogonadism, a condition marked by decreased function of the testicles. Testosterone levels may naturally become lower as a man ages.

"Loss of sex hormone results in accelerated bone loss in whomever it occurs, whenever it occurs, for whatever reason," says Michael

Kleerekoper, M.D., deputy associate chairman of internal medicine at Wayne State University. "Whether that translates to osteoporosis depends on how much bone you have when the loss begins and how quickly you lose it." Women find relief from osteoporosis with estrogen therapy, and some men respond to testosterone injections. But successes with hormone therapy come most often from "seeing young men in the early stages" of the condition, Kleerekoper says.

Another therapy shown to slow bone breakdown and reduce pain associated with fractures attributed to osteoporosis is the drug calcitonin, marketed as Miacalcin or Calcimar. FDA has not approved these drugs specifically for men, though some doctors prescribe them to males if they feel the patient will benefit. Currently under study for osteoporosis treatment are sodium fluoride, which some researchers think may help increase bone mass; vitamin D, which helps the body absorb calcium; and a nasal spray version of calcitonin.

Dan, the Michigan osteoporosis patient, receives biweekly testosterone injections and takes daily supplements of 1,500 milligrams of calcium with vitamin D. He also exercises in a swimming pool, where water provides a beneficial resistance to movement. He says his two fractured vertebrae three years ago made him realize that osteoporosis gives no warnings.

Factors that raise the risk of osteoporosis include cigarette smoking, alcohol consumption in excess of two drinks a day, advanced age, and an inactive lifestyle.

Eric, 45, says years of inactivity helped bring on his osteoporosis. In his early twenties, the New York resident (who asked that his last name not be used) had several sports accidents that seriously impaired his mobility. An eating disorder in college also encouraged development of the condition, he suspects. Now, his bone loss is so severe that "anytime I have an x-ray, the doctors go into shock," he says. He risks injury by simply taking a walk and cannot stand barefoot on a hard floor without excruciating pain. He is taking calcitonin, which he hopes will stabilize his bone loss and allow him to do more walking.

Though osteoporosis cannot be cured, it can be slowed down and steps can be taken to prevent it. The National Osteoporosis Foundation suggests these preventive measures:

- Eat a balanced diet rich in calcium.

- Exercise regularly, especially in weight-bearing activities.

- Don't smoke.

- If you drink alcohol, do so in moderation.

Breast Cancer

Primarily associated with women, breast cancer also occurs in men, although rarely. According to the American Cancer Society (ACS), men will make up 1,400 of the 183,400 new cases of breast cancer expected in 1995.

Men typically do not perform breast self-examinations to detect tumors, and doctors do not ordinarily examine men for breast cancer during physicals. Unlike women, men do not get routine mammograms Consequently, a tumor may be present and go undiscovered.

As with breast cancer in women, symptoms include the presence of a breast lump that is usually firm and painless. The nipple can have an abnormality such as retraction, crusting, or a discharge. Patients frequently are over 60.

Seymour Kramer was 70 when a gooey, bloodlike discharge from his nipple prompted him to seek medical attention. After analyzing the secretion, doctors told him he had breast cancer and recommended a lumpectomy, in which the nipple and a small amount of breast tissue are taken out. He also had several lymph nodes removed, and he underwent five weeks of radiation therapy to help ensure that residual cancer cells were killed. Though his prognosis appears very good, Kramer won't say he's been cured. But he expresses optimism: "Just because I had cancer doesn't mean my life is over."

The ACS says risk factors for male breast cancer include:

- **hyperestrogenism**, or abnormal secretion of the hormone estrogen.

- **Klinefelter's syndrome**, a male disorder characterized by reduced or absent sperm production, small testicles, and enlarged breasts

- **gynecomastia**, or enlargement of the male breast. Though medical professionals typically don't recommend detection exams for the general male population, doctors may advise men with gynecomastia to perform periodic breast self-examinations.

Because in men the disease is often detected at an advanced stage when the tumor has spread, radical mastectomy—removal of breast tissue and pectoral muscle—is often the initial treatment. But if the cancer is found before it spreads to surrounding tissue or to the lymph nodes, a lumpectomy can be performed. Radiation sometimes is used without surgery, but the verdict is still out on its effectiveness. As in

Kramer's case, radiation also can be employed after surgery to reduce the chance of local recurrence and to relieve symptoms in advanced cases. If cancer has spread into the lymph nodes, some physicians use chemotherapy. A therapeutic "tumor vaccine" for men and women to treat breast cancer that has already spread is in clinical trials now.

Possible complications after surgery or radiation include decreased shoulder function, fluid retention in the arm, and pain or stiffness in the operated or radiated area. The ACS emphasizes that besides tending to the physical consequences of breast cancer therapy, "attention should be paid to the psychological aftereffects."

Patients also need follow-up monitoring—including regular exams, blood chemistry, imaging (such as magnetic resonance imaging), and bone scans—to discover any recurring tumors quickly.

Kramer says his experience of being blindsided by the disease put him on "a crusade" to inform men and medical professionals about breast cancer in males. "During a routine physical exam, I think doctors should run their hands across a man's breast to see if there's anything irregular," he says. "I'm not saying men have to go out and get wholesale mammograms. But [as a rule] doctors don't do this [touch test] and men don't inspect themselves. Those men who are not aware need to be shocked into the fact that, 'Hey, guys, this could happen to you.'"

Eating Disorders

Though many people associate eating disorders with women, these illnesses also occur in males. In one disorder, anorexia nervosa, the person limits food intake to the point of starvation. In another, bulimia nervosa, sufferers alternate between eating large amounts of food and ridding the body of it through vomiting or laxative use. About half of those with anorexia also have bulimia symptoms.

According to the National Association of Anorexia Nervosa and Associated Disorders (ANAD), men make up about one million of the eight million Americans with eating disorders.

"It's a myth that these are illnesses of rich, white, perfectionist women," says Chris Athas, ANAD vice president. "Just as a man or woman may become an alcoholic, either may fall victim to an eating disorder."

Medical professionals say the disorders most often surface during the teen years, but in rare cases, men as old as 60 and boys as young as 8 can be afflicted. In both sexes, the illnesses can lead to lifelong medical and psychological complications. An estimated 6 percent of cases result in death. Most people find it difficult to halt the behavior without professional assistance. Though some men ultimately seek help, many continue untreated with the disorders, often for years, and sometimes for a decade or more.

Diagnosis is complicated by a reluctance some men have to seek medical help for disorders that are "still primarily women's," Athas says. "We live in a 'macho' society. Many men simply are ashamed to have an illness of this type." Thus, they suffer in silence.

Another problem, says Athas, is that a great number of doctors and healthcare professionals are not trained to identify or treat male eating disorders, especially anorexia. Families, too, often fail to see the diseases' symptoms. The illnesses then can progress to a more advanced stage where they are harder to treat.

During recovery, men sometimes are unwilling to participate in support-group sessions because the groups are mostly female. "Men as a whole are not comfortable in eating disorder support groups," says Athas. "But we encourage them to go anyways."

Unlike many women, who acquire eating disorders because they "feel" fat, men often are medically obese at some point in the illness and feel pressure to be thin. Sometimes athletic activities induce this struggle to be lean, prompting not only the eating disorder but also compulsive exercising. Men also may adopt disease behaviors when teased or criticized about being fat at critical development stages, such as puberty.

Treatment can be very effective, according to Arnold Andersen, M.D., an expert on eating disorders in men who has written a book on the subject. He describes a regimen of inpatient or outpatient hospital treatment, depending on the illness severity. Conditions such as anemia or depression are treated, and patients gradually relearn proper eating habits. Treatment also usually includes psychotherapy, which helps patients understand why they have the illness.

One antidepressant drug, Prozac (fluoxetine hydrochloride), is under review by FDA as a treatment for bulimia. Other antidepressants also are being studied. One, Wellbutrin (bupropion), was shown to induce seizures in both anorexia and bulimia patients. Doctors sometimes prescribe tricyclic drugs—a class that includes Elavil (amitriptyline), Tofranil (imipramine), and Norpramin (desipramine). FDA has approved tricyclics for other uses but not specifically for eating disorders. However, doctors may prescribe approved drugs for "off-label" uses if, in their judgment, the patient will benefit.

Patients also undergo what Andersen calls "nutritional rehabilitation," which allows them to regain a desirable body weight. Treatment is followed by weeks, months, even years of follow-up to ensure complete recovery.

Men in support groups for eating disorders, as well as those for breast cancer and osteoporosis, say the public gradually is becoming more aware that these disorders can occur in men. They also say there's a long way to go. Some think doctors need to be enlightened. Others bemoan the lack of research. But most seem to agree that men should be educated about the disorders and how to detect them.

As breast cancer patient Seymour Kramer says: "Men need to get the word that, yes, this is a woman's disease. But you're not immune. It can happen to you."

For More Information

Sources of information and support for the disorders described in this article include:

- National Association of Anorexia Nervosa and Associated Disorders, Box 7, Highland Park, IL 60035—Offers free programs to help victims and families, including counseling, support groups, health-care referrals, and a newsletter; telephone (708) 831-3438.

- National Osteoporosis Foundation, 1150 17th St., N.W., Suite 500, Washington, D.C. 20036—Will send information packet and can refer patients to support groups; telephone (1-800) 223-9994.

- The Cancer Information Service, 550 N. Broadway, Suite 300, Baltimore, MD 21205-2004—Will provide information on male breast cancer and can refer callers to cancer centers and support groups; telephone (1-800)4-CANCER.

—John Henkel

John Henkel is a staff writer for FDA Consumer.

Chapter 26

Male Breast Cancer

Carcinoma of the male breast is an uncommon phenomenon, accounting for less than 1 percent of all breast cancers. It is estimated that 1,000 new cases will be diagnosed in the United States in 1996 and will account for 300 deaths.[1]

Breast cancer in men has been traditionally thought to be substantially different from that in women. As more becomes known of this relatively rare entity, the similarities of the disease between genders become more striking than the differences. Cause, predisposition based on family history, prognosis, and response to treatment are remarkably similar between the sexes.

Family history of breast cancer is present in about 30 percent of males with breast cancer.[2-4] Multiple cases of male breast cancer within a family are unusual but have been reported to occur among siblings[2] and between uncle and nephew.[3] A review of familial breast cancer in males has described 10 families with sufficient evidence to suggest a familial distribution. The most common scenario in this group was female breast cancer, but rare male involvement was noted.[5] This finding suggests that a familial form of breast cancer exists in which both males and females show an increased risk for developing breast cancer. Inclusion, of male breast cancer has not routinely been considered as a component of such familial syndromes as the Li-Fraumeni syndrome.[6] As BRCA1 and other breast cancer genes become more widely applicable, the genetic relations of male breast may be better understood.

The risk for breast cancer increases with age in males but lacks the early premenopausal peak seen in females.[7] For this reason, the greatest incidence occurs 5 to 10 years later in males with the peak at 60 years of age. The annual incidence increases steadily from 35 years of age, with 0.1 case per 100,000 men to 11.1 cases at age 85 years or greater.

Various factors specific to males have been implicated as possibly contributing to the development of male breast cancer.[8-13] These include undescended testes orchiectomy, orchitis, late puberty, infertility, obesity, hypercholesterolemia, estrogen use, and environmental exposure.[10,11] Some evidence suggests that male breast cancer may develop in persons with relative androgen deficiency.

The global distribution of male breast cancer is similar to that of female breast cancer, with areas virtually devoid of both male and female disease and an increased reported incidence among males in those areas with higher rates for females. Certain exceptions exist. For example, in Egypt, male breast cancer is quite common and is related to schistosomiasis.

Radiation exposure may be related to an increased risk for the disease, with cancer developing 12 to 36 years after exposure.[13-16] The risk in men seems similar to the risk in women; exposure to radiation doses greater than 50 to 100 cGy increases the risk for cancer, and the risk increases if the exposure occurs at a young age.[13,17] Occupational or environmental exposure may exert an effect on the development of male breast cancer. A review of the occupation of males with breast cancer has shown a disproportionate frequency of chronic work exposure to heat, suggesting that increased environmental temperatures may potentiate the development of breast cancer in men.[18]B Potential etiologies may involve testicular dysfunction secondary to heat exposure and are consistent with the theory that male breast cancer may develop in response to relative androgen deficiency.[10]

Because of the unusual nature of male breast cancer and the potential of an endocrinologic basis, several studies have evaluated estrogen metabolism. The studies have used small sample sizes and lack an agreement or trend in their results.[19-23] Ballerini and colleagues[19] reported no difference in testosterone, estradiol, prolactin, folliclestimulating hormone (FSH) and luteinizing hormone (LH) between 10 men with breast cancer and matched controls. Excretion of estrogen metabolites was no different in 19 patients with cancer compared with controls.[20] Olsson and coworkers[23] reported increased prolactin and decreased FSH levels with no difference in LH, estradiol, or testosterone levels in 15 men with breast cancer compared with controls. Several additional studies, again involving small sample sizes, reported elevated estriol production, lower levels of estrone, and estrogen breakdown products in men with breast cancer.[21,22]

Exogenous hormone therapy clearly promotes breast cancer in several susceptible species of experimental animals, but similar data in human males are lacking. Breast cancer is rarely reported in men undergoing estrogen therapy for prostate cancer, and a breast mass in such a patient is more often metastatic than primary.[24] Anecdotal reports have described breast cancer in male-to-female transsexuals taking estrogen to promote secondary sexual characteristics.[25,26]

Excess circulating estrogen secondary to compromised hepatic metabolism may explain the increased incidence of male breast cancer seen in several parts of the world. In parts of Africa, hepatic dysfunction is common, secondary to bilharziasis, cirrhosis, and chronic malnutrition, and is associated with an increased incidence of male breast cancer. Schistosomiasis (and related hepatic dysfunction) is associated with an increased rate of male breast cancer in Egypt.

Patients with Klinefelter syndrome have a risk for breast cancer that approaches that of females.[27] The breasts of these men are hypertrophic, secondary not only to gynecomastia but also to the development of acini and lobules. Although Klinefelter syndrome is associated with an increased risk for breast cancer, it is rare and therefore accounts for less than 1 percent of male breast cancer.

Pathology

The distribution of the histopathologic findings of breast cancer differs between males and females primarily because lobules are routinely not developed in the male breast. An early series from Memorial Hospital documented the absence of infiltrating lobular carcinoma in males.[28] Nance and Reddick[29] described infiltrating carcinoma of the male breast, and Heller and colleagues reported an updated series from Memorial and similar to females infiltrating ductal carcinoma accounted for over 80 percent of all lesions. Intraductal carcinoma was more common in females (5 percent, versus 3.8 percent), and this difference increases as screening mammography detects more ductal carcinoma in situ (DCIS) in the screened female population.[30] Infiltrating lobular carcinoma in males is quite unusual and has been only reported in rare instances.[29] Lobular carcinoma in situ has not been reported. All other types of breast cancer—including medullary, papillary, colloid, and Paget disease—have been reported in men.

Hormone Receptors

Estrogen receptor protein is present in male breast cancer in a higher percentage of patients than in women with breast cancer.[31-36] Rosen and colleagues[32] described positive estrogen receptor protein results in 75 percent of 8 male cancers, and Mercer and coworkers[34] found 94 percent of the lesions to be positive for estrogen receptor protein and 93 percent to be positive for progesterone receptor protein. Other series have confirmed these findings, and no correlation seems to exist between patient age, histologic grade of the lesion, stage, or nodal status. In a collected series of 47 patients, 80 percent were estrogen receptor protein-positive, and over 30 percent with metastatic disease responded to hormonal manipulation.[31]

Diagnosis and Natural History

The most common presentation of male breast cancer is a painless, unilateral breast mass. It is most often eccentric, slightly irregular, and quite firm. Mammographically detected lesions in asymptomatic men or in those presenting with a normal breast examination and ipsilateral axillary node are quite rare.[37,38] Nipple discharge is an unusual presentation of the disease and, if present, is often bloody or serosanguineous. Treves and colleagues[39] reported that such discharge was associated with cancer 80 percent of the time and accounted for nearly 14 percent of the male breast cancers.

Differential diagnosis of a breast mass in a male routinely must distinguish between gynecomastia and cancer. Gynecomastia remains the most common cause of either unilateral or bilateral breast mass. Although more commonly bilateral and symmetric with well-defined discoid margins, histopathologic confirmation is the only sure differential between benign and malignant disease. Fine-needle aspiration cytology depends highly on the experience of both the clinician and the cytopathologist. Although this technique may become more useful as experience increases, fine-needle aspiration cytology is not widely used in the differentiation of a male breast lesion. Mammography may be useful in differential diagnosis, but the gold standard remains biopsy.[37] Although gynecomastia remains the most common differential of a breast mass, it is not thought to be related to an increased risk for breast cancer.

Treatment

The historical treatment of choice for male breast cancer had been radical mastectomy. This approach had been advocated because of the theoretical or realized proximity of the lesion to the pectoralis major muscle. In addition, the stage at presentation may be more advanced in men than women and thus may necessitate a radical mastectomy. The current trend is toward modified radical mastectomy. Kinne and colleagues[40] described 36 consecutive cases at Memorial Hospital, 27 of whom were treated by modified radical mastectomy. Similar findings were reported by Hodson and also showed similar survival and local control between radical and modified radical mastectomy.[41] A review of 104 patients treated at several institutions since 1975 showed that 67 percent were treated with modified mastectomy.[33] Breast conservation has not been an issue in male breast cancer.

Prognosis and Survival

Carcinoma of the male breast is staged similarly to female breast cancer, using the American Joint Committee Clinical Staging System. As in women, axillary nodal status is the strongest predictor of outcome. A multivariate analysis of prognostic factors in 166 male breast cancers showed that age at diagnosis, tumor size, and nodal status were significant prognosticators, with nodal status proving strongest.[42] Prognosis in 335 cases was reported by Guinee and coworkers[43] and showed that both clinical axillary nodal status and clinical tumor size were predictive of outcome. A patient with palpable axillary nodes had double the risk for disease-related death, and an increase in tumor diameter of 3 cm carried a similarly increased risk for treatment failure. Although fixation to the skin or chest wall, as well as ulceration of tumor are more commonly reported in males than females, neither finding was predictive of outcome in multivariate analysis.[42]

Overall survival is often stated to be worse for men than for women with breast cancer.[44] When corrected for disease stage, survival seems to be similar, although men more commonly have advanced disease. A recent analysis of male breast cancer showed that 30 percent of men had advanced disease at presentation. A collection of men with breast cancer described 335 cases with an 84 percent 10-year survival rate in node-negative patients and a 44 percent survival rate for node-positive patients. They concluded that the prognosis of breast cancer is the same in male and female patients when compared stage for stage.[43] A similar analysis of compiled cases reported 5-year survival rates at 100 percent for node-negative disease and 60 percent for node-positive disease.[33] Again it was concluded that the survival rates were quite similar to those of female breast cancer (Table 26.1).

Table 26.1. Survival in Male Breast Cancer

	5-Year Survival	
Investigators	Node-Negative Disease	Node-Positive Disease
	n	
Crichlow, 1972[44]	79	28
Heller et al, 1978[30]	90	NA
Yap et al, 1979[45]	77	38
Ramantanis et al, 1980[46]	57	31
Appleqvist & Salmo, 1982[47]	67	57
Erlichman et al, 1984[48]	77	37
Borgen et al, 1992[33]	100	60
Guinee et al, 1990[49]	90	74

NA, not available.

Adjuvant Therapy

Adjuvant radiotherapy has been used in the treatment of male breast cancer. Although local control may be slightly improved, no improvement exists in overall survival. Improvement in local control may reflect advanced disease stage in men, rather than a biological difference in the disease between genders.

Hormonal ablation in the treatment of metastatic disease dates to the report of Farrow and colleagues from Memorial Hospital in New York. They observed response from orchiectomy to symptomatic metastatic disease. Since the time of their report, orchiectomy has become the standard of care for metastatic disease. Recently, tamoxifen has been used as first-line treatment in receptor-positive disease and has shown response rates from 50 percent to 80 percent.[35,42,49,51,52]

Multiple reports have described the utility of adjuvant chemotherapy, but the disease is too uncommon to allow randomized clinical trials of systemic therapy.[53] General recommendations regarding patient selection for treatment resemble those for female patients. All patients with positive nodes and those selected node-negative patients who are at high risk for recurrence are treated with systemic therapy.

Several small series have described the efficacy of hormonal manipulation or chemotherapy in the treatment of male breast cancer. A review of hormone manipulation reported an overall response rate of 51 percent, but a rate of 71 percent was noted if the patient was positive for estrogen receptor protein. Patients who respond to first-line hormonal manipulation are more likely (70 percent) to respond to a second attempt.[40] The efficacy of adjuvant chemotherapy in male breast cancer has also been reported. Because of the relative rarity of the disease, benefit is usually determined in comparison with historic controls and is fraught with the usual inaccuracies of such studies. A study from the M.D. Anderson Cancer Center reported such results in seven patients with stage II and four with stage III cancers and concluded that adjuvant therapy reduced the risk for recurrence and favorably influenced survival.[51,53] Similar results were reported from the National Cancer Institute, where 24 node-positive patients were treated with cyclophosphamide, methotrexate, and 5-fluorouracil. The 5-year survival rate of 80 percent exceeded that of historic controls, and the investigators concluded that adjuvant chemotherapy was beneficial in the treatment of node-positive disease.[54]

References

1. Boreng C, Squires T, Tong T, et al. Cancer statistics 1994. CA Cancer J. Clin 1994;44:18.

2. LaRaja R, Pagnozzi J, Rodhenberg R. Cancer of the breast in three siblings. Cancer 85;55:2709.

3. Rosenblatt K, Thomas D, McTiernan A, et al. Breast cancer in men: aspects of familial aggregation. J Natl Cancer Inst 1991; 83:849.

4. Kozak FK, Hall JG, Baird PA. Familial breast cancer in males: a case report and review of the literature. Cancer 1986; 58:2736.

5. Kozak F, Hall J, Band P. Familial breast cancer in males: a case report and review of the literature. Cancer 1986;58:2736.

6. Malkin D. The Li-Fraumeni syndrome. Princ Pract Oncol Updates 1993;7:1.

7. Young I, Percy C, Asire A. Surveillance, epidemiology and end results: incidence and mortality data. (NIH Pub 81-2330). Natl Cancer Inst Monogr 1981;57:74.

8. Lenfant-Pejovic MH, Mlika-Cabanne N, Bouchardy C, et al. Risk factors for male breast cancer: a Franco-Swiss case-control study. Int J Cancer 1990;45:661.

9. Mabuchi K, Bross DS, Kessler I. Risk factors for male breast cancer. J Natl Cancer Inst 1985;74:371.

10. Thomas DB, Jiminez LM, McTiernan A, et al. Breast cancer in men: risk factors with hormonal implications. Am J Epidemiol 1992; 135:734.

11. Casagrande J, Hanische R, Pike M. A case-control study of male breast cancer. Cancer Res 1988;48:1326.

12. Mani S, Ahmad YH, Papac RJ. Male breast cancer: risk factors and clinical features. Proc Annu Meet Am Soc Clin Oncol 1992; 11 :A157.

13. Eldar S, Nash E, Abrahamson J. Radiation carcinogenesis in the male breast. Eur J Surg Oncol 1989;15:274.

14. Greene M, Goedert J, Bech-Hansen N. Radiogenic male breast cancer with in vitro sensitivity to ionizing radiation and bleomycin. Cancer Invest 1983;1:379.

15. Hauser A, Lemer I, King R. Familial male breast cancer. Am J Med Genet 1992;44:839.

16. Jauchum J. Occupational exposure to electromagnetic fields and breast cancer in men. Am J Epidemiol 1992; 135:1423.

17. Yahalom J, Petrek JA, Biddinger PW, et al. Breast cancer in patients irradiated for Hodgkin's disease: a clinical and pathologic analysis of 45 Events in 37 patients. J Clin Oncol 1992; 10:1674.

18. Mabuchi A, Bross D, Kessler I. Risk factors in male breast cancer J Natl Cancer Inst 1985;74:371.

19. Ballerini P, Recchione C, Cavalleri A, et al. Hormones in male breast cancer. Tumori 1990;76:26.

20. Scheike O, Svenstrup B, Frandson B. Metabolism of estradiol 17-ß in men with breast cancer. J Steroid Biochem 1973;4:489.

21. Zumoff B, Fishman J, Cassouto J, et al. Estradiol transformation in men with breast cancer. J Clin Endocrinol Metab 1966;26:960.

22. Dao T, Morreal C, Nemoto T. Urinary estrogen excretion in men with breast cancer. N Engl J Med 1973;289:138.

23. Olsson H, Alm P, Aspegren K, et al. Increased plasma prolactin levels in a group of men with breast cancer: a preliminary study. Anticancer Res 1990;10:59.

24. Schlappack OK, Braun O, Maier U. Report of two cases of male breast cancer after prolonged estrogen treatment for prostatic carcinoma. Cancer Detect Prev 1986;9:319.

25. Pritchard T, Pankowsky D, Crowe J, et al. Breast cancer in a male to female transsexual. JAMA 1988;259:2278.

26. Symmers W. Carcinoma of the breast in trans-sexual individuals after surgery and hormonal interference with primary and secondary sex characteristics. Br Med J 1968; 2:83.

27. Evans D, Crichlow R. Carcinoma of the male breast and Klinefelter's syndrome: is there an association? CA Cancer J Clin 1987;37:2

28. Holleb A, Freeman H, Farrow J. Cancer of the male breast. NY State Med 1968;68:836.

29. Nance KV, Reddick RL. In situ and infiltrating lobular carcinoma of the male breast. Hum Pathol 1989;20:1220.

30. Heller K, Rosen P, Schottenfeld D. Male breast cancer: a clinicopathologic study of 97 cases. Ann Surg 1978; 188:60.

31. Friedman M, Hoffman P, Dandolos E. Estrogen receptors in male breast cancer. Cancer 1981;47:134.

32. Rosen P, Botet C, Nisselbaum. Estrogen receptor protein in lesions of the male breast. Cancer 1976;37:1866.

33. Borgen P, Wong G, Vlamis V, et al. Current management of breast cancer: a review of 104 cases. Annals Surg 1992;215:451.

34. Mercer RJ, Bryan RM, Bennett RC. Hormone receptors in male breast cancer. Aust NZ Surg 1984;54:215.

35. Ribeiro G, Swindell R. Adjuvant tamoxifen for male breast cancer. Br J Cancer 1992;65:252.

36. Pacheco MM, Oshima CF, Lopes MP. Steroid hormone receptors in male breast diseases. Anticancer Res 1986;6:1013.

37. Dershaw DD, Borgen Pl, Deutch BM, et al. Mammographic findings in men with breast cancer. Am J Roentgenol 1993;160:267.

38. Balich SM, Khandekhar JD, Sener SF. Cancer of the male breast presenting as an axillary mass. J Surg Oncol 1993; 53:68.

39. Treves N, Robbins G, Amoroso W. Serous and serosanguineous discharge from the male nipple. Arch Surg 1956;73:319.

40. Kinne D, Hakes T. Male breast cancer. In: Harris J, Hellman S. Henderson IC, et al, eds. Breast diseases. Philadelphia, JB Lippincott, 1991:782.

41. Hodson GR, Urdaneta LF, Al-Jurf AS, et al. Male breast carcinoma Am Surgeon 1985; 51:47.

42. Hulthorn R, Friberg S, Hulthorn KA. Male breast carcinoma II. A study of the total material reported to the Swedish Cancer Registry 1958-1967 with respect to treatment, prognostic factors and survival. Acta Oncol 1987;26:327.

43. Guinee VF, Olsson H, Moller T, et al. The prognosis of breast cancer in males. Cancer 1993;71:154.

44. Crichlow R. Carcinoma of the male breast. Surg Gynecol Obstet 1972; 134:1011.

45. Yap H, Tashima C, Blumenschein G, et al. Male breast cancer: a natural history study. Cancer 1979;44:748.

46. Rarnantanis G, Besbeas S, Garas J. Breast cancer in the male: a report; of 138 cases. World J Surg 1980;4:621.

47. Appleqvist P, Salmo M. Prognosis in carcinoma of the male breast. Acta Chir Scand 1982; 148:499.

48. Erlichman C, Murphy K, Elhakim T. Male breast cancer: a 13-year review of 89 patients. J Clin Oncol 1984;2:903.

49. Guinee VF, Moller T, Olsson H, et al. Clinical prognostic factors in male breast cancer: eleven-center study, international cancer patient dare exchange system. Proc Annu Meet Am Soc Clin Oncol 1990;9:A138.

50. Farrow J, Adair F. Effects of orchiectomy on skeletal metastases from cancer of the male breast. Science 1942;95:654.

51. Jaiyesimi 1, Buzdar A, Sahin A, et al. Carcinoma of the male breast. Ann Intem Med 1992; 117:771.

52. Chi JC, Juler GL, Rosen AO. Treatment modalities and survival in male breast carcinoma. Proc Annu Meet Atn Soc Clin Oncol 1988;7:A94

53. Patel HZ, Burdar AU, Hortobagi GN. Role of adjuvant chemotherapy in male breast cancer. Cancer 1989;64:1583.

54. Bagley C, Wesley M, Young R, et al. Adjuvant chemotherapy in males with cancer of the breast. Am J Clin Oncol 1987; 10:55.

—Michael P. Moore

Chapter 27

Osteoporosis in Men

Chapter Contents

Section 27.1

Bone Basics for Men of All Ages

©1995 National Osteoporosis Foundation. Reprinted with permission.

Understanding Osteoporosis in Men

You might be surprised to learn that 20 percent of the 25 million Americans who have osteoporosis are men. In fact, osteoporosis affects nearly half of all people—women and men—over the age of 75. Although this disease has been studied more often in women, there are steps that can be taken to prevent and treat osteoporosis in men.

Understanding Your Bones

Bones are not lifeless structures, but are, in fact, living tissue. Bone constantly changes, with bits of old bone being removed to be replaced by new bone. During childhood, more bone is produced than removed, so the skeleton grows in both size and strength. The amount of tissue or bone mass in the skeleton reaches its maximum amount by the mid-30s. At this point, the amount of bone in the skeleton typically begins to decline slowly as removal exceed deposits of new bone.

While women lose bone mass rapidly in the years after menopause, by age 65 or 70, women and men lose bone mass at the same rate, and calcium absorption decreases in both sexes. Adequate calcium intake, proper exercise, and good health habits are essential throughout life to ensure that the body has enough bone tissue to draw from in the later years.

What Is Osteoporosis?

Osteoporosis is a painful and disfiguring disease that weakens bones and makes them more likely to fracture. Osteoporosis occurs because of inadequate bone formation, excessive bone removal or both.

Fractures resulting from osteoporosis typically occur in the hip, spine, and wrist, and can be permanently disabling.

Risk Factors for Men

There are several risk factors which have been linked to osteoporosis in men. One such factor relates to the male hormone testosterone, which plays an important role in bone health. Decreases in male hormones, or hypogonadism, can cause reduced bone mass and lead to fractures. Although men do not undergo the equivalent of menopause, gonadal function does decline in some elderly men and in younger men who have medical conditions which affect their ability to produce testosterone. Another risk factor is glucocorticoid medications, which are used for such conditions as asthma, arthritis, and Crohn's disease. These medications have side effects which interfere with bone and calcium metabolism. Men who are treated with glucocorticoids may develop osteoporosis.

Excessive use of alcohol also plays an important role in weakening bones, even in relatively young or middle-aged men. For example, alcohol has been found to reduce circulating levels of testosterone. Studies have found that some men with osteoporosis have higher alcohol and cigarette consumption.

Calcium: A Necessity at Any Age

To prevent osteoporosis, you need to eat a balanced diet rich in calcium throughout your lifetime. Adult men need 1,000 ma. of calcium a day. It's easy to add calcium to your diet. Try having a dairy product at every meal. Grate cheese over your salad, drink skim milk, or add a slice of low-fat cheese to your sandwich. Try low-fat yogurt, frozen yogurt, or ice milk for dessert or snacks. Enjoy high calcium foods like broccoli, tofu, and calcium-fortified fruit juice.

Some people have difficulty digesting milk products, a condition known as lactose intolerance. People who are lactose intolerant can satisfy their daily calcium requirements in a number of ways: by incorporating non-dairy, calcium-rich foods into the diet, by taking calcium supplements, and by using lactase pills or drops which make milk products digestible.

Exercise for Strong Bones

Regular weight-bearing exercise, which causes muscles to work against gravity, can help build bone density. Jogging is an excellent weight-bearing exercise, as are walking, tennis, and dancing. Experts believe that other forms of exercise, like swimming, bicycling, and rowing, while they are not weight-bearing, have cardiovascular benefits. And keeping active allows you to eat more without gaining weight, making it easier to maintain an adequate intake of calcium and other nutrients.

Adopt an active lifestyle. Walk short distances instead of driving. Do housework and yardwork. If you spend a lot of time at a desk in your office, it's especially important that you exercise. Use the stairs instead of the elevator and whenever possible, walk to appointments.

Healthy Habits Make Healthy Bones

Certain substances are toxic to bones, such as nicotine and alcohol. Smoking is toxic to bone cells, and extra calcium can't make up for the damage. Alcohol abuse is also harmful. Not only is it directly toxic to bones, but it also interferes with proper nutrition. To help protect your bone density, avoid smoking and practice moderation with alcoholic beverages.

Bone Density Testing

Once bone mass has been lost, it cannot be replaced. That is why the best "treatment" for osteoporosis is preventing it in the first place! Since osteoporosis can develop silently for decades until a fracture occurs, early diagnosis is essential in order to begin treatment as soon as possible to prevent further bone loss. Safe, accurate, and non-invasive tests are available for measuring bone mass. Use of these techniques is the only accurate way to measure bone mass and to assess the risk of fracture.

Bone mass measurement can be critical for preventing fractures. With the results of these measurements, physicians can identify areas in the body with low bone mass and determine the type of therapy to be used to prevent further bone loss. If you are interested in learning more about bone density testing, your doctor can further explain the test, and refer you to an exam site.

Living with Osteoporosis

If you have osteoporosis, you can live actively and comfortably if you seek proper medical care and make some lifestyle adjustments. Your doctor may prescribe a treatment program that includes calcium, exercise, or medication. For example, calcitonin, a hormone produced naturally in the thyroid gland, is involved in calcium regulation, and has been shown to slow bone breakdown. If hypogonadism is determined to be a cause of your osteoporosis, your doctor may prescribe treatment that provides the body with the male hormone testosterone.

Section 27.2

Osteoporosis in Men: A Major Health Problem

"Clinical Update" Reprinted from *The Osteoporosis Report,* Spring 1992.

Osteoporosis in men can be a major health problem. Although less common than in women, it is estimated that one-seventh of all vertebral fractures and one-fifth of all hip fractures occur in men. Seventeen percent of men will suffer a hip fracture before they reach age 90, leading to significant physical and emotional problems.

Osteoporosis develops less commonly in men than women because men have larger skeletons, bone loss starts later and progresses more slowly, and there is no period of rapid hormonal changes and accompanying rapid bone loss. Other factors may also be important. There are many causes of osteoporosis in men. For example, 40-45 percent of men with spinal osteoporosis and vertebral compression fractures have disorders or conditions which can produce bone loss and cause osteoporosis. These include hypogonadism, hyperthyroidism, neoplastic diseases, and genetic disorders (e.g., osteogenesis imperfecta) as well as steroid therapy (e.g., chronic prednisone therapy), immobilization, and gastric surgery. Hypogonadism in men can be due to disorders which produce primary testicular failure, hyperprolactinemia, Klinefelter's syndrome, anorexia nervosa, and hypothalamic-pituitary dysfunction. Delayed puberty can also lead to thin bones later in life. Additional risk factors in men with spinal osteoporosis include smoking and alcohol use.

Idiopathic osteoporosis (i.e., of unknown cause) is found in young men generally between the ages of 20 and 50. Patients usually present with back pain and multiple vertebral fractures. The axial skeleton (spine) is primarily affected. Idiopathic juvenile osteoporosis is usually seen in children before puberty. Multiple fractures can occur but the disease tends to disappear spontaneously, and neither its cause nor its reason for remission is understood.

Osteoporosis in older men may be related to testosterone deficiency, to the many causes of bone loss noted above, to abnormalities in the cellular repair of microfractures, and to other physiologic changes due to aging. With advancing age men (and women), when compared to younger individuals, ingest and absorb less calcium. They also are less able to increase their intestinal absorption efficiency for calcium and may have lower blood levels of the active form of vitamin D (1,25-dihydroxyvitamin D).

The evaluation of osteoporosis in men is similar to that in women. Assessment of the risks and other causes should be made through a detailed history and physical examination, in which such factors as alcohol use and gonadal function are evaluated. Blood and urine tests can help uncover secondary causes of osteoporosis, some of which can be specifically treated. Bone density measurements of the spine, hip, and forearm can provide quantitive information which can be helpful in assessing future risk for sustaining a fracture. Bone density tests can also help monitor the effectiveness of therapeutic intervention.

The treatment of osteoporosis in men consists of identifying and treating specific causes, maintaining a balanced diet and an adequate intake of calcium and vitamin D, avoiding immobilization, and following an adequate and appropriate physical therapy and exercise program. If testosterone deficiency is found, then testosterone replacement should be considered. Other agents which are being investigated for use in men include salmon calcitonin, the bisphosphonates, sodium fluoride, human parathyroid hormone, and others.

Preventing bone loss and fractures in men should also be emphasized. The same general principles, as stated above, may be helpful: identify risk factors, eat a balanced diet, and get proper exercise. In addition, the prevention of falls is very important, as are modifying and avoiding household hazards, and avoiding medications that dull the senses and produce drowsiness.

As we learn more from basic science concerning the biology of bone cells and the remodelling process, we will be able to develop new means to diagnose, prevent and treat osteoporosis. The future looks promising.

References

1. Jackson JA, Kleerekoper M. Osteoporosis in men: pathophysiology and prevention. Medicine 69:137152, 1990.

2. Seeman E, Melton LJ, O'Fallon WM, Riggs BL. Risk factors for spinal osteoporosis in men. Am J Med 75:977-983, 1983.

3. Francis RM, Peacock M, Marshall DH, Horsman A, Aaron JE. Spinal osteoporosis in men. Bone and Mineral 5:347-357, 1989.

4. Slovik DM, Rosenthal DI, Doppelt SH, Potts JT, Daly MA, Campbell JA, Neer RM. Restoration of spinal bone in osteoporotic men by treatment with human parathyroid hormone (1-34) and 1,25-dihydroxyvitamin D. J Bone Miner Res 1:377-381, 1986.

—David Slovik, M.D.

Section 27.3

Steps Men Should Take to Avoid Osteoporosis

©1996 *Tufts University Diet & Nutrition Letter*.
Reprinted with Permission.

Osteoporosis in men "has been under-diagnosed, under-reported, and inadequately researched,"says the National Osteoporosis Foundation in a new campaign to help men avoid the bone-shattering disease. Take a look at the statistics:

• American men over the age of 50 have a greater chance of suffering an osteoporosis-related fracture than of developing clinical prostate cancer. One out of eight men over 50 will break a bone due to osteoporosis.

- Each year, 100,000 men suffer hip fractures. A third of them die within a year, usually because of complications such as blood clots in the lung related to either the fracture, surgery to repair the break, or confinement to bed. The immobility reduces lung-clearing capacity, paving the way for life-threatening conditions such as pneumonia.

The incidence of osteoporosis in men is expected to rise as more men live into their 70s, 80s, and 90s. In a study of more than 800 men in Australia, those in their late 70s suffered 3 times as many fractures as those in their early 60s. Men in their 80s experienced 7 times as many fractures as men in their 60s.

In the years directly after menopause, women lose bone much more quickly than men of the same age. But by age 65 or 70, men and women lose bone mass at the same rate. Calcium absorption also decreases in both sexes with advancing age.

Bone-saving Measures

While no one can keep from growing older, there's plenty men (and women, too) can do to cut down on the risk of breaking a bone.

1. Eat plenty of high-calcium foods. The National Osteoporosis Foundation advises men younger than 65 to consume 1,000 milligrams of calcium a day. Men over 65 should consume 1,500 milligrams of calcium daily. Some good sources of calcium: 1 cup skim or 1-percent-fat milk (300 milligrams), 6 ounces nonfat yogurt (150-300 milligrams), 1 ounce Swiss or cheddar cheese (200 milligrams), 6 ounces calcium-fortified orange juice (200 milligrams), and 3 ounces canned salmon with bones (200 milligrams).

2. Keep alcohol consumption moderate. An Indiana study of more than 100 men that began when they were in their 40s and ended when they were in their 60s showed that those who averaged more than 11/2 drinks a day lost almost 70 percent more bone than nondrinkers.

3. Don't smoke. In the Indiana study, the more cigarettes smoked, the more bone was lost.

4. Maintain or improve the strength of the quadriceps—the muscles at the front of the upper thighs. In the Australian study, the weaker the quadriceps, the greater was the risk for

fractures. It may be because strong quadriceps help prevent falls that can result in broken bones.

Quadriceps strength can decrease as much as 30 percent between the ages of 60 and 80, but such a dramatic loss of power in the thigh muscles is not inevitable. Strength-training exercises such as knee extensions will keep the quadriceps in shape (see below). Other activities that stress and thereby strengthen the thighs include walking, jogging, bicycling, and playing sports such as tennis or basketball. Those activities will strengthen muscles and bones not just in the upper legs but in many parts of the body.

5. Speak with your doctor if you take steroids (for example, to treat asthma or arthritis), anticonvulsants, or aluminum-containing antacids such as Maalex or Mylanta. All of these medications can have a negative impact on bone density, so your physician might advise you to have a bone scan and exercise more or consume more calcium. Certain cancer drugs, such as methotrexate, and other medications like the cholesterol reducer cholestyramine can also have a negative effect on bone.

6. Keep your home fall proof. Falls greatly increase the chances of a fracture, and 1 out of 3 people 65 or older fall each year. Most falls occur at home, often because people trip while walking or slip when getting up from a chair or couch. Make sure floors are free from clutter, and tuck away all loose wires and electrical cords. In addition, keep frequently used items in closets and kitchen cupboards within easy reach rather than on hard-to-get-to shelves.

The National Osteoporosis Foundation has additional suggestions for making your home fall safe and is offering them as part of osteoporosis prevention and treatment kits. Seven different kits are targeted to particular groups: men, older women, mid-life women, young women, adolescents, children, and health professionals. To order a free kit, call 1-888 442-9473.

Knee Extension: Working the Quadriceps (The Front of the Upper Thigh)

Strap weights to your ankles. Put a rolled-up towel or a small cushion on the front part of the seat of a straight-back chair. Sit comfortably in the chair with the backs of your knees resting against the seat. Just the balls of your feet should touch the floor.

Extend one leg out in front of you until it is as straight as possible. Do not grip the chair as you lift, but gently hold onto the seat to help stabilize yourself. Slowly lower your leg until your foot is resting on the floor. Repeat with the other leg.

One set equals 8 to 12 repetitions on both sides. Do 2 sets in a row, 2 or 3 times a week.

Section 27.4

Men with Osteoporosis: In Their Own Words

Osteoporosis, the bone thinning disease that leads to painful, debilitating bone fractures, affects five million American men. While there has been increased national recognition of osteoporosis as a major women's health problem, the impact of this disease on men has been under-diagnosed, under-reported, and inadequately researched.

Did you know that:

- More than 1.5 million American men suffer from osteoporosis.

- An additional 3.5 million men are at risk for developing osteoporosis.

- One in every 8 men over age 50 will have an osteoporosis-related fracture.

- Each year, 100,000 men suffer a hip fracture and one-third of these men die within a year.

- Tens of thousands of men also fracture bones in their spine, wrists, or ribs as a result of osteoporosis.

Osteoporosis causes the skeleton to weaken and bones to break under the slightest strain or during routine activity. Any bone can be affected, but of special concern are fractures of the hip and spine. A hip fracture almost always requires hospitalization and major surgery. It can impair a person's ability to walk and may cause prolonged or permanent disability or even death. Spinal or vertebral fractures also have serious consequences, including loss of height, severe back pain, and deformity.

In an effort to better understand osteoporosis as a men's health issue, the National Osteoporosis Foundation surveyed men between the ages of 30 and 89 who have been diagnosed with osteoporosis. This section presents, in their own words, their thoughts and feelings on living with osteoporosis, as well as the latest information on this disease.

"I swung my golf club and felt intense pain in my back. The doctor at the hospital said I had a vertebral fracture from osteoporosis. Osteoporosis! I'm a 52-year-old healthy man, and I thought osteoporosis was a disease that only affected older women!"

(Bob J., age 52)

What Is Bone?

Bone is living tissue that is constantly undergoing a process called remodeling, which involves removal of old bone tissue that is then replaced with new bone tissue. During youth, bone grows in both length and density. During the teen years, maximum height is reached, but bones continue to grow more dense until about age 30; thereafter, bone removal exceeds formation and bone density declines.

Osteoporosis develops when not enough new bone is formed or when too much old bone is removed, or both. Bone tissue can also be affected at any time by heredity, diet, sex hormones, physical activity, lifestyle choices, and the use of certain medications.

"My mind is strong vital, and youthful, but my bones are prematurely old. "

(Barry C., age 50)

Are You at Risk for Osteoporosis?

Be sure to tell your doctor if you have any of the following risks for developing osteoporosis:

- Prolonged exposure to certain medications, such as steroids used to treat asthma, arthritis, or other diseases, anticonvulsants certain cancer treatments and aluminum-containing antacids.[1]

- Chronic diseases that affect the kidneys, lungs, stomach, and intestines, or alter hormone levels.[1]

- Undiagnosed low levels of the sex hormone testosterone.

- Unhealthy lifestyle habits (e.g., smoking, excessive alcohol use, low calcium intake, inadequate physical exercise).

- Age: The older you are the greater your risk.

- Heredity.

- Race: Caucasian men appear to be at greatest risk, but all men can develop this disease.

There may be other risk factors that have not yet been identified. Men who do not have any risk factors for this disease are not protected from developing osteoporosis.

"I have severe asthma and have been on the medication, prednisone for many years. This medication makes it easier for me to breathe but I have developed severe osteoporosis as a result of using it."

(Lou J., ago 66)

How Is Osteoporosis Diagnosed?

Osteoporosis can be prevented and effectively treated if it is detected before significant bone loss has occurred. However, because osteoporosis is a silent disease, it progresses without symptoms until a fracture occurs. For this reason, it is important to inform your doctor if you have risk factors for developing osteoporosis, notice a loss of height or change in posture, suffer a fracture, or have sudden back pain. A medical workup to diagnose osteoporosis will include a complete medical history, x-rays, and urine and blood tests.

In addition, your doctor may order a Bone Mineral Density Test (BMD) or bone mass measurement. A special type of x-ray, the BMD tests are accurate, quick, and painless and can detect low bone density, predict risk for future fractures, and diagnose osteoporosis.[2]

How Can Osteoporosis Be Prevented and Treated?

There have been few medical research studies on osteoporosis in men. However, experts agree that all people should take the following steps to preserve bone health.

- Change unhealthy habits such as smoking, excessive alcohol intake, and inactivity.

- Ensure a daily calcium intake of 1,000 ma/ day to age 65 and 1,500 mg/day over age 65.

- Ensure an adequate vitamin D intake. Normally, we make enough vitamin D from exposure to as little as 10 minutes of sunlight a day. If exposure to sunlight is inadequate, dietary vitamin D intake should be at least 400 IU but not more than 800 IU/day, the amount that is found in one cup of fortified milk and most multivitamins.

- Engage in a regular regimen of weight-bearing exercises where bones and muscles work against gravity. This includes walking, jogging, racquet sports, stair-climbing, and team sports. Also, lifting weights or using resistance machines appears to help preserve bone density. If you have already been diagnosed with osteoporosis, any exercise program should be evaluated for safety by your doctor before you begin. Twisting motions and impact activities such as those used in golf, tennis, or basketball may need to be curtailed depending on the severity of your condition.

- Recognize and treat any underlying medical conditions that affect bone health.[1]

- Discuss with your doctor the use of medications that are known to cause bone loss.[1]

"I called an 800 number regarding a research project that wanted participants with osteoporosis. The operator told me only women were eligible, but I have osteoporosis. We need the research effort to focus on us, too!"

(Stan V., age 67)

If you have already been diagnosed with osteoporosis, your doctor may prescribe one of the medications approved by the Food and Drug Administration (FDA) for use in women with this disease. These include calcitonin by injection or nasal spray or the bisphosphonate, alendronate. If your osteoporosis is the result of testosterone deficiency, your doctor may prescribe testosterone replacement therapy.

Living with Osteoporosis

The men who responded to the NOF survey expressed strong feelings and concerns about their future. The survey participants described the pain associated with their fractures and their fear of future fractures. Some of the participants gave up social activities and hobbies; others retired at an early age. The men were also frustrated by the lack of information on osteoporosis as it relates to them.

At the same time, the survey participants expressed the belief that by taking steps to preserve their bone health and by having a positive mental attitude, their outlook and quality of life improved.

"I am so angry that I have osteoporosis and have to worry about the future. I'm single. How do I explain to a special woman that I have to be careful because my bones are really fragile?"

(Warren J., age 46)

Research: the Key to Prevention and Treatment

Only recently have researchers begun to investigate the causes and consequences of osteoporosis in men. An expanded research effort is urgently needed to address this major public health problem.

"The severity of my osteoporosis may force me to take early disability retirement from a job I love. Even love-making is anxiety producing as I'm afraid of fractures."

(Don M, age 53)

Footnotes

1. For information on illness and medications that cause bone loss, contact NOF for the booklet *Medications and Bone Loss*.

2. For information on bone density testing, contact NOF for the booklet *How Strong Are Your Bones*.

Chapter 28

Binge Eating Disorder

Binge eating disorder is a newly recognized condition that probably affects millions of Americans. People with binge eating disorder frequently eat large amounts of food while feeling a loss of control over their eating. This disorder is different from binge-purge syndrome (bulimia nervosa) because people with binge eating disorder usually do not purge afterward by vomiting or using laxatives.

How does someone know if he or she has binge eating disorder?

Most of us overeat from time to time, and many people feel they frequently eat more than they should. Eating large amounts of food, however, does not mean that a person has binge eating disorder. Doctors are still debating the best ways to determine if someone has binge eating disorder. But most people with serious binge eating problems have:

- Frequent episodes of eating what others would consider an abnormally large amount of food.

- Frequent feelings of being unable to control what or how much is being eaten.

NIH Publication No. 94-3589. November 1993. This epub is not copyrighted. Readers are encouraged to duplicate and distribute as many copies as needed.

- Several of these behaviors or feelings:

  1. Eating much more rapidly than usual.
  2. Eating until uncomfortably full.
  3. Eating large amounts of food, even when not physically hungry.
  4. Eating alone out of embarrassment at the quantity of food being eaten.
  5. Feelings of disgust, depression, or guilt after overeating.

Episodes of binge eating also occur in the eating disorder bulimia nervosa. Persons with bulimia, however, regularly purge, fast, or engage in strenuous exercise after an episode of binge eating. Purging means vomiting or using diuretics (water pills) or laxatives in greater-than-recommended doses to avoid gaining weight. Fasting is not eating for at least 24 hours. Strenuous exercise, in this case, is defined as exercising for more than an hour solely to avoid gaining weight after binge eating. Purging, fasting, and strenuous exercise are dangerous ways to attempt weight control.

How common is binge eating disorder, and who is at risk?

Although it has only recently been recognized as a distinct condition, binge eating disorder is probably the most common eating disorder. Most people with binge eating disorder are obese (more than 20 percent above a healthy body weight), but normal-weight people also can be affected. Binge eating disorder probably affects 2 percent of all adults, or about one million to two million Americans. Among mildly obese people in self-help or commercial weight loss programs, 10 to 15 percent have binge eating disorder. The disorder is even more common in those with severe obesity.

Binge eating disorder is slightly more common in women, with three women affected for every two men. The disorder affects blacks as often as whites; its frequency in other ethnic groups is not yet known. Obese people with binge eating disorder often became overweight at a younger age than those without the disorder. They also may have more frequent episodes of losing and regaining weight (yo-yo dieting).

What causes binge eating disorder?

The causes of binge eating disorder are still unknown. Up to half of all people with binge eating disorder have a history of depression. Whether depression is a cause or effect of binge eating disorder is unclear. It may be unrelated. Many people report that anger, sadness, boredom, anxiety or other negative emotions can trigger a binge episode. Impulsive behavior and certain other psychological problems may be more common in people with binge eating disorder.

Dieting's effect on binge eating disorder is also unclear. While findings vary, early research suggests that about half of all people with binge eating disorder had binge episodes before they started to diet. Still, strict dieting may worsen binge eating in some people.

Researchers also are looking into how brain chemicals and metabolism (the way the body burns calories) affect binge eating disorder. These areas of research are still in the early stages.

What are the complications of binge eating disorder?

The major complications of binge eating disorder are the diseases that accompany obesity. These include diabetes, high blood pressure, high cholesterol levels, gallbladder disease, heart disease, and certain types of cancer.

People with binge eating disorder are extremely distressed by their binge eating. Most have tried to control it on their own but have not succeeded for very long. Some people miss work, school, or social activities to binge eat. Obese people with binge eating disorder often feel bad about themselves, are preoccupied with their appearance, and may avoid social gatherings. Most feel ashamed and try to hide their problem. Often they are so successful that close family members and friends don't know they binge eat.

Should people with binge eating disorder try to diet?

People who are not overweight or only mildly obese should probably avoid dieting, since strict dieting may worsen binge eating. However, many people with binge eating disorder are severely obese and have medical problems related to their weight. For these people, losing weight and keeping it off are important treatment goals. Most people with binge eating disorder, whether or not they want to lose weight, may benefit from treatment that addresses their eating behavior.

What treatment is available for people with binge eating disorder?

Several studies have found that people with binge eating disorder may find it harder than other people to stay in weight loss treatment. Binge eaters also may be more likely to regain weight quickly. For these reasons, people with the disorder may require treatment that focuses on their binge eating before they try to lose weight.

Even those who are not overweight are frequently distressed by their binge eating and may benefit from treatment.

Several methods are being used to treat binge eating disorder.

- **Cognitive-behavioral therapy** teaches patients techniques to monitor and change their eating habits as well as to change the way they respond to difficult situations.

- **Interpersonal psychotherapy** helps people examine their relationships with friends and family and to make changes in problem areas.

- **Treatment with medications** such as antidepressants may be helpful for some individuals.

- **Self-help groups** also may be a source of support.

Researchers are still trying to determine which method or combination of methods is the most effective in controlling binge eating disorder. The type of treatment that is best for an individual is a matter for discussion between the patient and his or her health care provider.

If you believe you have binge eating disorder, it's important you realize that you are not alone. Most people who have the disorder have tried unsuccessfully to control it on their own. You may want to seek professional treatment.

Additional Readings

Marcus MD. "Binge Eating in Obesity." In: Fairburn CG, Wilson GT (eds).

Binge eating: nature, assessment, and treatment. New York: Guilford Press. This chapter reviews the scientific knowledge about binge eating disorder. It is geared to health professionals who do research on and treat patients with binge eating problems. The book is scheduled for publication in Spring 1993.

de Zwaan MD, Mitchell JE. "Binge Eating in the Obese." *Annals of Medicine.* Vol. 24, pp. 303-308, 1992. This review article is written for health professionals. It describes previous studies of binge eating in obese individuals and how they differ from obese people who do not binge eat.

Stunkard AJ. "Eating Patterns and Obesity." *Psychiatric Quarterly*, 1959, Vol. 33, pp. 284-295. This classic paper provides one of the first descriptions of binge eating in obese individuals.

Binge Eating Disorder Programs

Behavioral Medicine
Stanford University School of Medicine
Department of Psychiatry TD209
Stanford, CA 94305
Tel: 415-723-5868

Binge Eating Program
Western Psychiatric Institute and Clinic
3811 O'Hara Street
Pittsburgh, PA 15213
Tel: 412-624-2823

Eating Disorders Clinic
New York State Psychiatric Institute
Columbia Presbyterian Medical Center
722 W. 168th Street
Unit #98
New York, NY 10032
Tel: 212-960-5739/5746

Eating Disorder Research Program
University of Minnesota
2701 University Avenue, S.E.
Suite 102
Minneapolis, MN 55414
Tel: 612-627-4494

Nutrition Research Clinic
Baylor College of Medicine
6535 Fannin Street
MS F700
Houston, TX 77030
Tel: 713-798-5757

Rutgers Eating Disorders Clinic
GSAPP, Rutgers University
Box 819
Piscataway, NJ 08854
Tel: 908-932-2292

Women's Recovery Center
110 N. Essex Avenue
Narberth, PA 19072
Tel: 215-664-5858

Yale Center For Eating and Weight Disorders
P.O. Box 11A, Yale Station
New Haven, CT 06520
Tel: 03-432-4610

Chapter 29

Urinary Tract Infections
in Men

Urinary tract infections? Don't they affect only women?

Yes and no. Women generally develop urinary tract infections
(UTIs) at an earlier age and have them more frequently throughout
their lives. But men also get UTIs.

The classic symptom is difficulty in voiding or a painful sensation
when you urinate. Even when you feel the urge, you can't pass urine
freely, or you release only a small amount. The urge quickly returns.

Most urinary tract infections aren't dangerous if you get proper
care. But if you also have pain in your abdomen or back, chills, fever
or vomiting, your kidneys may be infected.

A kidney infection is a serious medical condition requiring prompt
treatment and, perhaps, hospitalization

What causes a UTI?

The most common cause is the *Escherichia coli* (E. coli) bacterium.
It resides in your intestinal tract and may migrate through your
lymph system to your bladder.

Inflammation of the bladder (*cystitis*) can result from infection with
E. coli. Other factors also promote urinary tract infections in men:

- **Prostate problems.** Your prostate is a walnut-sized gland below your bladder and surrounding your urethra. A UTI can occur if an enlarged prostate constricts your urethra, preventing your bladder from emptying completely. Leftover urine can create a breeding ground for bacteria.

  Enlargement of the prostate gland is a normal part of aging, but infection is not.

  Also, your prostate gland secretes proteins into your seminal fluid. These proteins have an antibacterial property.

  Little or no production of these proteins by your prostate can make you more susceptible to infection.

- **Invasive medical procedures.** A urinary catheter can introduce bacteria, especially if the catheter stays in place for several days. Infection-causing bacteria also may be introduced when a catheter is first inserted.

- **Narrowed urethra.** Frequent inflammation of your urethra (urethritis) can scar and narrow your urethra. This is called a urethral stricture.

  In years past, physicians believed strictures usually were caused by recurrent bouts with a sexually transmitted disease, such as gonorrhea. Today, strictures are more commonly associated with catheters or use of instruments used to explore or treat urologic problems.

- **Dehydration.** An inadequate intake of fluids can foster stagnant (concentrated) urine. Hot weather can lead to dehydration.

Medications Work Quickly

Your doctor can diagnose a UTI from symptoms and tests, including urinalysis and a urine culture.

Don't "push" fluids before a test. Fluids can dilute your urine sample and reduce the accuracy of tests.

Your physician will prescribe a broad-spectrum antibiotic or a sulfa-type drug.

Symptoms usually subside after several days, but be sure to take all your prescribed medication.

Chapter 30

Hormone Replacement Therapy for Men: Has the Time Come?

Hormonal changes in older women are well-documented, and their effects widely studied. No one can dispute the complications of heart disease and osteoporosis associated with estrogen loss after menopause. We know less, however, about the effects of declining serum hormone levels in aging men. Is it possible that the age-related loss of growth hormone and testosterone has similar consequences in men? If so, might hormone replacement therapy help men age more "successfully?"

The late Daniel Rudman, MD, was devoted to finding answers to these questions. An endocrinologist, Dr. Rudman developed an interest in human growth hormone early in his career. In 1971, he and his colleagues published the definitive study on human growth hormone replacement therapy in children with growth hormone deficiency.[1] When he became chief of geriatric medicine at the North Chicago VA Hospital, he turned his attention to geriatric endocrinology in general and to the biology of growth hormone metabolism in particular. In 1990, he and colleagues published a ground-breaking study describing the beneficial effects of human growth hormone treatment in men over age 60.[2] Dr. Rudman, one of AFAR's most prestigious grantees, died unexpectedly in April 1994 at the age of 67.

Early in 1994, Dr. Rudman had agreed to be interviewed for this series and had provided numerous background materials. This article, written posthumously, highlights Dr. Rudman's studies and examines their potential clinical implications for older men. The questions and answers are based on Dr. Rudman's writings and have been reviewed by his colleagues—Edmund H. Duthie, Jr., MD, and Kaup R. Shetty, MD, at the Medical College of Wisconsin, Milwaukee.

Why consider hormone therapy for older men?

Many of the age-associated changes in elderly men—loss of muscle and bone mass, increased adipose tissue, mild anemia, and reduced aerobic work capacity—can result from deficient secretion of growth hormone and luteinizing hormone by the hypothalamic/pituitary system. Such neuroendocrine deficiencies lead to low serum levels of insulin growth factor 1 (IGF-1) and testosterone. When we examined men over age 60, we found that 80 percent had serum levels of IGF-1 and testosterone that were two standard deviations below the levels of young healthy men. Whether these levels are pathologic or physiologic in elderly men is still not known. When deficiency of growth hormone or testosterone occurs in young or middle-aged men, however, hormone replacement is usually given because of its beneficial effects. Thus, we thought it reasonable to consider replacement therapy for hormone-deficient older men, and this has been the focus of our work.

Has replacement therapy for hormonally deficient elderly men been found beneficial?

Our first study[2] looked at men between the ages of 61 and 81 who had serum levels of IGF-1 significantly below those found in young healthy men (<0.35 U/ml). Twelve men were treated for 6 months with recombinant human growth hormone (rHGH), and nine age-matched men were untreated. The treated group showed a 9 percent increase in lean body mass, a 14 percent decrease in adipose mass, and a small but significant increase in lumbar vertebral bone density without adverse reactions. The untreated men showed no significant changes in these parameters.

We subsequently published the results of a larger, 12-month study[3] of elderly men (mean age, 69) with serum IGF-1 levels below 0.35 U/ml who were treated with rHGH. After 12 months, treated men showed a 6 percent increase in lean body mass and a 16 percent decrease in adipose mass. The most favorable results were observed in subjects whose mean serum IGF-1 during replacement therapy was between 0.5 and 1.0 U/ml. The normal physiologic range for young healthy men is 0.5 to 1.5 U/ml. Untreated men continued to lose lean body mass throughout the study period. Adverse results (most commonly gynecomastia and/or carpal tunnel syndrome) occurred, with one exception, in subjects with mean serum IGF-1 levels above 1 U/ml.

A recent report[4] suggested beneficial effects of weekly administration of 100 mg of testosterone in elderly men (mean age, 69) with low or borderline low serum testosterone levels (<13.9 nmol/L). On replacement therapy, serum testosterone levels rose. After 3 months of therapy, lean body mass, hematocrit, and prostate specific antigen (PSA) levels increased significantly, whereas LDL cholesterol and urinary hydroxyproline excretion (a possible indicator of reduced bone reabsorption) decreased. There are much less data on the effect of pharmacologic doses of human growth hormone or testosterone in humans without hormone deficiency, although the use of androgens to augment athletic performance is widely reported in the press, and clinical trials of supraphysiologic therapy are now underway.

Do you recommend hormone replacement therapy for hormone-deficient older men?

Not yet. We are encouraged by our clinical studies of replacement therapy with rHGH in older men, but it has not been FDA-approved. Although rHGH has been shown to increase muscle strength and physical fitness in young IGF-1-deficient individuals, we do not yet know if the rHGH-stimulated increase in lean body mass in elderly men will also lead to increased muscle strength and physical well-being. We anticipate that rHGH (or stimulants of rHGH secretion) will first be used in frail and debilitated patients where the risk-benefit ratio is higher.

Although testosterone has been approved for use in hypogonadal men, its use in older men remains experimental, as the benefits have yet to be proven. Concerns also remain about the potential risks of long-term therapy on prostatic hypertrophy, prostatic carcinoma, and serum lipoproteins.

What is your therapeutic approach to hormonally deficient elderly men?

The goal of growth hormone therapy is to raise serum IGF-1 into the normal range of 0.5 to 1.0 U/ml, and patients who are maintained in this range have the best clinical results. Our recent studies in patients with post-polio syndrome indicate that these levels can be achieved with one-fourth to one-half the standard dosage of growth hormone (0.03 mg/kg of body weight three times weekly).[5] It is reasonable to start therapy with a daily injection of 0.25 to 0.50 mg of growth hormone daily at bedtime and increase the dose as necessary until the desired serum level of IGF-1 is achieved.

The goal of testosterone therapy is less well defined, but serum testosterone levels between 240 and 460 ng/ml are a reasonable target. A more physiologic treatment regimen would be the daily injection of testosterone or its continuous administration using a skin patch in order to achieve a more constant level of hormone. Conventional treatment with depot testosterone injections initially gives high serum levels, which then decline.

For how long should replacement therapy be given to the older man?

Both short-term and chronic therapy with rHGH and/or testosterone may be indicated. Short-term therapy may be indicated to maintain lean body mass when impaired nutrition or catabolic states develop. Such an approach might well facilitate wound healing in a debilitated elderly patient. Chronic replacement therapy in elderly men, as we have shown, might limit age-associated loss of lean body and bone mass.

What adverse effects occur in hormonally deficient men given replacement therapy?

Some studies have reported that as many as one-third of elderly patients given growth hormone developed carpal tunnel syndrome, approximately 10 percent developed gynecomastia, and a small percentage, hyperglycemia.[3] We found that the patients who developed these side effects had mean serum IGF-1 levels above 1.0 U/ml. Those whose IGF-1 levels were maintained in the range of 0.5 to 1.0 U/ml had the greatest level of desired responses and few or no adverse effects.

A number of adverse reactions have been reported in testosterone-treated elderly patients, including fluid retention, increased cardiovascular risk associated with changes in lipoproteins, erythrocytosis, sleep apnea, and increased PSA levels. These effects have been seen within 6 to 12 months of therapy. As prostatic hypertrophy and cancer do not occur in the absence of androgens, the risk of increasing these conditions by testosterone therapy is a cause for concern. A trial currently in progress is examining the beneficial and adverse effects of androgens among testosterone-deficient men, especially their effects on the prostate.

Similarly, there is a theoretical concern about the development of cancer in patients on long-term growth hormone therapy. Not only is IGF-1 a mitogen for cells of many lineages, but acromegalic patients with elevated IGF-1 levels have an increased incidence of colon and breast cancer. Whether there is a significant risk of cancer in patients given physiologic doses of growth hormone is not known. Finally, there is also a theoretical risk of prostatic hypertrophy and arthritis.

Could women also benefit from growth hormone or androgen replacement therapy?

This is certainly a theoretical possibility. The level of IGF-1 in women also declines with age, and growth hormone-deficient young women do benefit from replacement therapy. No one would consider treating women with testosterone because of its virilizing actions. However, the use of another weak androgenic hormone, dehydroepiandrosterone (DHEA), has been considered.

DHEA declines with age, and at every age the risk of breast cancer is highest in women with the lowest serum concentration of DHEA. Subsequently, low DHEA levels in serum have been found to be associated with increased death from all causes. A 28-day randomized, double-blind trial of DHEA therapy in young men was reported to produce a significant decrease in adipose mass and LDL cholesterol.[6] It is not known, at present, whether replacement therapy with growth hormone or DHEA in either older men or women with low serum concentration of these hormones would convey clinical benefit.

In summary, there is reason to believe that hormone replacement therapy will come to play an important role in maintaining the health of our older population—both women and men.

References

1. Rudman D, Patterson JH, Gibbas DL. Responsiveness of growth hormone-deficient children to human growth hormone. Effect of replacement therapy for one year. J Clin Invest 1973; 52:1108-1212.

2. Rudman D, Feller AG, Nagraj HS, et al. Effects of human growth hormone in men over 60 years old. N Engl J Med 1990; 323:1-6.

3. Cohn L, Feller AG, Draper MW, Rudman IW, Rudman D. Carpal tunnel syndrome and gynaecomastia during growth hormone treatment of elderly men with low circulating IFG-1 concentrations. Clin Endocrinol 1993; 39.417-25.

4. Tenover JS. Effects of testosterone supplementation in the aging male. J Clin Endocrinol Metab 1992; 75:1092-8

5. Gupta KL, Shetty KR, Agre JC, Cuisinier MC, Rudman IW, Rudman D. Human growth hormone effect on serum IGF-l and muscle function in poliomyelitis survivors. Arch Phys Med Rehabil 1994; 75:889-94.

6. Nestler JE, Barlascini CO, Clore JN, Blackard WG. Dehydroepiandrosterone reduces serum low density lipoprotein levels and body fat but does not alter insulin sensitivity in normal men. J Clin Endocrinol Metab 1988; 66:57-61.

—Marc E. Weksler, MD

Weksler is president emeritus, American Federation for Aging Research, New York, and Irving S. Wright professor of medicine and director, geriatrics and gerontology, Cornell University Medical College New York.

Chapter 31

Headache

Description

Headache is a common and frequently recurrent disorder that can seriously disrupt a person's life. Headache pain may be generalized (all over) or localized (in one area) and may range from mild to severe. Some headaches have a known cause while others, like migraine headaches, do not. Postural changes, prolonged coughing, sneezing, or exposure to sunlight may contribute to headache. Sometimes a headache may be a symptom of a serious underlying problem (such as stroke or brain tumor) and may call for prompt medical care. Serious headaches include those that are sudden and severe, associated with convulsions or seizures, accompanied by confusion or loss of consciousness, associated with a blow on the head or pain in the eye or ear, or persistent in a person who was previously headache-free. Recurring headaches in children, those associated with fever, or those that interfere with normal life should be checked by a doctor. The most common types of headaches include migraine, cluster, and tension-type. Migraines produce throbbing pain on one or both sides of the head. Symptoms, besides pain, may include nausea, vomiting, light and noise sensitivity, fever, chills, flu-like achiness, and sweating. Some sufferers have warnings before a migraine, such as visual disturbances.

National Institutes of Health, epub – (http://www.ninds.nih.gov/healinfo/ DISORDER/Headache/headache.htm) June 1997. Last updated October 23, 1997. National Institute of Neurological Disorders and Stroke, Bethesda, Maryland 20892.

Migraine attacks may last from a few hours to days, and may recur several times a week or once every few years. Cluster headaches, which mainly occur in men, occur as a series of one-sided headaches that are sudden and excruciating and may continue for 15 minutes to 4 hours. Symptoms on the painful side may include nasal congestion, drooping eyelid, and irritated, watery (teary) eye. Tension-type headaches, which are the most common headache type, produce a dull, achy pain that feels like pressure is being applied to the head or neck. These headaches may be associated with muscle tenderness and increased electromyogram (EMG) activity.

Treatment

For many people, analgesics may provide relief. Antidepressants may be used to relieve stress-related headaches. Muscle relaxants may benefit chronic tension headache sufferers. Ergotamine tartrate or sumatriptin taken at the beginning of a migraine headache may reduce the severity of the headache. Other therapeutic options may include supportive measures such as regular exercise, biofeedback, and physical therapy. Chronic and repetitive use of headache treatments may increase headache frequency in some individuals. Monitoring by a physician experienced with treating headache is helpful.

Research

The NINDS supports and conducts research aimed at improving the diagnosis of headaches and finding ways to prevent and treat them.

These articles, available from a medical library, are sources of in-depth information on headache:

Farley, D. "Headache Misery May Yield to Proper Treatment." FDA Consumer, Food and Drug Administration, Rockville, MD, pp. 26-31 (September 1992).

Mathew, N. "Cluster Headache." Neurology, 42 (Suppl 2):3; 22-31 (March 1992).

Silberstein, S. "Tension-type and Chronic Daily Headache." Neurology, 43:9; 1644- 1649 (September 1993).

Stewart, W, et al. "Prevalence of Migraine Headache in the United States." Journal of the American Medical Association, 267:1; 64-69 (January 1, 1992).

Welch, K. "Drug Therapy of Migraine." The New England Journal of Medicine, 329:20; 1476-1483 (November 11, 1993).

Information is available from the following organizations:

American Council for Headache Education (ACHE)
875 Kings Highway, Ste. 200
Woodbury, NJ 08096
(609) 845-0322
(800) 255-2243

American Chronic Pain Association
P.O. Box 850
Rocklin, CA 95677
(916) 632-0922

National Headache Foundation
428 West St. James Place
Chicago, IL 60614
(773) 388-6399
(800) 843-2256

National Chronic Pain Outreach Association, Inc.
P.O. Box 274
Millboro, VA 24460
(540) 997-5004

Part Eight

Other Common Concerns

Chapter 32

Facts about Kidney and Urologic Disorders

Kidney Problems

Kidney Conditions (Infection, Kidney Stones, Cancer, Missing Kidney, Other)

- Prevalence (1994): 3.512 million conditions (in civilian non-institutionalized population)[1]

Polycystic Kidney Disease

- Prevalence: Between 1 in 1,000 and 1 in 400 people (closer to latter)[3]

End-stage Renal Disease (ESRD)

- Prevalence (period, 1993): 257,351[3] people, resulting from three primary diseases:

Diabetes	73,681
Hypertension	63,440
Glomerulonephritis	41,532

NIH Publication No. 96-3895, April 1996, etext updated: 30 October 1996. This epub is not subject to copyright restrictions. The clearinghouse encourages users of this etext to duplicate and distribute as many copies as desired.

681

- Incidence (new beneficiaries of treatment, 1993): 56,600 people,[3] resulting from these primary diseases:

Diabetes	19,013
Hypertension	15,064
Glomerulonephritis	5,655

- Deaths in treated patients (1993): 40,916 people[3]

- Amount spent (public and private, 1994): $11.1 billion[3]

ESRD treatment

- Use of dialysis (1995): 200,162 people[4]

In-center therapy:

Hemodialysis	166,173
IPD	90
CAPD	194
CCPD	114

Home therapy:

Hemodialysis	2,086
IPD	137
CAPD	21,369
CCPD	9,999

- Number of kidney transplants (by year):[4]

1995	11,902
1994	11,312
1985	7,695

- Number of kidney transplants (by type, 1995):[4]

From cadaver	8,486
From living related donor	2,992
From living unrelated donor	424

- People awaiting transplants (August 31, 1996):[5] 34,798

Kidney (only)	33,399
Kidney and pancreas	1,399

- Dialysis survival (percent of patients surviving):[3]

1 year (1993)	77.30
2 years (1992-1993)	60.32
5 years (1989-1993)	28.14
10 years (1984-1993)	9.65

- Cadaver-donor transplant survival (percent of recipients surviving):[3]

1 year (1993)	93.57
2 years (1992-1993)	90.27
5 years (1989-1993)	78.63
10 years (1984-1993)	55.07

- Living-related-donor transplant survival (percent of recipients surviving):

1 year (1993)	97.53
2 years (1992-1993)	95.72
5 years (1989-1993)	89.81
10 years (1984-1993)	77.16

Urologic Problems

Acute Urinary Conditions

(infections of the kidneys and urinary tract, nephrotic syndrome, urethral stricture, cystitis, other)

- Incidence (1994): 8.140 million conditions (in civilian non-institutionalized population)[1]

Bladder Disorders

- Prevalence (1994): 3.747 million disorders (in civilian non-institutionalized population)[1]

Kidney and Ureter Stones

Doctor visits (1991)	895,467 visits[6]
Cost (total direct and indirect, 1993)	$1.83 billion[7]
Hospitalizations (1993)	302,000[8]

Urinary Tract Infections

Doctor visits (1991)	9.642 million visits[6]
Hospitalizations (1991)	1.547 million[9]

Urinary Incontinence

- Prevalence: About 13 million adults[10]

Interstitial Cystitis

- Prevalence: About 500,000 people (90 percent of those are women)[11]

Other Related Problems

Diseases of the Prostate

- Prevalence (1992): 2.048 million men (in non-institutionalized population)[1]

Enlarged Prostate (BPH)

- Prevalence: More than 50 percent of men past age 60; 80 to 90 percent of men past age 80[12]

- Hospital discharges for BPH (1993): 375,000 hospitalizations[8]

Prostate Cancer

- Incidence (1991): 120,000 men develop it each year[13]

- Mortality (1991): 30,000 men die of it each year[13]

Impotence/erectile Dysfunction

- Prevalence: 10 to 15 million men[14]

Sources

1. *Current Estimates from the National Health Interview Survey, 1994.* National Center for Health Statistics, Centers for Disease Control and Prevention (CDC), U.S. Dept. of Health and Human Services (HHS), December 1995.

2. Torres, V. E., et al. General features of autosomal dominant polycystic kidney disease: Epidemiology. In: *Problems in Diagnosis and Management of Polycystic Kidney Disease,* Grantham, J. J., and Gardner, K. D., eds. Polycystic Kidney Research Foundation, Kansas City, MO (1985).

3. *United States Renal Data System 1996 Annual Data Report,* National Institute of Diabetes and Digestive and Kidney Diseases, NIH, HHS, 1996.

4. *End Stage Renal Disease Program Highlights 1995* (fact sheet), Health Care Financing Administration, HHS, August 1996.

5. United Network for Organ Sharing. For updates contact the UNOS Data Request Fax Line at (804) 323-3794 or visit the UNOS homepage at http://www.ew3.att.net/unos/.

6. Unpublished data from 1991 National Ambulatory Medical Care Survey (National Center for Health Statistics).

7. Clark, J. Y., et al., Economic impact of urolithiasis in the United States. *Journal of Urology,* vol. 154, pp. 2020-2024, December 1995.

8. *National Hospital Discharge Survey: Annual Summary, 1993,* CDC, HHS, 1995.

9. *Detailed Diagnoses and Procedures, National Hospital Discharge Survey, 1991,* National Center for Health Statistics, CDC, HHS, February 1994.

10. *Urinary Incontinence in Adults: Clinical Practice Guideline Update.* Agency for Health Care Policy and Research, HHS, 1996.

11. *Interstitial Cystitis,* National Institute of Diabetes and Digestive and Kidney Diseases, National Institutes of Health, HHS, 1994.

12. Prostate Enlargement: Benign Prostatic Hyperplasia, National Institute of Diabetes and Digestive and Kidney Diseases, NIH, 1991.

13. *Prostate Cancer: What Every Man Over 40 Should Know,*
     Prostate Health Council, c/o American Foundation for Uro-
     logic Disease, Inc., Baltimore, MD.

14. Impotence(fact sheet), National Institute of Diabetes and Di-
     gestive and Kidney Diseases, NIH, HHS, 1995.

ESRD numbers are based on Medicare enrollments and refer to
about 92 percent of total U.S. ESRD patients.

There is probably an undercount of patients with these diseases
reported to the Health Care Financing Administration during the
third quarter of 1993.

IPD=intermittent peritoneal dialysis; CAPD=continuous ambulatory peritoneal dialysis; CCPD=continuous cyclic peritoneal dialysis.

National Kidney and Urologic Diseases Information Clearinghouse
3 Information Way
Bethesda, MD 20892-3580
E-mail: kudic@aerie.com

Chapter 33

Backache

What's Behind Back Pain and What You Can Do to Prevent it

Your back hurts. The pain comes whenever you stoop to tie your shoes or pump the brakes in your car. Maybe you've "thrown out" your back lifting something heavy. Or maybe you can't remember when or how it started, but now it seems like the pain won't go away. Your back reminds you it's there. And it hurts.

You're not alone. Back pain is ranked second only to headaches as the most frequent cause of pain. Four out of five adults will experience a bout of back pain at some time in their lives.

In fact, back injuries were the nation's most common form of disabling work injury in 1992. And, even though back trouble is rarely life-threatening, it costs an estimated $40 billion a year in medical bills, lost wages and insurance claims in the United States.

With numbers like these, it may surprise you that you can ward off back problems with simple steps such as exercise and adopting a new way to sit or stand. Even if you've injured your back before, you can learn techniques to help you avoid recurrent injuries. Back pain is common, particularly as you get older. But it's not inevitable.

687

Back Basics

If you're like most people, you don't think much about your back—at least not until it hurts. What does your back actually do for you?

The answer is a matter of balance. Cars have four wheels; chairs have four legs. And fellow mammals from mice to monkeys walk on four feet. Four points make balance easy.

But humans stand and move about on two legs—a remarkable piece of engineering. Muscles contract and relax to enable you to stand and move. Tendons fasten muscles to the bones in your back (vertebrae). Ligaments—tough, fibrous bands—hold your vertebrae together. Your backbone also protects the spinal cord, the main pathway for your central nervous system.

It takes this delicately balanced interworking of bones, muscles, ligaments, tendons and nerves to balance and bear the weight of your body and the loads you carry.

Common Kinds of Backaches

Even minor damage to any one component of your back's structure can upset the delicate balance and make movement painful. Back pain can occur for no apparent reason and at any point on your spine. The most common site for pain, however, is your lower back because it bears the majority of your weight.

Lack of muscle tone and excess weight, especially around your middle, commonly cause and aggravate back pain. Poor posture adds stress, too. When you slouch or stand with a swayback, you exaggerate your back's natural curves. Any imbalance can stress muscles and joints, causing fatigue and injury from overuse.

Add the daily stresses and strains you put on your back, such as carrying out the trash, mowing the lawn, leaning over close handwork for long periods, or even applying the brakes in your car. And all too often the result is the familiar complaint, "Oh, my aching back."

From the simple backache to more serious back problems, here are common sources of back pain:

- **Muscle strains and spasms.** Once commonly called "lumbago," aches and pains usually signal strained muscles, tendons or ligaments, or inflamed joints along your backbone. If you strain your back, you may feel the pain immediately or develop soreness or stiffness later. Muscle spasm may occur after an injury. Spasm is your back's response to injury, designed to immobilize you and prevent further damage.

- **Osteoarthritis.** Commonly referred to as arthritis, this disorder affects nearly everyone past age 60. Excessive use, injury or aging slowly deteriorates cartilage, the protective tissue that covers the surface of vertebral joints. Discs between vertebrae become worn and the spaces between the bones narrow. Bony outgrowths called spurs (osteophytes) also develop. Gradually, your spine stiffens and loses flexibility. As vertebral joints rub together with greater force than normal, the surfaces where they meet, called facets, compress and become irregular. Cartilage becomes inflamed, and the result is pain.

- **Sciatica.** One to two people in 100 with back pain may experience "sciatica" (sy-AT-ic-a), named after the sciatic nerve that extends down each leg from your hip to your heel. Nerve inflammation or compression of a nerve root in your lower back can cause sciatica. You may feel the pain radiating from your back down through your buttock to your lower leg. Tingling, numbness or muscle weakness may also accompany nerve compression. Coughing, sneezing and other activities that exert pressure on your spine can worsen sciatica. Usually, the pain resolves on its own. However, severe nerve compression can cause progressive muscle weakness.

- **Osteoporosis.** The amount of calcium in your bones decreases as you age. Loss of calcium weakens your bone structure. In some cases, the vertebrae become compressed, resulting in back pain. One in three women older than 50 is affected by compression fractures caused by osteoporosis. Progressive compression of vertebrae often leads to a gradual loss of height in women, starting after menopause. Frequently, structural changes also occur in the spinal column that may cause many women to develop a crooked stance or a stooped-shoulder posture called "dowager's hump."

- **Herniated disc.** A "slipped disc" is how you might describe this problem. While they don't actually "slip," normal wear and tear or strain may cause a disc to bulge or to rupture (herniate). Discs have a strong, fibrous outer structure that contains a gel on the inside. When a disc herniates, its soft, jelly-like interior protrudes from its normal position between your vertebrae. Pain can result when a fragment of the herniated disc places pressure on an adjacent nerve.

- **Injuries and accidents.** A decrease in muscle tone as you age makes you prone to back pain, especially that caused by muscle injuries. A shifting in your center of gravity due to increased fat around your abdomen also may offset your balance and increase your risk of an injury or accident.

- **Fibromyalgia (fye-bro-my-AL-gee-ah).** This syndrome is characterized by achy pain, tenderness and stiffness in muscles and areas where tendons insert into bones. Pain often worsens after you're inactive and tends to improve with movement. It's uncertain how many people have fibromyalgia. Doctors have only recently identified the syndrome and the cause is not well understood. At Mayo Clinic, physicians diagnose about 5,000 people a year with fibromyalgia.

Less Common Causes of Back Pain

A less common cause of back pain in older adults is **spinal or lumbar stenosis**. Stenosis means a narrowing of the spinal canal. Narrowing compresses nerves in your lower back and can cause numbness, pain and weakness in your back and legs. Symptoms often worsen when you walk and subside when you sit or bend forward.

Ankylosing spondylitis (AN-ki-LO-sing SPON-dill-I-tis), a serious form of arthritis, is an uncommon type of back pain that typically affects young men. At first, it causes pain and stiffness in the joints of your spine. With time, the disease causes your vertebrae to fuse together, limiting movement in your back.

Rarely, **infections** can develop in your vertebrae. **Tumors** may spread from other parts of your body, such as your breasts or esophagus, to cause pain. But it's not common. Also, tumors typically don't originate in your spine and, if they do, are usually benign.

Sometimes your brain mistakes pain signals from other organs as pain originating in your back. Problems with your kidneys, uterus or prostate, or cancers in other parts of your body are common sources of "**referred pain**."

Lifestyle factors such as stress and smoking also may play a role in back pain, although the mechanisms aren't proven.

Back Care

Try simple measures first

Because most back problems aren't life-threatening, many doctors recommend home treatment first. Episodes of back pain usually resolve within two weeks with simple measures like rest and over-the-counter pain relievers. And regardless of the type of treatment, 80 to 90 percent of back pain resolves within six weeks.

If you have strained ligaments or severe muscle strain, your recovery could take as long as 12 weeks. But with time and proper care, even a herniated disc can repair itself.

Here are guidelines for treating back pain at home:

- **Apply cold, then heat.** Sources of heat and cold, such as a hot bath and hot or cold compresses, can soothe sore and inflamed muscles. Use cold treatment first.

  1. Immediately after an injury, apply ice several times a day, but for no longer than 20 minutes at a time. Put ice in a plastic bag, then wrap the bag in a cloth or towel to keep a thin barrier between it and your skin.

  2. After acute pain subsides, usually within the first one to two days, apply heat from a heating pad or heat lamp. Limit each heat application to 20 minutes. To avoid burns, keep the heating pad on a low setting and away from areas of reduced sensation.

- **Use over-the-counter medications.** Pain relievers like acetaminophen may help control pain. Nonsteroidal anti-inflammatory drugs like aspirin and ibuprofen can also reduce inflammation that affects muscles and joints. Be sure to check with your doctor if you're taking medications for other health problems.

For persistent pain, get professional care

In rare cases, back pain can signal serious medical problems. Don't hesitate to contact your doctor immediately if your back pain is the result of a fall or blow to your back. Also, be on the lookout for weakness or numbness in one or both legs, and new bladder or bowel control problems.

If you've tried home remedies for several weeks but still have pain, your family doctor or internist may be able to pinpoint the source of your pain and recommend additional therapy. During a typical visit, your doctor will ask how the pain began, how long it has lasted and what aggravates or relieves it. He or she will probably watch your muscles and joints as you stand, walk and move your back.

Your doctor may also recommend special tests. If your doctor refers you to a physician specialist, such as a physiatrist, neurologist, orthopedic surgeon or neurosurgeon, you may be prescribed additional treatment including:

- **Prescription medications.** For relief of pain, your doctor may prescribe an anti-inflammatory medication along with a "muscle relaxant." For some people, corticosteroid injections may also help relieve localized inflammation, but they're usually reserved for short-term use.

- **Heat, cold and massage.** When performed by a licensed professional, applications of heat, cold and gentle massage may relieve back pain due to muscle spasms.

A word of caution: Manipulation of your spine may aggravate a disc problem or cause compression fractures if you have osteoporosis. Ask your primary-care doctor if spinal manipulation is safe and helpful for you.

- **Electrical stimulation.** A procedure called transcutaneous electrical nerve stimulation (TENS) may help stop pain by blocking nerve signals from reaching your brain. A physical therapist places electrodes on your skin near the painful area. TENS is a reasonable approach, but it may have minimal benefit for chronic back pain.

- **Back schools.** Available in many communities, these programs are geared toward managing back pain and preventing its recurrence. Classroom study generally involves back anatomy and function, followed by practice sessions on how to protect your back at home and work. Depending on the program, you may need a physician's referral.

- **Exercise and physical therapy.** Exercise can play a vital role in your recovery. Two days of rest in bed on a firm surface or mattress help ease pain caused by strains or most disc problems. But because you need to move regularly to maintain muscle tone, doctors warn against longer periods of strict bed rest.

Once acute pain improves, your doctor or a physical therapist can design a rehabilitation program to help prevent recurrent injuries.

Rehabilitation typically includes exercises to help correct your posture, improve your flexibility and strengthen the muscles supporting your back.

Sometimes surgery is the answer

Odds are you won't need surgery for back pain. The pain and disability caused by a herniated disc or spinal stenosis frequently diminish with conservative treatment. However, if you have unrelenting pain or muscle weakness caused by nerve compression, you may need surgery.

Using a procedure called lumbar laminectomy, your surgeon can remove disc fragments that press on nerve roots within your spine. Unfortunately, it's difficult to predict whether surgery will relieve all your symptoms. Talk to your doctor about the type of relief laminectomy may offer you.

Some people with nerve compression may benefit from aspiration percutaneous lumbar diskectomy (APLD). During this procedure, the surgeon loosens and removes the damaged disc with a device that fits into a large needle inserted through your skin. This technique may offer a less painful recovery period than laminectomy, but the long-term benefits are less certain.

Before you agree to back surgery, consider getting a second opinion. Surgery to repair a herniated disc is among the most frequently performed procedures in the United States. Yet the outcome is often the same whether you have surgery or choose a less-invasive treatment.

Exercise is the cornerstone of pain prevention

Regular exercise is your most potent weapon against back problems. Activity can increase your aerobic capacity, improve your overall fitness and help you shed excess pounds that stress your back.

Stretching and toning your back and other supporting muscles can help reduce wear and tear on your back. Stretching reduces your risk of injury by warming up your muscles. It also increases your long-term flexibility.

Strength training can make your arms, legs and lower body stronger. In turn, your risk for falls and other injuries decreases. Strong arms, legs and especially abdominal muscles also help relieve back strain. If you have osteoporosis, back strengthening exercises may help prevent additional compression fractures (see *Mayo Clinic Health Letter*, October 1993).

Ask your doctor or a physical therapist for advice before beginning an exercise program, especially if you've hurt your back before, or if you have other health problems such as significant osteoporosis. Then follow these general suggestions:

- **Start slowly.** If you're out of condition from lack of activity, your back muscles may be weak and susceptible to injury. Pace yourself and don't overdo. As you become stronger, work up to 15 minutes of exercise daily.

- **Make smart moves.** Generally, swimming and other water exercises are safest for your back. Because they're non-weight-bearing, these activities place minimal strain on your lower back. Workouts on a stationary bike, treadmill or cross-country ski machine are less jarring to your back than running on hard surfaces. Bicycling is a good option, too. However, be sure to adjust the heights of the seat and handlebars so that you assume proper posture while pedaling. If you golf, protect your back by shortening your back swing.

- **Avoid high-risk moves.** You may need to avoid or modify activities, especially if you've had back problems. Avoid movements that cause you to exaggerate the stretch of your muscles. For example, don't try to touch your toes with your legs straight. Activities that involve a lot of twisting, quick stops and starts, and impact on hard surfaces, such as tennis, racquetball, basketball and contact sports, pose the greatest risks to your back.

Back-saving body mechanics

To practice sound body mechanics, pay attention to how you move. By maintaining your spine's normal curves throughout daily activity, you save energy and reduce strain on your back.

Use these tips to help prevent injuries and use your back wisely:

- **Plan ahead.** Think through and reorganize your work or leisure activities to eliminate high-risk movements.

- **Listen to your body.** If your back hurts, stop what you're doing and rest. If you must sit or stand for a prolonged period, change your position often. Avoid unnecessary bending, twisting and reaching.

- **Prevent falls.** Falls can seriously injure your back, especially if you have osteoporosis.

- **Stand tall.** Poor posture is exhausting work for your back. Good posture is more relaxing. It takes minimal effort to balance your body and maintain the three natural curves in your back.

- **Sit comfortably.** Sitting is stressful for your back. To minimize stress, choose a seat that supports your lower back. Or place a pillow or a rolled towel in the small of your back to maintain the normal curve. When you drive, adjust your seat to keep your knees and hips level. Move your seat forward to avoid over-reaching for the pedals.

- **Sleep smart.** Because you spend about one-third of your life in bed, lie in a good position on a firm mattress. Use pillows for support, but don't use one that forces your neck up at a severe angle.

- **Lift with your legs.** Before you lift a load, decide where you'll place it and how you'll get there. Pushing is safer than pulling. Always bend your knees so your arms are level with the object. Avoid lifting overhead. Use a footstool to reach high objects. Place heavy objects on casters.

Keep Your Back Strong and Healthy

Take stock of your back and how you use it. Then "invest" in prevention—regular exercise, healthy weight, good posture and, perhaps most important, back-saving lifting techniques. Keep your mind on your back each time you take out the trash, pick up a suitcase, swing a golf club or just lean over to brush your teeth.

If you have periodic bouts of back pain, remember to rest and take an over-the-counter pain reliever for the temporary discomfort. This type of simple self-care together with sensible daily living can help keep you and your back strong, healthy partners.

Index

Index

699

teenagers *see* adolescents
Tegretol 148
Tenex (guanfacine) 63
Tenormin (atenolol) 62
terazosin 63, 101, 111
terbutaline 233, 241
TESS *see* toxic exposure surveillance
  system (TESS)
testes (testicles)
  defined 463
  described 138
  enlarged 139
  formation 3
  removal (orchiectomy) 134, 141
  self-examination 142–43
  shrunken, vasectomy reversal 456
  under-sized 395, 398
testicles *see* testes (testicles)
testicular cancer 137–43
  diagnosis 139–40
  staging 140–41
  treatment 141–42
    side effects 141–42
  vasectomy 445
Testing and Materials, American Society for
  Medical and Dental Equipment
    Standards 274
Testoderm patch 6
testosterone
  finasteride (Proscar) side effects
    101, 112
  hair follicles 534, 540
  hormone replacement therapy 393,
    669–74
    Klinefelter syndrome 396, 404,
      405–7
  low levels effects 372, 630
    diminished libido 5
    diminished potency 5
    diminished sperm production 5
    strength levels 5
  masculinity hormone 3–6
  synthetic 583, 585
tests
  angiography 149
  asthma 239
  blood glucose levels 302

tests, continued
  chlamydia 286
  colorectal cancer 96–97
  digital rectal examinations 125–26,
    131
  fecal occult blood tests 91, 95
  fertility 384–86
    endometrial biopsy 385
    hysterosalpingogram 385
    laparoscopy 385
  hamster-egg penetrance assay 385
  HIV infection 264, 272–73, 292
    Amplicor HIV-1 Monitor Test 273
    anonymity 272
    Coulter HIV-1 p24 Antigen Assay
      273, 276
    ELISA 264, 273
    Western blot 264, 272
  impotence 373
  mucus penetrance test 385
  prostate disorders 108–9, 130
  prostate massage 126
  pulmonary function tests 231–33
    aterial blood gas test 232
    peak flow test 232
    pulse oximetry test 232
    spirometry 232
    x-ray 233
  sleep apnea 517–18
  three-glass urine collection test 126
  transrectal ultrasound (TRUS) 132–
    33
tetracyline 284, 286
Thalitone (chlorthalidone) 62
theophylline 234, 242
therapeutic recreation specialists, described 161
thirst, increased, diabetes mellitus
  299, 300
thoractomy 78
thorax 66
thorazine 363
three-glass urine collection test 126
3TC (lamivudine) 265, 276
thromboses, cause of death 38
thymus 66
thyroiditis, autoimmune
  XXY males 409

Environmentally Induced Disorders Sourcebook

Basic Information about Diseases and Syndromes Linked to Exposure to Pollutants and Other Substances in Outdoor and Indoor Environments Such As Lead, Asbestos, Formaldehyde, Mercury, Emissions, Noise, and More

Edited by Allan R. Cook. 620 pages. 1997. 0-7808-0083-4. $75.

Fitness & Exercise Sourcebook

Basic Information on Fitness and Exercise, Including Fitness Activities for Specific Age Groups, Exercise for People with Specific Medical Conditions, How to Begin a Fitness Program in Running, Walking, Swimming, Cycling, and Other Athletic Activities, and Recent Research in Fitness and Exercise

Edited by Dan R. Harris. 663 pages. 1996. 0-7808-0186-5. $75.

Food & Animal Borne Diseases Sourcebook

Basic Information about Diseases That Can Be Spread to Humans through the Ingestion of Contaminated Food or Water or by Contact with Infected Animals and Insects, Such As Botulism, E. Coli, Hepatitis A, Trichinosis, Lyme Disease, and Rabies, along with Information Regarding Prevention and Treatment Methods, and a Special Section for International Travelers Describing Diseases Such as Cholera, Malaria, Travelers' Diarrhea, and Yellow Fever, and Offering Recommendations for Avoiding Illness

Edited by Karen Bellenir and Peter D. Dresser. 535 pages. 1995. 0-7808-0033-8. $75.

"A comprehensive collection of authoritative information." — *Emergency Medical Services, Oct '95*

"Targeting general readers and providing them with a single, comprehensive source of information on selected topics, this book continues, with the excellent caliber of its predecessors, to catalog topical information on health matters of general interest. Readable and thorough, this valuable resource is highly recommended for all libraries." — *Academic Library Book Review, Summer '96*

Gastrointestinal Diseases & Disorders Sourcebook

Basic Information about Gastroesophageal Reflux Disease (Heartburn), Ulcers, Diverticulosis, Irritable Bowel Syndrome, Crohn's Disease, Ulcerative Colitis, Diarrhea, Constipation, Lactose Intolerance, Hemorrhoids, Hepatitis, Cirrhosis and Other Digestive Problems, Featuring Statistics, Descriptions of Symptoms, and Current Treatment Methods of Interest for Persons Living with Upper and Lower Gastrointestinal Maladies

Edited by Linda M. Ross. 413 pages. 1996. 0-7808-0078-8. $75.

". . . very readable form. The successful editorial work that brought this material together into a useful and understandable reference makes accessible to all readers information that can help them more effectively understand and obtain help for digestive tract problems." — *Choice, Feb '97*

Genetic Disorders Sourcebook

Basic Information about Heritable Diseases and Disorders Such As Down Syndrome, PKU, Hemophilia, Von Willebrand Disease, Gaucher Disease, Tay-Sachs Disease, and Sickle-Cell Disease, along with Information about Genetic Screening, Gene Therapy, Home Care, and Including Source Listings for Further Help and Information on More Than 300 Disorders

Edited by Karen Bellenir. 642 pages. 1996. 0-7808-0034-6. $75.

". . . geared toward the lay public. It would be well placed in all public libraries and in those hospital and medical libraries in which access to genetic references is limited." — *Doody's Health Sciences Book Review, Oct '96*

"Provides essential medical information to both the general public and those diagnosed with a serious or fatal genetic disease or disorder." — *Choice, Jan '97*

Head Trauma Sourcebook

Basic Information for the Layperson about Open-Head and Closed-Head Injuries, Treatment Advances, Recovery, and Rehabilitation, along with Reports on Current Research Initiatives

Edited by Karen Bellenir. 414 pages. 1997. 0-7808-0208-X. $75.

Health Insurance Sourcebook

Basic Information about Managed Care Organizations, Traditional Fee-for-Service Insurance, Insurance Portability and Pre-Existing Conditions Clauses, Medicare, Medicaid, Social Security, and Military Health Care, along with Information about Insurance Fraud

Edited by Wendy Wilcox. 530 pages. 1997. 0-7808-0222-5. $75.

Continues next page

Immune System Disorders Sourcebook

Basic Information about Lupus, Multiple Sclerosis, Guillain-Barré Syndrome, Chronic Granulomatous Disease, and More, along with Statistical and Demographic Data and Reports on Current Research Initiatives

Edited by Allan R. Cook. 608 pages. 1997. 0-7808-0209-8. $75.

■

Kidney & Urinary Tract Diseases &Disorders Sourcebook

Basic Information about Kidney Stones, Urinary Incontinence, Bladder Disease, End-Stage Renal Disease, Dialysis, and More, along with Statistical and Demographic Data and Reports on Current Research Initiatives

Edited by Linda M. Ross. 602 pages. 1997. 0-7808-0079-6. $75.

■

Learning Disabilities Sourcebook

Basic Information about Disorders Such As Autism, Dyslexia, Hyperactivity, and Attention Deficit Disorder, along with Statistical and Demographic Data and Reports on Current Research Initiatives

Edited by Linda M. Ross. 600 pages. 1998. 0-7808-0210-1. $75.

■

Men's Health Concerns Sourcebook

Basic Information about Topics of Special Interest to Men, Including Prostate Enlargement, Impotence and Other Sexual Dysfunctions, Vasectomies, Condoms, Snoring, Sleep Apnea, Hair Loss, and More

Edited by Allan R. Cook. 600 pages. 1998. 0-7808-0212-8. $75.

■

Mental Health Disorders Sourcebook

Basic Information about Schizophrenia, Depression, Bipolar Disorder, Panic Disorder, Obsessive-Compulsive Disorder, Phobias and Other Anxiety Disorders, Paranoia and Other Personality Disorders, Eating Disorders, and Sleep Disorders, along with Information about Treatment and Therapies

Edited by Karen Bellenir. 548 pages. 1995. 0-7808-0040-0. $75.

". . . provides information on a wide range of mental disorders, presented in nontechnical language."
— Exceptional Child Education Resources, Spring '96

"The text is well organized and adequately written for its target audience." — Choice, Jun '96

"The great strengths of the book are its readability and its inclusion of places to find more information. Especially recommended." — RQ, Winter '96

"Recommended for public and academic libraries."
— Reference Book Review, '96

". . . useful for public and academic libraries and consumer health collections."
— Medical Reference Services Quarterly, Spring '97

■

Ophthalmic Disorders Sourcebook

Basic Information about Glaucoma, Cataracts, Macular Degeneration, Strabismus, Refractive Disorders, and More, along with Statistical and Demographic Data and Reports on Current Research Initiatives

Edited by Linda M. Ross. 631 pages. 1996. 0-7808-0081-8. $75.

■

Oral Health Sourcebook

Basic Information about Diseases and Conditions Affecting Oral Health, Including Cavities, Gum Disease, Dry Mouth, Oral Cancers, Fever Blisters, Canker Sores, Oral Thrush, Bad Breath, Temporomandibular Disorders, and other Craniofacial Syndromes, along with Statistical Data on the Oral Health of Americans, Oral Hygiene, Emergency First Aid, Information on Treatment Procedures and Methods of Replacing Lost Teeth

Edited by Allan R. Cook. 560 pages. 1997. 0-7808-0082-6. $75.

■

Pain Sourcebook

Basic Information about Specific Forms of Acute and Chronic Pain, Including Headaches, Back Pain, Muscular Pain, Neuralgia, Surgical Pain, and Cancer Pain, along with Pain Relief Options Such As Analgesics, Narcotics, Nerve Blocks, Transcutaneous Nerve Stimulation, and Alternative Forms of Pain Control, Including Biofeedback, Imaging, Behavior Modification, and Relaxation Techniques

Edited by Allan R. Cook. 608 pages. 1997. 0-7808-0213-6. $75.

■

Pregnancy & Birth Sourcebook

Basic Information about Planning for Pregnancy, Fetal Growth and Development, Labor and Delivery, Postpartum and Perinatal Care, Pregnancy in Mothers with Special Concerns, and Disorders of Pregnancy, Including Genetic Counseling, Nutrition and Exercise, Obstetrical Tests, Pregnancy Discomfort, Multiple Births, Cesarean Sections, Medical Testing of Newborns, Breastfeeding, Gestational Diabetes, and Ectopic Pregnancy

Edited by Heather Aldred. 752 pages. 1997. 0-7808-0216-0. $75.